MECHANICS OF MUSCLE: SECOND EDITION

**NEW YORK UNIVERSITY
BIOMEDICAL ENGINEERING SERIES**

General Editor: Walter Welkowitz

MECHANICS OF MUSCLE: SECOND EDITION

Daniel J. Schneck
Virginia Polytechnic Institute and State University

NEW YORK UNIVERSITY PRESS
New York *and* London

Manufactured in the United States of America

Library of Congress Cataloging-in-Publication Data
Schneck, Daniel J.
Mechanics of muscle / Daniel J. Schneck.—2nd ed.
p. cm.—(New York University biomedical engineering series)
Includes bibliographical references and index.
ISBN 0-8147-7935-2 (alk. paper)
1. Muscle contraction.   2. Striated muscle—Mechanical properties.
3. Muscles—Physiology. I. Title. II. Series.
[DNLM: 1. Biomechanics. 2. Models, Biological. 3. Muscle
Contraction—physiology. 4. Muscles—physiology.   WE 103 S3575]
QP321.S34   1991
612.7'4—dc20
DNLM/DLC
for Library of Congress   91-27603
                                                                  CIP

New York University Press books are printed on acid-free paper,
and their binding materials are chosen for strength and durability.

To Judi, Cyndi, and Patti,

Because they were always there when I needed them ...

Table of Contents

List of Figures

List of Tables

List of Symbols

a No-load, cross-sectional area of muscle fiber at rest $= \dfrac{\pi (dx)^2}{4}$

a_0 $\dfrac{v_{max}}{3} = \dfrac{1}{3\tau_F} [L(\infty) - L(0)]$

a_1 $B + F$

a_j Series of constants in the expansion [4-26] for f_2

a^* Constant in the exponential expression [4-27] for f_1

b Ordinate-axis intercept of straight line segment (see Problem 2-3a)

b_1 $\dfrac{v}{v_{max}} + \dfrac{1}{3}$

b_i Series of polynomial-expansion coefficients (see Problem 2-3b)

b^* Interfilamentary-Overlap coefficient (see Problem 4-5); $0 \leq b^* \leq 1$

c Dashpot constant in viscoelastic model of muscle

c_1 $\dfrac{1}{3}(P + B)$

c^* Constant of proportionality in the relaxation-time function [3-53]

d_i Location of centers of gravity of limb segments in Nubar's Total Body Model; $i = 1, 2, 3, 4, 5$

e_h Efficiency associated with the process whereby work appears as the result of the breakdown of high-energy phosphates

e_p Efficiency associated with the oxidative synthesis of High-Energy Phosphates

f Tensile force in muscle fiber

$f(\ell^*_i)$ Tensile force in group of fibers having given length ℓ^*_i

$f_{1/2}$ Alpha-motoneuron firing frequency at which $[Ca^{++}] = \dfrac{1}{2}[Ca^{++}]_\infty$

f_1 Tensile force in dashpot-contractile-element-series-spring-element loop of viscoelastic model of muscle

f_2 Tensile force in parallel-spring-element loop of viscoelastic model of muscle

$f^*_a(\dot{\zeta})$	$\dfrac{s_8}{s_9 + e^{-s_{10}F_{10}(\dot{\zeta})}}$
f_x	Tensile force in annulus (ring) of muscle fibers all located a radial distance x from the longitudinal axis of the muscle
$f_{(\text{sub})}$	Firing frequencies (impulses per second) of afferent and efferent nerve fibers innervating either the muscle spindle or the motor end plate; (sub) = Ia, II, α, γ, i (i'th fiber), b, I_b, Λ-II-β, Λ-III-δ, C-IV-δ, t (threshold), and so on
$f_{L,U}$	Upper (U) and Lower (L) break-point or corner frequencies, respectively
$f^*_0, f^*_1, ...$	Coefficients of components of Hamiltonian Function
f_ω	Linear frequency, in cycles per second
$g_{1,2}\left(\dfrac{\Delta\ell}{\ell}\right)$	Coefficients in the second-order differential equation [2-5] defining the quantity p^*
$\bar{g}(s)$	LaPlace Transform of the arbitrary function, $g(t)$
h	Total Contraction Heat, $H + a_1\xi$
$h_{(i)}$	Musculoskeletal Constraint Functions, $i = 1, 2, 3, ...$
i	Integer index, 0, 1, 2, ... , or, Subscript index, α, Ia, II, ... ; Also, where indicated, $\sqrt{-1}$; Also, where indicated, a subscript designating "initial"
j	Integer index, 0, 1, 2, ...
k	$1 + \dfrac{k_s}{k_p}$
k_b	Elasticity of muscle spindle equatorial region
k_e	Elasticity of tendinous attachment of muscle spindles to extrafusal muscle fibers
k_f	Elasticity of muscle poles (intrafusal fiber region)
k_o	Rate-constant in Logistic Equation [1-1]
k_p	Parallel spring constant in viscoelastic model of muscle
$k_p^{(j)}$	Parallel spring constants ($j = 1, 2, 3, ...$) in the network of Kelvin Elements that are linked together in series arrangement to model the viscoelastic behavior of muscle tissue
k_s	Series spring constant in viscoelastic model of muscle
$k^*(\zeta^*)$	$e^{-\left\{\dfrac{\zeta^* - 1}{s_k}\right\}^2}$
ℓ	Total no-load length of single muscle fiber at rest
ℓ_b	"Bias" length (pre-stretch) of muscle spindle equator

ℓ_c	Critical length of muscle spindle equator (end of response range)
ℓ_e	Instantaneous (actual) length of muscle spindle equator
$\ell*_i$	Initial lengths of individual muscle fibers $(i = 1, 2, 3, ...)$ in Decraemer's statistical model for muscular contraction
ℓ_r	Arbitrary reference length of muscle spindle equator
ℓ_t	Threshold length of muscle spindle equator (beginning of response range)
m	Slope of straight-line segment; Also, used to designate muscle mass in viscoelastic models
$m_{1,2}$	$-\rho_2 \pm \sqrt{\rho_2{}^2 - 1}$ (subscript 1 = + root; subscript 2 = − root)
n_o	Number of Sarcomeres in muscle fiber
$n(\ell*_i)$	The number of muscle fibers in the muscle as a whole which will have the instantaneous length $\ell*_i$ at any given time
o	Except where otherwise defined in the text, a subscript designating passive (unstimulated) states of muscle
p	Total lateral strain due to passive stretching; also, used as a suffix for the parallel spring constant in the viscoelastic model for muscle; Also designates a probability density function
$p(\ell*_i)$	Probability Density Function for $\ell*_i$
p_i	Generalized Poisson Ratios $(i = 1, 2, 3)$
$p*$	$\dfrac{dq*(\cdot)}{d[Ca^{++}]}$
q	Total Lateral Strain Due to Active Contraction
q_i	Active Stimulation Coefficients $(i = o, 1, 2, 3)$
$q*(\cdot)$	Normalized Active State Function of Several Variables
$q*_o$	$q*(\cdot)$ in the muscle at rest $= q*(0)$
q_s	Generalized angular position coordinate of skeletal limb relative to joint s $(s = 1, 2, 3, ...)$
r	Number of Constraints in Minimum-Energy Analysis
r_1	$q_1 - p_1(1 + q_o)$
r_2	$q_2 - p_2(1 + q_o) - p_1 q_1$
r_3	$q_3 - p_3(1 + q_o) - p_2 q_1 - p_1 q_2$
r_4	$\dfrac{\pi}{12}(2 + q_o)q_o = \dfrac{\pi}{12} B_1$
r_5	$\dfrac{\pi}{12}\left[\dfrac{3}{2} + (2 + q_o)q_o - 2r_1(1 + q_o)\right]$

r_6	The Numerical Ratio, $\dfrac{G}{E_1}$
$\dot{r}_6$	The Time Rate-of-Change of r_6
r_{11}	$\rho_1{}^2(\zeta^*)$
r_{12}	$2\rho_2\rho_1(\zeta^*)$
s	Suffix for series spring constant in viscoelastic muscle model; Also, LaPlace variable; Also, generalized angular position coordinate suffix
s_i	Muscle-specific constants in Hatze's formulation ($i = 1, 2, 3, 4, 5, 6, 7, 8, 9, 10, 11$); See equations [4-33, 34, 35, 38, 39] and Table 4-I
s_k	"Peakedness" parameter characterizing the normal distribution curve of the statistically-distributed muscle fibers in Hatze's formulation (see equation [4-37])
s_o	Fixed leg-separation in Nubar's minimum-energy model
t	time coordinate, in general
t_o	specific reference instant of time
t^*	Arbitrary dummy time variable for purposes of integration
u	Output, or monitored, or controlled signal of feedback control system
u_a	"Overshoot" coefficient of feedback control system
u_c	Controlling signal of feedback control system
u_d	Disturbing or Input signal of feedback control system
u_m	Manipulating signal of feedback control system
u_o	Primary command signal of feedback control system
u_p	Primary feedback signal of feedback control system
u_r	Reference signal of feedback control system
$u - u_r$	Error signal of comparator in feedback control system
u_w	Signals that warn of impending breakdowns in feedback control systems
$u^*(t)$	Nonhomogeneous forcing function driving a feedback control system (c.f., equation [7-51])
v	$\dot{L} =$ The velocity of muscular contraction; Also, where indicated, membrane conduction velocity (c.f., Table 6-III)
w	$w_1(x, y, z) + \lambda w_2(x, y, z)$
$w_{1,2}$	Arbitrary energy functions
x	Radial distance measured relative to longitudinal axis of muscle; radial location of unloaded muscle fiber at rest; Also, arbitrary rectangular coordinate

x' Radial location of stimulated, loaded muscle fiber, measured relative to the longitudinal axis of the muscle

x_d Length of viscous element in viscoelastic model of muscle

x_{os} Undeflected resting length of series spring element in viscoelastic model of muscle

x_s Length, at any given time, of series spring element in viscoelastic model of muscle

x_{ts} Some reference tetanic isometric length for the series spring element in viscoelastic model of muscle

y Rectangular coordinate

z Longitudinal coordinate axis of whole muscle, along centerline from tendon to tendon

A Reference cross-sectional area of muscle, as defined in the text (e.g., at rest, $A = \pi D^2/4$)

A_o Passive (unstimulated) cross-sectional area of muscle

A_1 Same as N

A_3 $\dfrac{8}{9}(r_1 + 2r_2\alpha + 3r_3\alpha^2)(N^2 - 1)$

A_i Coefficients in the series-expansion representation for β' (c.f., equation [2-14] and Problem 2-4)

A' Cross-sectional area of muscle stimulated to contract under loaded conditions

B $AE_1\left[\dfrac{3}{2}\dfrac{G}{E_1} - \dfrac{D^2}{L^2}r_4 + \alpha\left(\dfrac{D^2}{L^2}r_5 - \dfrac{\pi}{8}\right)\right]$

B_1 $q_0(2 + q_0)$

B_2 $2[r_1(1 + q_0) + p_1]$

B_3 $r_1{}^2 + 2r_2(1 + q_0) - p_1{}^2 + 2p_2$

B_4 $2[r_1r_2 + r_3(1 + q_0) - p_1p_2 + p_3]$

B_b Dashpot constant for Voigt Model of Muscle Spindle

B_f Dashpot constant for viscoelastic Model of Muscle Spindle Poles

C Magnification Factor $= \sqrt{\left(\dfrac{k_s}{c\omega}\right)^2 + \left[1 + \dfrac{k_s}{k_p}\right]^2} \div \sqrt{1 + \left(\dfrac{k_s}{c\omega}\right)^2}$

C_o $-\sin\phi_o - \dfrac{u_r}{u_a}$

C_1 $d_1W_1 + \ell_1[W_2 + W_3 + W_4 + W_5]$

C_2 d_2W_2

C_3 $d_3W_3 + \ell_3[W_4 + W_5]$

C_4　　　　$d_4 W_4$

C_5　　　　$d_5 W_5$

C^*_m　　　Membrane Capacitance

Ck_p　　　Gain

$\mathfrak{C}$　　　　Creep Compliance

D　　　　Maximum Diameter of Muscle in some reference state

D_1　　　　$\dfrac{\sqrt{D_2{}^2 + D_3{}^2}}{D_4 D_5}$

D_2　　　　$1095.0484\omega - \omega^3$

D_3　　　　$88.85\omega^2 + 66.02298$

D_4　　　　$220.8196 + \omega^2$

D_5　　　　$5483.4025 + \omega^2$

D_6　　　　$1 + 32.500861\omega^2 + 11.02695456\omega^4 + 0.019072463\omega^6$

D_7　　　　$1.726\omega + 7.86753469\omega^3 + 0.415033942\omega^5$

D_8　　　　$1 + 25.250729\omega^2 + 6.26840725\omega^4 + 0.00455625\omega^6$

D_9　　　　$\dfrac{1}{D_8}\sqrt{D_6{}^2 + D_7{}^2}$

D'　　　　Maximum Diameter of Muscle Stimulated to Contract Under Loaded Conditions

E　　　　Young's Modulus in a Hookean Elastic Sense for a given muscle

E_i　　　　Generalized Young's Modulus ($i = 1, 2, 3$)

$E_{(sub)}$　　Various Moduli of Elasticity for Muscle Tissue: (sub) = "complex"; "dynamic" (magnitude of "complex"); "secant" (secant modulus of passive stress-strain curve); "static" ("Relaxed" elastic modulus, passive); "storage" (real part of "complex"); "tangent" (tangent modulus of nonlinear passive stress-strain curve); "viscous" (imaginary part of "complex")

$E^*_{complex}$　　Nondimensional Complex Modulus of Elasticity $= \dfrac{E_{complex}}{E_{static}}$

E_μ　　　Mechanical Impedance Function

F　　　　Total Force, or Tension generated at the tendons of a muscle; $F(L_f)$ if variable with total muscle length; $F(t)$ if variable with time

$F_a(\dot{\zeta})$　　Average force output of a typical actomyosin cross-bridge

$F^e(t^*)$　　State of Muscle Tone at the start ($t = t^*$) of the loading cycle (see equation [4-13])

F_m　　　Maximum force in muscle tissue, associated with a sinusoidal dis-

	placement input at the tendons
F_o	Passive (unstimulated) force in a muscle, at any given time
F_T	Active (stimulated) isotonic force in a muscle
F_u	Total force generated by one motor unit
F_1	Value of finite, constant, passive, step-force input to muscle tendon at $t = 0$
F_2	Total Force in Muscle Spindle
$F_{10}(\dot{\zeta})$	$\text{Sinh } (s_{11} \dfrac{\dot{\zeta}}{\dot{\zeta}_m} + \dfrac{s_{11}}{2})$
$F^*(t)$	Nondimensionalized Relaxation Force $= \dfrac{F(t)}{F_{t \to \infty}}$
$F^*_a(\dot{\zeta})$	Normalized velocity-of-shortening function (see equation [4-29])
F^*_m	Active force generated in viscoelastic model of muscle spindle as a result of γ-nerve innervation
$\bar{F}$	Faraday Constant, 96,500 coulombs per mole of univalent ions
G	Lateral pressure distribution function $= G^*4(\dfrac{L}{D})^2$
$G(t)$	Relaxation Function in stochastic constitutive model for muscle tissue
G_i	Constraint equations in Nubar's Least Energy Analysis $(i = 1, 2, 3, ..., r)$
G_n	Geometric Ratio $= \dfrac{\pi D^2}{4L}$
G^*	Lateral Pressure Distribution (force per unit circumferential area)
$G^r_{complex}$	Complex Reduced Relaxation Function
$G_r(t - t^*)$	$\dfrac{G(t - t^*)}{G(0)}$
$G'_r(\omega)$	Storage (elastic) part of the complex reduced relaxation function
$G''_r(\omega)$	Loss (viscous) part of the complex reduced relaxation function, c.f., equation [4-21]
H	Heat of Activation $= \dfrac{6FGL}{\pi E_1}$
H^*	Hamiltonian Function
$H(t - t^*)$	Heaviside Function $= 0$ for $t < t^*$; $= 1$ for $t \geq t^*$
J	Complex Muscular Compliance $= (1/E_{complex})$
K	Reciprocal of the Retardation Time Constant $= \dfrac{k_s k_p}{c(k_s + k_p)}$; Also,

	Generalized Feedback Control System Transfer Function
K_1	Loop Gain of Feedback Control System
K_2	Baran Constant $= k_e/B_b$
$\lvert \overline{K}(i\omega) \rvert$	Gain $= Ck_p$
$\overline{K}(s)$	LaPlace Transfer Function
$\overline{K}_x(s)$	Passive LaPlace Transfer Function for Muscle Spindle Equator
$\overline{K}_F(s)$	Active LaPlace Transfer Function for Muscle Spindle Equator
$K(i\omega)$	Feedback Control System Transfer Function
$K_{(\text{sub})}$	Transfer Function; (sub) $= t$ (transducer or Controlled Element of Feedback Control System), c (Comparator and Controlling Element of Feedback Control System), $\gamma = \partial u/\partial f_\gamma$, $\xi = \partial u/\partial \xi$, $\alpha = -\partial u/\partial f_\alpha$, $X = 1 - \dfrac{X_2}{X_m}$, $F = -\dfrac{X_2}{F^*_m}$, $o =$ Gain of Reflex Pathway in Stein and Oğuztöreli model for the muscle spindle (see equation [7-37]), also, Gain of Reflex Pathway in Houk and Simon model for the Golgi Tendon Organ (see equation [7-38]), $i = 1, 2, 3, 4, \ldots, p =$ Feedback Element, and $r =$ Reference Element.
L	Total length of muscle; also, as a subscript, means, "lower"
$L_{2,3}$	Second and Third (respectively) Lumbar Vertebrae
L_f	Final extension length of total muscle in Decraemer Model
L_{op}	Undeflected resting length of parallel spring element loop in viscoelastic model for muscle
M	Molar Concentration (moles/liter); or, Molecular Weight
M_i	Torque generated at the i'th joint, $i = 1, 2, 3, \ldots S$
M_∞	Sarcoplasmic Calcium Concentration corresponding to the tetanic state of muscle tissue
N	$\dfrac{1 + q_0 + r_1\alpha + r_2\alpha^2 + r_3\alpha^3}{1 + \alpha}$; also, arbitrary integer superscript on the Laplace variable s in equation [7-17]
N_o	$\dfrac{1 - p_1\alpha - p_2\alpha^2 - p_3\alpha^3}{1 + \alpha}$
N_∞	Total number of muscle fibers in the entire muscle
N_B	Total number of cross-bridges present in a half-sarcomere
P	Force generated by the contractile elements of muscle; also used (where indicated in the text) as a symbol for Permeability Coefficients, with an appropriate subscript to indicate which one, and for what species of biochemical constituent

Q	$\frac{8}{3}(1 + \alpha)(N^2 - 1)$
Q_o	$\frac{8}{3}(1 + \alpha)(N_o{}^2 - 1)$
R	The Universal Gas Constant
$R^*{}_m$	Membrane Resistance
$\mathscr{R}$	Relaxation Modulus
S	Total number of joints involved in musculoskeletal motion
T	Absolute Temperature
T_1	First Thoracic Vertebra
T_3	Tri-iodothyronine
T_4	Thyroxine
T_b	Build-up, or Rise Time of a feedback control system
T_d	Decay Time of a feedback control system
T_i	Corner-frequency Time-periods of a generalized Transfer Function for a feedback control system, $i = 1, 2, 3, \dots, A, B, C, \dots$
T_t	Period of the damped response of a feedback control system
T_ω	Period of Oscillation $= \dfrac{1}{f_\omega}$
T^*	Kinetic Energy Function
U	Total Strain Energy $= U_1 + U_2$
U_1	Longitudinal Strain Energy
U_2	Transverse Strain Energy
$U_1{}^{(x)}$	Longitudinal Strain Energy in a ring of muscle fibers located a distance x from the axis of the muscle
U^*	Energy Function $= (\beta_1 M_1{}^2 + \beta_2 M_2{}^2 + \beta_3 M_4{}^2 + \beta_4 M_5{}^2)\Delta t$
$\overline{V}$	Potential Energy Function $= V^* - \lambda h_{(i)}$
V_m	Mechanical or Structural Parameter $= G_n V_n$
V_n	Normalized Parameter characteristic of the basic properties of the biological muscle tissue
$V_N \alpha^*(t)$	Nerve impulse arriving at the motor end plate of a muscle fiber
$V_T \beta^*(t)$	Depolarizing Potential of the T-system
V^*	Potential Energy Function
W	Weight Fraction of Elastic Material per cubic centimeter of muscle volume

W_i Respective weight of individual limbs ($i = 1, 2, 3, \ldots$) in articulated total body model

X Dummy variable for integration in the radial direction

X_1 Deflection of spindle tendons

X_2 Deflection of spindle tendons plus spindle poles

X_m Total Deflection of entire spindle, i.e., spindle poles plus spindle tendons plus spindle equator

Y Carrier molecule in sodium pump

ΔY_o $\dfrac{\Delta F(t,t_o)}{G(t - t_o)}$ (c.f., equations [4-8] and [4-9])

$[Y_m]$ Concentration of Y in sarcolemma

Z Degree-of-freedom exponent in equation [4-34]

Z^* Faraday Constant $= \bar{F}$

α Prefix designating receptors in tissues that can be activated by norepinephrine and/or epinephrine (adrenergic), and whose excitatory activity can be further blocked or activated by specific chemical compounds, such as Phenoxybenzamine (an α-blocker) and Methoxamine (an α-activator); Also, a prefix designating the motor neuron (6-17μ-diameter) primarily responsible for activating contraction of a striated skeletal muscle; Also, used to designate Total Muscle Strain $= \Delta L/L$

α_1 Phase lead/lag parameter such that $\sin \phi_{max} = \dfrac{1 - \alpha}{1 + \alpha}$

$\dot{\alpha}$ Time rate of change of $\alpha = \dfrac{d\alpha}{dt}$

$\alpha^*(t)$ End-plate potential function $= \sin 1000\pi(t - t^*_i)$

α_i Body segment orientation angles in Nubar's Saggital-Plane Model of the Total Body

β Prefix designating receptors in tissues that can be activated by norepinephrine and/or epinephrine (adrenergic), and whose inhibitory activity can be further blocked or activated by specific chemical compounds, such as Propranolol (a β-blocker) and Isoproterenol (a β-activator); Also, used to designate nondimensionalized muscle fiber location, x/L

β_i Sensitivity coefficients ($i = 1, 2, 3, \ldots$) in Nubar's Energy Function (see U^*)

β' Nondimensionalized location, $\dfrac{x'}{L + \Delta L}$

$\beta^*(t)$ Depolarizing Potential Weighting Function (c.f., equation [4-33])

γ The Joule Coefficient $= \left(\dfrac{\partial F}{\partial T}\right)_L$

γ_1 or γ_p Efferent Motor Nerve Fibers (5-7μ-Diameter) that innervate discrete motor end plates on the larger nuclear bag intrafusal contractile fibers of striated skeletal muscle spindles

γ_2 or γ_l — Efferent Motor Nerve Fibers ($3\text{-}5\mu$-Diameter) that innervate the smaller nuclear chain intrafusal contractile fibers of striated skeletal muscle spindle poles

δ — Dirac Function (c.f., equation [7-54]); Also, designates cutaneous, myelinated, $1\text{-}6\mu$-Diameter afferent sensory nerve fibers

δ_m — Average membrane thickness

ε — Total Isometric Muscle Strain

$\varepsilon(\ell^{*}{}_i)$ — Total strain in a *group* of muscle fibers $= \dfrac{l_f - \ell^{*}{}_i}{\ell^{*}{}_i}$

$\dot{\varepsilon}(\ell^{*}{}_i)$ — Strain Rate

ε_3 — Dissociation Rate Constant of Sodium Pump

ε_z — Longitudinal strain of *single* muscle fiber $= \dfrac{\Delta\ell}{\ell}$

$\zeta(t)$ — Instantaneous length of a sarcomere at any given time, t

$\dot{\zeta}(t)$ — Velocity of interfilamentary movement $= \dfrac{d\zeta}{dt}$

ζ_o — Initial length of sarcomere $= \zeta(0)$

$\bar{\zeta}$ — That Sarcomere length at which the force output of the fully stimulated and isometrically contracting Contractile Element attains a maximum value

$\bar{\zeta}_m$ — Maximum shortening velocity of the myofilament structures at optimum length, $\bar{\zeta}$

ζ^{*} — Normalized Sarcomere Length $= \dfrac{\zeta}{\bar{\zeta}}$

ζ — Experimentally determined constant in expression [4-34] for normalized calcium density function $\rho^{*}(\zeta^{*})$

η — Viscosity coefficient for fluid in viscoelastic dashpot element in time-dependent model of muscle, $= \dfrac{E_{viscous}}{\omega}$

θ — Brain wave activity associated with dreaming

κ — Linear Thermal Expansion Coefficient of a material $= \dfrac{1}{L}\left(\dfrac{\partial L}{\partial T}\right)_F$

$\lambda, \lambda^{(i)}$ — LaGrange Multiplier(s), $i = 1, 2, 3, \ldots$

μ — Symbol for the unit "micron" $= 10^{-6}$ meters

μ_d — Dynamic Viscosity

ν — The ratio $\dfrac{k_s}{k_p} = \dfrac{\tau_\sigma}{\tau_\varepsilon} - 1$

ξ — Total deformation of the entire muscle relative to its resting state $= L - L_{op} = L\alpha = \xi(t)$

$\xi(t)$ Where so defined, refers to a time strain function for Creep

ξ_m Amplitude of Sinusoidal Displacement forcing function

ξ_o Finite deformation at $t = 0$

$\xi^*(t)$ The nondimensional ratio $\dfrac{\xi(t)}{\xi_{t \to \infty}}$

ρ Standard deviation of mean value, ℓ, for initial length of muscle fiber in Decraemer's statistical model for muscular contraction

$\rho_1(\zeta^*)$ $\sqrt{r_{11}}$

$\rho_2(\zeta^*)$ $\dfrac{r_{12}}{2\rho_1(\zeta^*)}$

$\rho^*(\zeta^*)$ Normalized calcium density function

σ Stress in muscle as a whole $= \dfrac{F}{A}$

$\sigma(\ell_i^*)$ Stress in the Hookean sense $= E_D\varepsilon(\ell_i^*)$

$\sigma(t)$ Stress function of time, which accounts for Relaxation Phenomena

σ^e Instantaneous, immediate $(t = t^*)$ stress response of muscle tissue $= F^e(t^*)/A$

$\sigma_1{}^e(\alpha)$ Amplitude of the fundamental harmonic in the Fourier series expansion of σ^e

σ_o Passive (unstimulated) stress in whole muscle $= F_o/A_o$; Also, step-stress input at $t = 0$.

$\sigma_1(\alpha, \omega)$ Amplitude of the fundamental harmonic in the Fourier series expansion of $\sigma(t) = \sigma[\alpha(t), \omega]$

τ Time constant for mass-spring-dashpot system; also, absolute nerve or muscle refractory period

τ_o Time delay of physiologic reflex pathway

τ_1 Velocity sensitivity of muscle spindle; also, time constant defining the location of one of the "zeroes" of a standard mechanical lead/lag viscoelastic network (in the LaPlace Phase Plane)

τ_2 Acceleration sensitivity of muscle spindle; also, time constant defining the location in the LaPlace Frequency Domain of one of the "Poles" of a standard mechanical lead/lag viscoelastic network

τ_3 Time constant defined by the quantity $\dfrac{B_f}{k_f}$

τ_d Decay Time-Response Constant of Feedback Control System

τ_F Isotonic Twitch Time Constant $= \dfrac{c(k_s + k_p)}{k_s k_p} = \dfrac{1}{K} =$ Strain Relaxation Time Constant

τ_L — Lower Breakpoint Frequency Time Constant

τ_P — Stress Retardation Time Constant $= \dfrac{c}{k_s}$

τ_S — Synaptic Time Constant for Acetylcholinesterase

τ_U — Upper Breakpoint Frequency Time Constant

τ_ε — Stress Relaxation Time Constant $= \dfrac{c}{k_s}$

τ_σ — Strain Retardation Time Constant, $\dfrac{1}{K}$

τ^* — Dummy variable for integration with respect to stress-relaxation time-constant (c.f., equation [3-52])

$\tau^*{}_o$ — Time interval necessary to bring membrane to threshold

$\tau^*{}_m$ — Membrane Time Constant $= R^*{}_m C^*{}_m$

ϕ — Phase Angle; $\tan \phi = (k_s/c\omega) \div (k_p/k_s)[(k_s/c\omega)^2 + (\dfrac{k_s}{k_p} + 1)]$

ϕ_o — Phase Angle defined by: $\sin \phi_o = \pm \dfrac{u_r}{u_a} \sqrt{\left(\dfrac{u_a}{u_r}\right)^2 - \dfrac{T_t{}^2}{4\pi^2 \tau_d{}^2}}$

ϕ_1 — Muscle Spindle Phase Angle

ϕ_2 — Golgi Tendon Organ Phase Angle

$\phi_1(\alpha, \omega)$ — Phase Angle defined by: $\tan \phi_1(\alpha, \omega) = \dfrac{G''_r(\omega)}{G'_r(\omega)}$

χ — Dummy Variable for purposes of integration

ψ — Hill Equation Exponent (c.f., equation [1-3])

ψ_o, ψ_1 — Components of Hamiltonian Function

ω — Circular Frequency $= 2\pi f$

ω_o — Driving (Forcing) Frequency

$\omega_{U,L}$ — Upper (U) and Lower (L) Circular Break-point or Corner Frequencies, respectively $= (1/\tau_U)$ and $(1/\tau_L)$

Φ — Nondimensionalized Active Muscle Tension $= B_1 \dfrac{F_{\text{total}} - F_{\text{passive}}}{F_{\text{isometric}}}$

Ω — Weighting Function designating the fraction of active cross-bridges in a half-sarcomere of a contracting muscle fiber

Foreword

The *New York University Biomedical Engineering* series is a series of books and monographs which will attempt to present a number of the more important contributions which engineering has recently made in the fields of medicine and biology. For many years the contributions of the physical sciences to medicine were primarily restricted to the field of radiology. However, with the explosive growth of engineering theory and technology in the last 40 years, the applications of engineering to medicine have become important in fields as diverse as cardiology, cardiac surgery, neurology, neurosurgery, orthopedics, ophthalmology, urology, respiratory medicine, and indeed in general medical diagnosis.

In these applications it has been desirable to draw upon many classical engineering disciplines, such as electrical engineering, electronics, computer engineering, computer science, mechanical engineering, mechanics, hydraulics, material science, and chemical engineering, as well as such recent disciplines as systems theory and information theory.

There has been a widespread impression that work in such interdisciplinary fields as biomedical engineering is impeded by the difficulties in communication among the physicians, life scientists, physical scientists, and engineers. This series of books is evidence that such a blockage in communications no longer exists and that the scientists involved in exploring this interdisciplinary field have learned each other's language.

The successes of engineering methodologies in medicine have been substantial in recent years. In cardiology we see patient monitoring, cardiac output measurement, noninvasive assessment, implantable cardiac pacemakers, intra-aortic balloon pumps, and artificial hearts. In imaging we see computer-aided tomography, ultrasonic analysis, digital fluorography, magnetic resonance imaging, and positron emission tomography. In biomaterials and biomechanical engineering we see artificial joints, artificial limbs, artificial skin, gait analysis, connective tissue studies, and myoelectrically controlled prostheses. Finally, in the neurological sciences we see electroencephalography, electromyography, electrooculography, evoked potentials, radionuclide brain imaging, vision analysis, and the study of visual fields and thresholds.

It is these successes and many others that are described in the books in this series, and in each case a careful engineering analysis is presented with appropriate mathematics to elucidate the various physiological and anatomical mechanisms discussed.

Walter Welkowitz
Rutgers University

Preface and Acknowledgments

Throughout history, the mechanics of striated skeletal muscle has fascinated and challenged humankind. In sports, coaches and trainers are constantly striving to optimize musculoskeletal performance -- to get athletes to run faster, to jump higher, to gain physical agility and strength, to swim farther, to hit harder, and so on. In the military, there is an ever-increasing need to define and expand upon the envelope of human performance capabilities as these relate to sophisticated combat technology and adverse theaters of operation. Indeed, it is well documented that physiologic limitations seriously restrict both the actual performance capabilities of man-machine-type combat vehicles, and the types of combat situations into which military personnel may be effectively engaged.

In medicine, physicians, scientists, and allied health-care practitioners are being perpetually challenged by the mysteries of neuromusculoskeletal diseases and other disabilities. And even in the arts (the visual and performing arts, including all forms of dance), muscles and bones play a prominent role as a means of expression and communication. Visual artists have painted them. Sculptors have carved and modelled them. Photographers have taken pictures of them. Choreographers have beautified them in graceful form and movement.

Throughout the years, this interest in muscles has resulted in the development of many theories that attempt to describe its chemistry, physics and mechanical behavior. A detailed review of several of these theories has been presented at VPI&SU annually since 1973 in a course entitled, "Mechanics of Muscles and Soft Tissues." In 1985, the class notes that had been prepared for this course, and developed over a 12-year period were assembled into the first edition of a textbook entitled, *Mechanics of Muscle.*

What follows is a revised, updated second edition of this textbook which includes additional material accumulated since 1985. The material presented, including a significant number of homework problem sets, is at a level suitable for fourth-year engineering students or first-year graduate students. As mentioned by a reviewer of the first edition, writing in the journal *Annals of Biomedical Engineering,* Vol. 15, No. 3/4, pp. 413-415, 1987, "This book would serve as an excellent textbook in any bioengineering curriculum. Furthermore, it is a useful reference for researchers interested in understanding muscular mechanics." Another reviewer called it, "The best textual reference on the subject of muscle mechanics ... a timely and excellent addition to the tutorial literature."

Chapter 1 provides an introduction to the anatomy and physiology of striated skeletal muscle, to the extent that an understanding of these is necessary in order to follow subsequent discussions related to the physics and chemistry of its mechanical behavior. In Chapters 2, 3, and 4, mathematical models are developed to describe quantitatively the response characteristics of muscle tissue. Chapter 2 addresses Nubar's elegant nonlinear elastic (time-independent) model; Chapter 3 examines Bahler's classic linear viscoelastic conceptualization; and Chapter 4 looks at two attempts (those of Decraemer, et al., and Hatze) that have been made more recently to explore the nonlinear behavior of muscle within the context of its statistical time-dependent properties. These particular models have been chosen for study because of their accurate prediction of what is known concerning muscular performance.

In Chapter 5, we take a look at the mechanics and energetics of muscular contraction -- both the kinematics and kinetics of this process; work, energy, efficiency of contraction, and so on. This is followed in Chapter 6 by an anatomical and physiological review of the mechanisms involved in *control* of muscular contraction; and, finally, in Chapter 7 by an introduction to concepts related to the mathematical modelling of such neuromuscular control systems.

Throughout the book, the mechanics of muscular contraction is always presented from a bioengineering point of view, but within the context of biochemical and biophysical considerations as we think we know them today. In all cases, the reader is first introduced to the basic fundamentals related to the topic to be discussed -- anatomical, physiological, and engineering -- and then the material is presented, complete with numerical examples and homework problems. This makes it particularly suited for classroom use. It is the author's opinion (and that of several reviewers, as mentioned earlier) that this book should also prove useful in a more general sense as a reference text for individuals working in the field of muscle mechanics. There is much useful information of a broader anatomical and physiological nature that can be readily assimilated by those who do not necessarily have a highly technical background.

Many kudos are in order here before I can take any of the credit for the work which follows. In fact, I could probably fill a textbook just thanking by individual citation all of the wonderful people who have helped to bring this venture to fruition. There are, of course, the three women in my life -- my wonderful wife, Judi, and my equally-delightful daughters, Patti and Cyndi -- without whom anything I do would mean nothing. They *exemplify* the meaning of the words love, tolerance, patience, and understanding, and I shall be forever grateful to them for putting up with me! I am also indebted to the New York University Press series in Biomedical Engineering -- edited by Dr. Walter Welkowitz -- and to director Colin Jones and acquisitions editor Jason Renker, for agreeing to include this book as a part of the series, and for their many helpful editorial suggestions. That's six people already!

Connie Callison, what would I do without you? Your ability to make a preliminary manuscript look so polished in final typeset format never ceases to amaze me -- as does the good-natured way in which you always seem to handle any impending crisis. And ditto to Paula Lee, who did all of the Tables; and to Beulah Prestrude for her wonderful artwork in all of the Figures. That's three more people. Then there is the administration within my Department (Engineering Science and Mechanics), my College (Engineering), and my University (VPI&SU), who encouraged and supported me all the way. Gosh, that's lots of people.

Then there are all of the authors, investigators, researchers, and teachers (appropriately referenced throughout the book) whose work contributed (directly or indirectly) to much of the material presented. That's literally hundreds of people who have provided me with tremendous amounts of resource "stuff" in order that I could develop our Muscle Mechanics course, and the textbook that eventually evolved from it. Not to mention my *own* students, perhaps a couple of hundred of them since 1973, who helped with proof-reading, providing "helpful" suggestions and inputs, trouble-shooting the problems, and telling me when what I was writing was not making any sense to *them*.

Wow, we are getting up in the neighborhood of around six or seven hundred individuals to this point ... so, in the interest of space, perhaps I should stop. You get the message, though. While only one name appears as the "author" of a book such as this, the credit deserves to be shared among all who contributed in whatever way -- and reducing it to only one "author" is just a matter of convenience. My heartfelt thanks goes out to *all* of you with much humility and sincerity.

Blacksburg, Virginia
Daniel J. Schneck
June 1, 1991.

Chapter 1

Introduction, Anatomy and Physiology of Striated Skeletal Muscle ... The Source of Human Power

Introduction

The broad science dedicated to the study of movement, and to the active and passive structures involved, is called *kinesiology*. This word is derived from the Greek, "kinesis", meaning "movement", and "-logia", pertaining to a complete body of knowledge. Kinesiology thus addresses such diverse subjects as:

1) the scientific study of the mechanisms involved in transforming chemically-bound potential energy into mechanical energy, in a process known as *Excitation-Contraction Coupling* (see later in this chapter);

2) the processes (biochemical, physiological and anatomical) by which motor skills are learned and developed, including mechanisms of adaptation, conditioning, and the general topic of *work physiology*;

3) the techniques that can be used to perfect motor skills and improve the efficiency of human movement -- an area which includes *exercise physiology*;

4) the behavioral patterns (psychological, environmental and cultural) that motivate biological systems to take action of some

kind -- i.e., *body language*, in the more popular sense of this terminology;

5) interactions that take place at human-machine interfaces, including concern for designating work stations to accommodate the
anatomical, physiological, and psychological characteristics and
limitations of the human organism in such a way as to enhance
human efficiency and well being. This activity is in the realm of
Ergonomics and *Human Factors Engineering*, which recognize
humans as the ultimate builders and users of "things", whatever
those "things" might be;

6) the effects of the environment, or of environmental extremes of
temperature, pressure, acceleration, gravity, and so on, on
musculoskeletal function -- an area generally designated as *environmental stress physiology*, and including aerospace medicine as
a sub-discipline; and,

7) the space and time response of biological organisms to distributed
systems of external and internal forces. This last topic comprises
the subject matter of the engineering science called *Biomechanics*.

Mechanics, in general, is the engineering science that concerns itself
with interactions among things in our universe -- the "things" being classified generically as *solids, fluids*, and/or substances exhibiting the behavior of either or both (e.g., *viscoelastic* materials); and the "interactions"
manifesting themselves as *forces*. Biomechanics of the musculoskeletal
system, then, deals more specifically with the action of the central nervous
system, motor nerves, skeletal muscles, bones, and joints, in causing
(and/or allowing) the human body to function effectively and efficiently
within the external and internal force environments to which it is exposed.
Forces external to the organism include, for example, gravity, magnetism,
electromagnetism, ground reactions, atmospheric drag, atmospheric pressure, inertia (acceleration), vibration, certain types of impact, and various
forms of buoyancy.

Forces internal to the organism are derived from a special mechanism which is designed to transform chemical free (or bond) energy into

mechanical work. This mechanism is the striated skeletal muscle, and the work done is, or the forces developed are transmitted to a type of engineering structure designed to convert muscular effort into the maintenance of postural balance or the locomotion of parts or all of the animal body. The latter is, of course, the skeletal system and its associated articulations (joints).

The study of muscle is called *Myology,* again after the Greek, "mys", meaning "muscle". There are three types of muscle:

1) Cardiac Muscle, which has the anatomic and physiologic characteristics of striated skeletal muscle, but which shows electrical stimulation and excitation-contraction behavior more typical of smooth muscle tissue;

2) Vascular and Visceral Smooth Muscle, which, together with Cardiac Muscle, maintain the *internal* environment ("tone" and "dynamics") of the human body; and,

3) Striated Skeletal (voluntary) muscles, attached to bones by tendons, and acting:

   a) To maintain postural balance by serving (together with ligaments) as tensile load-bearing members -- in equilibrium with bones acting as rigid compressive members -- of the physiologic system; and,

   b) To cause locomotion of parts or all of the animal body by pulling on the bones to which they are attached, thereby creating a lever-type action around joints serving as pivot points.

Skeletal muscle is the single largest tissue in the body, accounting for up to 40-43% of total body weight in men and 23-25% in women. It contains 33% of the total protein content of the organism; and it is responsible for some 50% of the resting metabolic energy consumption of the physiologic system. For the most part, these mechanical transducers are capable of performing their functions by quickly and reversibly shortening in a process called *contraction.* This represents the ability that muscle has to alter its length and/or its lengthwise tension in a unidirectional fashion. That is, one end of the muscle, its *origin,* remains essentially stationary (fixed), while the other end, its *insertion* (usually spanning across a joint), moves -- and contraction always takes place *from* insertion *towards* origin, pulling the distal (insertion-end) bone towards (flexion) or away from (extension) the proximal (origin-end) bone.

It should be noted that -- properly used -- the term, "contraction", only indicates *shortening,* but does not describe the actual generation of a *force.* The latter results only from the muscle's attempt to contract against a resistance, in which case the contraction *generates* a force by virtue of the fact that the resistance pulls back against the contractile mechanism. When contraction takes place in the *absence* of any resistance, *no* force is generated, and the shortening takes place at *maximum* speed. This is known as a "no-load-contraction", or, an *Atonic Contraction.* When contraction takes place against the *maximum* resistance, *maximum* muscular force is generated and the shortening takes place at *zero* speed, i.e., there is no measurable change in muscle length. This is known as an *Isometric Contraction.* In-between these two extremes, one can define an *Isotonic* (constant-force) and/or an *Isokinetic* (constant-velocity) contraction, both of which we shall get back to later in this text.

To understand the process of muscular contraction, one must have at least a working knowledge of the fine structure of muscle. Many excellent texts are available on this subject and no attempt will be made here to add to the vast and comprehensive literature already at the reader's disposal. However, some essential features of the anatomy and physiology of striated skeletal muscle will be presented to the extent that they will be useful in understanding the material which follows in subsequent chapters.

Anatomy of Muscle

Molecular Ultramicroscopic Structure of Contractile Elements

By weight, muscle is composed of about 20% protein, 75% water, and 5% "extractives" and inorganic salts. The protein *Myosin* (molecular weight up to around 490,000 Daltons, where 1 Dalton = 1.66024×10^{-24} grams) accounts for more than half (some 50-60%) of the total protein in muscle tissue. This protein assumes the shape of a molecular rod, about 1500Å long by 15-20 Å wide, with a short globular region at one end that "bends" the overall configuration into an L-shaped structure. The "corner" of the L is called a *hinge*. When treated with the enzyme Trypsin, the "horizontal-leg" of the "L" splits off from the "vertical-spine" or "tail" at the hinge, producing two quite-different molecules. The heavier of the two molecules has a molecular weight up to about 350,000 and is known as *Heavy Meromyosin*, HMM. This molecule has ATP-ase activity (i.e., it can catalyze the hydrolysis of Adenosine Triphosphate to release energy for muscular contraction), an affinity for the protein Actin (i.e., it can form a "cross-bridge" configuration with Actin as described later), and appears in the electron microscope to consist of a short (200 Å), rod-like, double-helical polypeptide chain known as Segment-2 (i.e., HMM-S-2), at the end of which lies a two-headed 60-70 Å-Diameter globular polypeptide region known as Segment-1 (i.e., HMM-S-1 or, the "head" of the molecule). HMM-S-2 and HMM-S-1 are also attached at a "hinge" (see Figure 1-1).

The two globular heads of HMM-S-1 are presumed to contain one binding site to which an energy-providing molecule of ATP is believed to become attached in the presence of Calcium ions, and one binding site to which the protein Actin apparently becomes attached during the contractile process. When the muscle tissue is at rest, the Actin binding sites are not occupied because the Troponin-Tropomyosin protein complex essentially acts as a passive "filler" to prevent the establishment of an Actomyosin Complex (see later). It is also believed that, at rest, ATP bound to the HMM-S-1 "head" of HMM further contributes to the dissociation of this segment (i.e., the "cross-bridge") from Actin molecules, thereby giving ATP a "Relaxation Role" in muscle metabolism.

The smaller of the two products formed by the trypsin-digestion of Myosin has a molecular weight of 96,000 to 140,000 and is known as Light Meromyosin, or LMM. This molecule has no ATP-ase activity, will not react with Actin, and appears under the electron microscope to be two rod-shaped polypeptide chains wrapped around each other in a double-helix and devoid of a terminal globular region. Thus, LMM acts as a "spine" or "tail" from which HMM-S-2 side chains emanate at periodic intervals. The "tails" of many (100 to 250) Myosin molecules become entwined around one another, as illustrated in Figure 1-1, establishing an overlapping, helical pattern in which a rather thick (100-120 Å) 0.15-micron-long H-zone separates end-regions from which as many as 250 HMM side-chains (or "cross-bridges") emanate. The significance of these side-chains shall be discussed later.

The protein *Actin* (total molecular weight up to 76,000) constitutes an additional 12, to as much as 25% by weight of the total muscle protein content. Actin has been identified in two combined forms: Globular, or G-Actin (molecular weight about 42,000 to 47,000), and a polymer of G-Actin, known as Fibrous, or F-Actin, which is presumed to be the backbone of the thin muscular filaments (see later). Fibrous Actin consists of two helical strands having a pitch of 700 Å (see Figure 1-2). The two strands are pieced together with 55 Å-length-attached-subunits, and are out of phase, so that they cross over each other at intervals of around 350 Å. It is believed that each G-Actin molecule contains one bound ADP (Adenosine Diphosphate) molecule which, as does ATP, contains ionized phosphate groups and thus carries a net negative charge. Myosin is presumed to bind to Actin at these ADP-sites. Figure 1-2 illustrates how the double-helical configuration of Actin may intertwine with the HMM-S-1 side-chains of Myosin, forming "potential" cross-bridge attachments between the two protein filaments. The word "potential" is used within quotation marks because these cross-bridge attachments are not manifest in the muscle at rest, for reasons discussed below.

The most important of the remaining proteins are *Troponin, Tropomyosin, Myoglobin,* and *Collagen.* Although present in relatively small amounts in mammalian muscle, Troponin and Tropomyosin are key elements in the contractile process. This is because, as previously mentioned, when striated skeletal muscles are in a resting state, the molecular

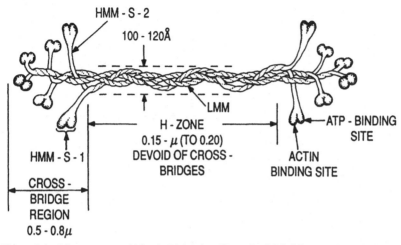

HMM - S - 2
100 - 120Å
LMM
H - ZONE
0.15 - μ (TO 0.20)
DEVOID OF CROSS -
BRIDGES
HMM - S - 1
CROSS -
BRIDGE
REGION
0.5 - 0.8μ
ATP - BINDING
SITE
ACTIN
BINDING SITE

Figure 1-1 Microstructure of Myosin Molecules, illustrating Light Meromyosin (LMM) inter-twined "spines" devoid of cross-bridges—forming the H-Zone of the structure—and Heavy Meromyosin (HMM) "appendages" forming the cross-bridge region of the structure. The HMM region consists of a short side-chain segment, HMM-S-2, at the end of which lies a globular cross-bridge sement, HMM-S-1. The latter has binding sites for Adenosine Triphosphate (ATP), and, during the contractile process, Actin.

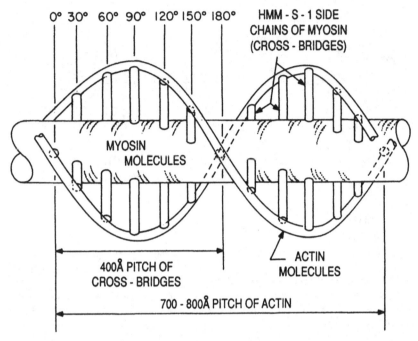

0° 30° 60° 90° 120° 150° 180°

HMM - S - 1 SIDE
CHAINS OF MYOSIN
(CROSS - BRIDGES)

MYOSIN
MOLECULES

400Å PITCH OF
CROSS - BRIDGES

ACTIN
MOLECULES

700 - 800Å PITCH OF ACTIN

Figure 1-2 Schematic illustration of one mechanism by which the double-helical configuration of thin Actin molecules may intertwine with the thicker Myosin molecules, forming cross-bridge attachments at the HMM-S-1 sites of the Heavy Meromyosin side chains—each 30° of circumferential increment, approximately every 60 to 70 Angstroms along the longitudinal axis of the thicker Myosin polymers—thus establishing the "Active-State" Actomyosin Complex of the contractile muscular Myofilaments.

sites at which the cross-bridges from the Myosin molecules would normally attach to Actin are occupied instead by the two proteins, Troponin (which has three subunits -- TnT, TnI, and TnC) and Tropomyosin. These are long (about 40 nm) polypeptide, rod-shaped molecules (MW = 70,000) that attach end-to-end, forming thin continuous strands that run along the length of the Actin filament. Each 40 nm-Troponin molecule contains calcium-binding sites (TnC) that are empty when the muscle is in a resting state, and Actin-binding sites (TnI) that "tie-up" seven Actin monomers (400 Å/55 Å $\approx$ 7) at a time with the muscle at rest. Thus, the Troponin-Tropomyosin complexes (attached to each other at the TnT binding sites) lie in the "grooves" between the Actin and Myosin chains, thereby inhibiting or actually blocking any potential interaction that could occur between the Actin molecules and the Myosin cross-bridges, and causing the myofilament complex to have a discontinuous structure at rest. The Troponin-Tropomyosin blockade of the establishment of an Acto-Myosin cross-bridge configuration with the muscle at rest is believed to allow for a "free-sliding" arrangement, so muscles can be stretched or otherwise deformed while at rest. Otherwise, the Actomyosin complex would keep the muscle filaments in a "locked" state at all times, such that muscles "at rest" would always be in a "cramped" or "rigor mortis" state, significantly impeding any freedom of movement.

The red-pigment protein Myoglobin, which has been observed in quantities ranging by weight of muscle from 0.10 to 1.00 percent, binds oxygen for immediate needs during muscular contraction. Collagen, the most abundant protein in the whole body (representing 30% of total body protein), comprises the insoluble fiber of the binding, supporting and connecting substance in muscle tissue.

The extractives of muscle consist of fats, electrolytes (the most important of which are Calcium, Sodium, Potassium, Magnesium, and Chlorine), nitrogenous wastes, nonnitrogenous wastes, pigments (organic coloring matter such as from myohemoglobin), enzymes, and carbohydrates -- the most important of which is the sugar, Glucose, or, in its stored form, Glycogen. Glycogen, together with the compounds Adenosine Triphosphate (ATP, manufactured in the Mitochondria of the muscle tissue) and Phosphocreatine form the "fuel element" of the muscle.

The proteins Actin and Myosin, when immersed in water, gel into long (300-400 connected molecules) complex threadlike molecular Actomyosin chains known as filaments or myofilaments. As shown in Figures 1-1 and 1-2, the longitudinal configuration of these myofilaments shows the actin molecules "wrapped" in a double-helix around the myosin molecules (Figure 1-2), which are themselves "twisted" around each other along a bridge-free zone where LMM strands overlap (the H-zone; Figure 1-1). Viewed in cross section, thick filaments (100-120 Angstrom diameter by 1.2 to 1.8 microns in length, containing up to 400 intertwined myosin molecules) are seen to be closely packed with thin filaments (60-70 Angstrom diameter by 1.0 micron long Actin chains), in a double-hexagonal array which forms the contracting ultrastructure (elastic element, EE) of the muscle. Generally, some 100 to 1500 myosin filaments are grouped together with about twice as many actin filaments to form a *myofibril* (see later).

The hexagonal cross-sectional array of the thick filaments measures some 250 ± 50 Angstroms on a side, while that of the thin filaments measures about 145 ± 30 Angstroms on a side. As is illustrated in Figure 1-2, and, in somewhat more detail in Figure 1-3, the two kinds of filaments can be linked together by an intricate double-helical system of 100-200 Å cross-bridges (formed in part by the head of the HMM portion of the myosin molecule), spaced 60-70 Angstroms apart along the axis of the filament and 30 degrees apart in a circumferential direction. That is, viewed from the side (Figure 1-2) the thin filaments are seen to be wrapped around the thick filaments in a spiraling configuration, with the pitch of the helix being about 400 Angstroms along the myosin chain and about 700-800 Å along the actin chain. Thus, to get from one cross-bridge to the next, one would have to travel in a helical fashion, 60 to 70 Angstroms longitudinally and 30 degrees circumferentially, so that after travelling about 400 Angstroms *along* the filament (about 6 bridges) the individual would be half-way around the myosin molecule, and after travelling about 800 Angstroms (about 12 bridges) the individual would arrive back to the same circumferential position from which he or she started.   The double-hexagonal cross-sectional array and the double-helical longitudinal configuration of the myofilaments results in each thin filament being surrounded by three thick filaments and each thick filament being surrounded by six thin filaments (see cross-sectional end-view in Figure 1-3).

Some 400 to 2500 (even up to as many as 4500) tiny muscle filaments are now packed tight in a 0.5 to as large as 3-micron-diameter bundle known as a fibril or *myofibril,* and covered by a membrane called the *endomysium.* The function of the endomysium is to support the nerve fibers, capillaries, and veins that connect the muscle fiber to the central supply system.   Myofibrils are bathed and surrounded by muscle cytoplasm (cell fluid), within which lie a large number of *mitochondria.* These are elongated cellular organelles (literally, "little organs") which are the sites of energy production through ATP-ADP metabolism (see Schneck, D. J., 1990).

A fibril is the smallest natural muscle unit from which a contraction has been obtained.   Hence, the term *contractile element,* CE is often used to describe this part of the muscle that generates the tension.   Moreover, although thick and thin myofilaments are segregated into separate rows, the rows overlap (see side-views in Figure 1-3) to yield light and dark segments which appear as striations when viewed under an electron microscope -- hence the name *striated* skeletal muscle.   Cardiac muscle also shows such striations; smooth muscle tissue does not.

The light areas, called the isotropic or I-bands (about 0.4 microns long), consist mainly of actin molecular chains having low indices of refraction.   The dark areas, called the anisotropic, or A-bands (1.2-1.8 microns long), consist mainly of myosin molecular chains having high indices of refraction.   The striations show a characteristic repeating pattern about every 0.002 millimeters, or 2 to $2 - \frac{1}{2}$ microns, such that the fibril appears to be composed of a series of disk-like partitions, called

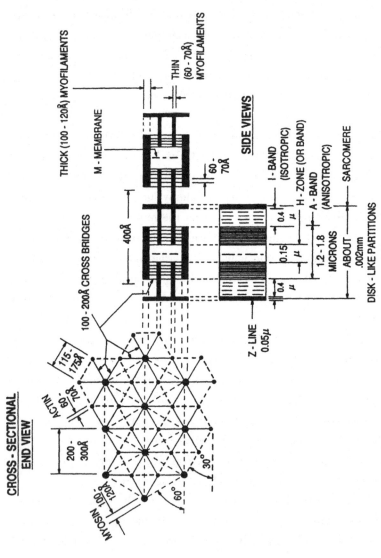

Figure 1-3 Schematic Representation Of The Anatomical Cross-Striated (Side Views), Double-Hexagonal (Cross-Sectional End View) Microstructure Of Striated Skeletal Muscle.

sarcomeres. The sarcomere boundaries are delineated by spacers called "Z-lines" (from the German, "Zwischenscheidung," meaning, "dividing band"). These are dense membranes believed to add structural rigidity and stability against buckling to the delicate actin molecular chains that are anchored to them. A similar, but lighter membrane (called the M-membrane, to which the myosin molecular chains are anchored) exists at the center of the A-band, which has been previously identified as the 0.15-micron-long H-zone representing the bridge-free region of LMM-overlap. The thick myosin and thin actin filaments overlap for about 0.5 to 0.8 microns at either end of the A-band, yielding relatively dark striations in a region that contains on the order of 250 cross-bridges. In effect, then, viewed under a light-microscope, the myofibril is seen as a long chain of sarcomeres (like a roll of coins), separated by Z-lines and wrapped with a connective tissue (the endomysium) which contains capillaries to furnish oxygen and vital nutrients to the tissue.

Microstructure of Motor Units

Myofibrils surrounded by muscle cytoplasm *(sarcoplasm)* are arranged into tightly packed bundles called *fasciculi*, which are wrapped by a fibrous structure of connective tissue called *fascia*. Embedded within the fascia are more nerves and blood vessels that both innervate and vascularize the fasciculi separated and bathed by the cytoplasmic fluid called *sarcoplasm.* Many bundles of fibrils are grouped together and covered by a thin (less than 10 nm thick) semipermeable membrane called the *sarcolemma.* This constitutes the basic *muscle fiber,* which is a cylindrical unit, 10 to 100 microns in diameter by 1 to as many as 400 millimeters long. The multifidus muscle fiber in the human spinal column, for example, is 5 mm long, while the Sartorius muscle fiber of the human thigh is about 400 mm long. More generally, muscle fibers tend to "average" around 45 mm in length, and to contain many hundreds, or even thousands of fibrils. Moreover, each striated skeletal muscle fiber is a *single* large cell, containing large numbers of mitochondria and as many as several hundred nuclei located at regular intervals near the surface of the fiber, just subjacent to the sarcolemma. The *number* of fibers in any given muscle is fixed at birth. The *size* of fibers, however, is not. Thus, exercise and conditioning can stimulate the production in muscle tissue of more Actin and Myosin filaments, a greater number of cross-bridges, additional blood vasculature, and corresponding connective tissue -- all resulting in an increase in both the size, strength and endurance of the muscle.

As illustrated in Figure 1-4, the muscle fiber at rest has a polarized sarcolemma due, for the most part, to the active transport mechanism known as the *Sodium-Potassium Electrogenic Pump* (see Chapter 3 of Schneck, D. J., 1990). This "pump" (actually, many pumps), located in the cell membrane actively transports *three* sodium ions *from* the inside of the muscle fiber *to* the outside, in exchange for *two* potassium ions transported from outside in. There is thus a net transfer of 50% more positive charges outward through the membrane than inward, creating a transmural electrical potential of about 0.10 Volts in the fiber at rest, as well as a chemical concentration gradient for sodium, potassium *and* (passively) chlorine ions. Activation for contraction is accomplished by depolarizing this membrane, as described below. The depolarization, in turn, is triggered from the central nervous system by attaching to a muscle fiber an efferent motor nerve (or α-moto-neuron, see Figure 1-4), which carries an *action potential excitatory impulse* to the *motor end plate* of a group of muscle fibers. The motor end plate is where several muscle fibers share some common portion of sarcolemma in a region near their respective center called the *myoneural junction.*

The smallest muscular unit (group of fibers) that can be controlled by an alpha-moto-neuron is called a *motor unit* (m.u.) and consists of anywhere from one-to-three short fibers up to 2000 long fibers, all innervated by a *single* motor axon emanating from the ventral (stomach-side) root of the spinal cord. The muscle fibers of one motor unit do not necessarily lie side by side in a contiguous region of the tissue, but, rather, tend to assemble in bundles of only a few fibers each, spread in "clusters"

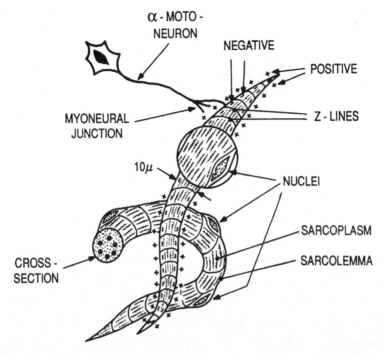

Figure 1-4 Polarized (inside about 90 millivolts negative relative to outside) Striated Skeletal Muscle Fibers. Each is a single multinucleated cell, innervated at the Myoneural Junction by an alpha-motoneuron originating in the Ventral Root of the Spinal Cord. For details of Cross-Section, see Figure 1-3.

throughout the entire muscle. Thus, "firing" one motor unit does not cause a strong (or concentrated) contraction at one *specific* location in a muscle, but, instead, tends to produce a weak (or diffuse) contraction *throughout* the entire muscle, generating a corresponding small force at the muscle tendons. It *is* true, however, that excitation of each fiber in a motor unit is an all-or-none response, i.e., the fiber contracts all the way, or it does not contract at all. Thus, the tension developed by any *single* muscle fiber, or the amount by which it shortens against a given external load will *not* be increased by increasing the *strength* (above some minimum *threshold* level, see later) of a single action potential stimulus. This quantum of response elicited from a *single* threshold stimulus administered to a *single* motor unit is known as a *muscle twitch;* and the "all-or-none" principle applies *only* to such a *single stimulus* applied to a *single muscle fiber*.

Increasing the strength or frequency of a stimulus applied *repeatedly* to a *whole* muscle *will* increase the force of contraction -- an effect called a *graded response*. This results from: a) an increased *frequency-dependent active state* of any *given* muscle fiber -- known as the *staircase-effect* up to a *tetanic contraction;* or, b) an increase in the *number* of muscle fibers and motor units activated by a continuously increasing frequency of stimulation of any given muscle -- known as *recruitment* up to a *tetanic contraction;* or, c) some combination of (a) and (b) plus, perhaps, the additional help of *other* muscles that come to the aid of the one in question in a process called *synergism*. All of these shall be discussed both later in this chapter and in subsequent chapters in this text, but the point to be made is that the *intensity* of any muscular contraction is controlled less by the *intensity* of the stimulus than by its *frequency*.

An α-moto-neuron may innervate more than one motor unit, but each motor unit is innervated by only *one* α-moto-neuron. Thus, the *Innervation Ratio* is defined to be the number of nerve fibers (i.e., 1), divided by the number of innervated muscle fiber(s). The *larger* this ratio (i.e., the *less* fibers innervated per nerve), the finer the muscle *control*. For example, the musculature of the eye has an innervation ratio of about

1:7, while this ratio for the quadriceps femoris musculature affecting knee extension is approximately 1:1000.

The action potential delivered by an α-motoneuron to the motor end plate region of a muscle fiber propagates both longitudinally *along* the fiber to depolarize the sarcolemma, and transversely *into* the fibers through inward conducting structures that are in the form of transverse tubules which originate as inward extensions (invaginations) of the sarcolemma at each Z-band (see Figure 1-5). These interconnecting transverse tubules appear almost as bands wrapped around the muscle filaments and fibrils, and are referred to collectively as the *T-system* of the muscle. The T-system, discovered in 1957, was found to be a membraneous structure in close proximity to, but not a part of *another* system of 400-Angstrom diameter, agranular anastomosing tubules that run *parallel* to (as opposed to *transverse* to) the myofibrils, and that form a "plumbing" network called the *Sarcoplasmic Reticulum* or *SR-system* of the Muscle (see Figure 1-5). As illustrated in Figure 1-5, each T-tubule, polarized to a potential in the range from 0.5 to 1.5 millivolts, runs between a pair of "sacs" formed by the fusion of the sarcoplasmic reticulum or SR-tubules at their ends. The sacs are large vesicular chambers lying in the spaces between the myofibrils, and are called *cisterns*. Each tubule (structure 3 in Figure 1-5), together with the two adjacent cisternae with which it is associated (structures 1 and 2 in Figure 1-5) make up what is known as a *Triad*. In human muscle tissue, there are a pair of T-tubule networks for each sarcomere, i.e., one originating at each Z-line located near the ends of the myosin filaments. Thus the tissue is optimally organized for rapid and efficient excitation.

The sarcoplasmic reticulum provides a fluid transport system between the cells inside and outside the muscle. Its polarized membrane helps carry electrical messages, while the sarcoplasmic matrix fluid it contains helps carry chemical constituents and fuel into and out of the muscle fibers. Within the terminal cisternae of the SR -- which *also* run transverse to the fibers (i.e., are parallel to the T-system) are trapped calcium ions, which cannot escape when the muscle is at rest because the

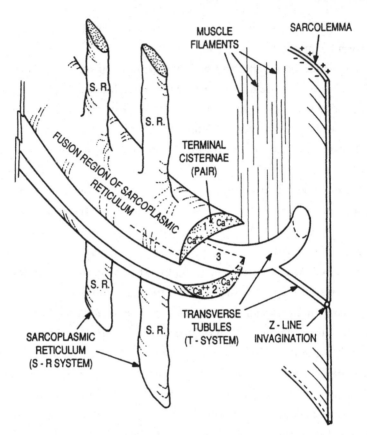

Figure 1-5 Transverse Tubule (3) sandwiched in-between a pair of calcium-containing Terminal Cisterns (1,2) in the fused region of the Sarcoplasmic Reticulum—the elements 1,2, and 3 forming what is known as a *Triad*. Note that the triad runs transverse to the muscle filaments and fibrils, which, themselves, run essentially parallel to the polarized sarcolemma. The T-System originates from invaginations of the Sarcolemma at the Z-Lines.

membrane of the sarcoplasmic reticulum is normally semipermeable to these ions -- allowing them passage into (via a calcium "pump"), but not out of these chambers.

In general, motor units are classified as being either of the low threshold *Tonic* or high threshold *Phasic* type. Short, Type I, Slow Oxidative (S.O.), *Tonic motor units* -- otherwise known as *red slow twitch* (S.T.) muscle fibers -- are innervated by small α-motoneuron axons, and activated by sustained *low frequency* muscle action potentials (m.a.p.) that are conducted slowly through the tissue, and produce *slow* twitches (60-120 msec "time-to-peak", see later) that generate *small* peak tensions in isolated muscle preparations. Such motor units are associated with movements requiring fine control (e.g., motion of the fingers, face, or eyes). They are highly fatigue-resistant because their high capillary density (which gives them their characteristic "red" appearance) and rich supply of the oxygen carrier, myoglobin, provides sufficient blood perfusion and oxygen to allow a great deal of aerobic activity. These motor units, however, do not function well under anaerobic conditions.

On the other hand, movements requiring *large* forces but not necessarily fine control, such as are typical of the arms and legs, are accomplished by long, Type II, *white fast twitch* (F.T.), *Phasic motor units,* which are innervated by large motor axons, and activated by intermittent bursts of *high frequency,* more intense muscle action potentials that are conducted relatively rapidly through the tissue, such that they produce *fast* twitches (15-50 msec "time-to-peak") generating *large* peak tensions in isolated muscle preparations. Type II fibers have been further classified as being either *fast oxidative glycolytic* (F.O.G., or type IIa), or, simply *fast glycolytic* (F.G., or type IIb). The latter have a very low capillary density (i.e., are the "whitest" of the white fibers). Being thus deprived of a substantial blood supply, F.G. fibers have a low aerobic capacity with the consequent result that they are the most easily fatiguable of all fibers. However, they *do* have the highest *anaerobic* capacity.

By contrast, the type IIa fibers -- which are physically the largest in *size* of *all* fibers -- have a higher capillary density than do type IIb fibers, but lower than type I fibers. Thus, their aerobic and anaerobic capabilities are in the medium range and they are moderately fatiguable. Any given person has a characteristic distribution of all three types of muscle fibers in his or her body, and hence may have a specific physical predisposition for certain types of athletic activities. For example, the marathon runner may be endowed with a disproportionate percentage of slow-twitch motor units, giving that individual great endurance as compared with the sprinter who may be endowed with a disproportionate quantity of fast twitch type IIb motor units, giving *that* individual a greater ability to perform intense activity for shorter periods of time.

Moreover, although all muscle fibers within one *motor unit* are generally of the same type, it is believed that motor units controlled by any motoneuron *pool* contain a continuous spectrum of sizes and excitabilities, which are progressively recruited from small to large fibers (i.e., lowest to highest threshold frequencies) as described later in this and subsequent chapters. The sequential recruitment of motor units according to their sizes is called, appropriately enough, the *Size Law for Motor Units,* or, more simply, *Weber's Law* for motor unit recruitment. As more and more fibers are recruited according to Weber's Law, the cumulative cross-sectional *area* occupied by the activated tissue of the *recruited* motor units, relative to the *total* cross-sectional area of the muscle involved, increases approximately exponentially. The exponent is proportional to the ratio of the number of *stimulated* motor units to the *total* number of motor units present in a specific muscle; and, the "size" of the recruited units grows in proportion to this exponential function.

The maximum rate of motor unit recruitment in human tissue is around 14 to 20 per second for the largest muscles. They are activated by increasing size, and *deactivated* in reverse order. Furthermore, the gradual recruitment of motor units with increasing stimulation frequency is called *rate coding*.

A word of caution is in order here. The time scales, 60 to 120 milliseconds or 15-50 msec, associated with "slow" or "fast" twitch fibers, respectively, are inherent characteristics of the tissue measured *in situ*.

That is, these time scales represent the *idealized* manner in which the respective fibers have been found to respond under *no-load* (maximum velocity) conditions in *isolated* muscle preparations studied in the laboratory. More realistically, as will be seen in later chapters, the response time of muscles *in vivo* is *much* slower, and depends also on such factors as the *load* against which the muscle is contracting, the extent to which it is externally *constrained* (tethered), the *"will"* of the operator, and other *environmental* conditions that will be addressed later. Thus, the reader should keep in mind the *relative* differences in contraction behavior of *"fast twitch"* versus *"slow twitch"* fibers, rather than specific *absolute* *"time-to-peak"* values.

Macrostructure of the Striated Skeletal Muscle

A dozen or more (up to as many as 150) muscle fibers constitute the so-called *primary bundle,* or *Fasciculus,* which is wrapped in a collagenous membrane called the *perimysium.* Several primary bundles form a tightly packed secondary bundle wrapped in some more connective tissue. Secondary bundles, in turn, are grouped to form tertiary bundles ... and so on until a tapered ellipsoidal ovoid of revolution, containing from a few to several hundred thousand muscle fibers, and up to 400 or more motor units, is generated. The latter, covered by a membrane called the *Epimysium* or Fascia wrapping constitutes the basic *striated skeletal muscle.* Epimysium tapers to a *tendon* at each end of the muscle, which attaches it directly to the *Periosteum* or outer membrane of bone. The bundles of muscle fibers show patterns of arrangement which allow four basic classifications:

1) *Fusiform,* in which the fibers lie essentially parallel to the long (longitudinal) axis or *"line of pull"* of the muscle (which corresponds to the direction of the force-transmitting tendons);

2) *Unipenniform,* in which the fibers still lie parallel to one another, but have an oblique orientation relative to the long axis of the muscle;

3) *Bipenniform,* in which two sets of fibers run in complementary parallel directions. The directions lie at an oblique angle to the long axis of the muscle, and one set of parallel fibers lies on each side of the muscle centerline (like the barbs on the shaft of a feather); and,

4) *Multipenniform,* in which the fibers can lie in a multitude of different directions oblique to the long axis of the ovoid of revolution.

These factors, together with the size, type (Phasic, Tonic, and so on), and shape of the muscle fibers themselves, affect the net force vector which a muscle can generate, the extent to which it can contract, and the resulting speed of the moving limb or part upon which the muscle exerts its power.

As mentioned earlier, muscular contraction is often defined in terms of its *isometric* behavior (wherein the tension in the muscle increases with time to an upper limit in the absence of any perceptible change in its overall external length from tendon to tendon); or, in terms of its *isotonic* behavior (wherein the tension in the muscle remains essentially constant as its length decreases significantly); or, in terms of its *isokinetic* behavior (wherein the linear or angular velocity of contraction is presumed to remain relatively constant at a given loading). One also frequently hears of *isoinertial* behavior (wherein muscular activities are exerted against a constant mass, such as lifting or lowering of weights); or, *concentric contractions* (wherein the muscle does *positive* work in the sense of the actual shortening taking place from muscle insertion towards muscle origin); or, *eccentric contractions* (wherein the muscle does *negative* work in the sense that the external loading against which the muscle is contracting actually pulls the insertion end in a direction *opposite* to that in which the contractile force is being generated). We shall get back to these definitions later in the text, but, again, the reader must be cautioned that in the "real life scenario" a given muscular contraction is never *really* absolutely isometric, isotonic, isokinetic, isoinertial, concentric, or eccentric in a pure sense, but, more likely it is the resultant of some complicated combination of *all* of these activities occurring at the same time. To consider the contraction as a function of length, velocity, acceleration, force generated, or direction of motion is merely a convenient abstraction which helps to explain the behavior of the tissue in terms of its corresponding anatomic and physiologic characteristics.

The average human body contains, depending on how one counts them, at least 639, to as many as 656 striated skeletal muscles. The discrepancy in number relates to the fact that some investigators list as separate muscles what others regard as common portions of adjacent muscles. Some of the major muscle groups (called by their Latin names) and associated tendons are illustrated in Figure 1-6, reproduced by permission from Keller, R., *Human Anatomy* (Maplewood, New Jersey, Hammond, Inc., 1968). Anatomically, the muscles are arranged in opposing groups -- *flexors* and *extensors* (or Protagonists and Antagonists). Flexors act to pull bones in such a way that the *joint angle*, i.e., the angle between the longitudinal axes of two bones attached at a joint, closes by having the distal (insertion-end) bone pulled *towards* the proximal (origin-end) bone. Extensors act to pull the bones back the other way, so as to open or increase a joint angle by pulling the distal bone away from the proximal bone.

The reason that two sets of muscles are required at each joint is that muscles can do nothing more than *contract* to *pull* on bones. Their subsequent relaxation and return to resting length is passive; i.e., they cannot "push" against bones. Thus, for every protagonist (or Agonist) muscle that bends a joint (flexion) or pulls a bone one way there is a corresponding antagonist that straightens the joint (extension) or pulls the bone the other way; and for every muscle that raises a bone, there is one that lowers it.

To summarize, then, a muscle at rest has four characteristic features:

1) a polarized Sarcolemma, Sarcoplasmic Reticulum (S-R System), and Transverse Tubular Network (T-System);

2) a discontinuous Actomyosin complex, in which the Troponin-Tropomyosin protein filaments prevent the formation of the Actin-Myosin cross-bridge configuration required for contraction;

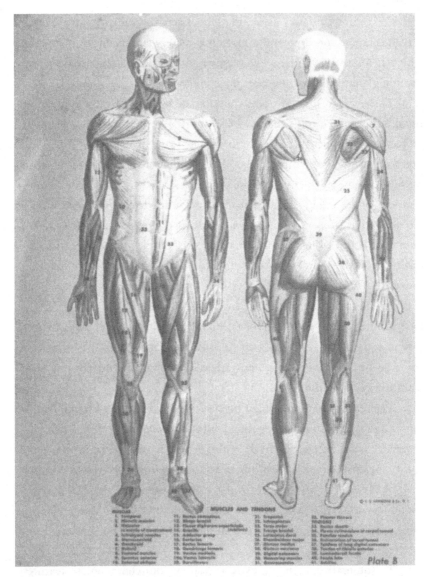

Figure 1-6 Some of the major muscles and muscle groups of the human body, as illustrated for the human male species (This Figure is reprinted by permission from Keller, R., *Human Anatomy*, Maplewood, New Jersey, Hammond, Incorporated, 1968.)

3) a situation in which Calcium ions are safely sequestered in the terminal cisternae of the Sarcoplasmic Reticulum; and,

4) a Myosin configuration to which is bound the Adenosine Triphosphate (ATP) "fuel" containing the chemical potential energy required for the contractile process.

Bearing this in mind, the physiological features of the contraction mechanism are described in the next section, to the extent that they will help the student to understand the energetics and thermodynamics of muscular mechanics.

Physiology of Muscular Contraction

Excitation and Establishment of an Active State

As discussed earlier, the sarcolemma has semipermeable characteristics which cause it to be polarized, such that the inside is about 90 to 100 millivolts negative relative to the outside. This allows contraction of striated skeletal muscle to be mainly voluntary and under the conscious control of the Somatic Nervous System. This control is manifest through the requirement that the sarcolemma (outer membrane of the fiber) must first be depolarized at least 40 millivolts from the resting value, to a *threshold potential* before the energy for contraction can be potentially released from ATP.

Depolarization is accomplished when an impulse (action potential) of sufficient threshold strength (coded into an electromyogram, see Schneck, D. J., 1990, and others) is delivered by an α-moto-neuron to the 300,000 or so 300-500 Å-Diameter synaptic vesicles located just proximal to the myoneural junction. This action potential, by activating the Ca^{2+}-controlled release of the neurotransmitter substance Acetylcholine (ACh) from some 300 of these nerve-ending vesicles (about 10^{-17} mole of ACh liberated per action potential), locally changes the sarcolemma permeability (see later), allowing Sodium ions to penetrate the membrane and to neutralize the interior negativity. This local depolarization, termed the *end plate potential* (EPP), propagates rapidly at a speed of about 5 meters per second along the muscle fiber membrane, altering the potential of the membrane and acting just like an electric current.

The depolarization wave (or "electric current") causes hydrolysis of water molecules, releasing Hydrogen and Hydroxyl ions which, in turn, proceed to attack the Adenosine Triphosphate (ATP) complex illustrated in Figure 1-7 and discussed in Schneck, D. J., (1990). This "attack" of the ATP bound to Myosin splits off a phosphate group in the presence of activated Myosin (ATP-ase) as a catalyst. That is, once "activated" by Calcium ions, the Myosin molecules to which ATP is attached in the muscle at rest actually *catalyze* the breakdown of ATP (i.e., Myosin is said to have "ATP-ase" activity). The result is the formation of Adenosine Diphosphate (ADP) and Phosphoric Acid (H_3PO_4) through an exergonic (energy-releasing) reaction that, in early studies, was believed to liberate a total of anywhere from 11,000 to 12,000 calories of energy per mole of ATP involved (Sienko and Plane, 1957). More recent studies suggest that the values for hydrolysis of the terminal (as well as the adjacent penultimate) phosphate bonds of ATP are closer to 7600 to 7800 calories per mole, with perhaps as little as 7300 actually being made available for the contractile process (Harper, H. A., 1967).

The calcium-activated, myosin-catalyzed breakdown of ATP is the reaction responsible for supplying the *primary* source of energy for contraction, and it can drive mechanical processes up to a maximum useful power output of some 800 calories per minute per kilogram of an individual's body weight. To get some "feel" for how much energy this is, note that the burning of a match liberates approximately 500 calories of heat (where the *thermodynamic* calorie is the amount of heat required to raise the temperature of one gram of water one degree centigrade; the *dietary* Calorie = 1000 thermodynamic calories, or, one kilocalorie). Moreover, 800 calories per minute is equivalent to some 0.075 horsepower, which is on the order of 55 watts. This is a rather substantial rate of energy discharge for a single motor unit. Thus, ATP serves well its function of being the "battery" that operates muscle fibers.

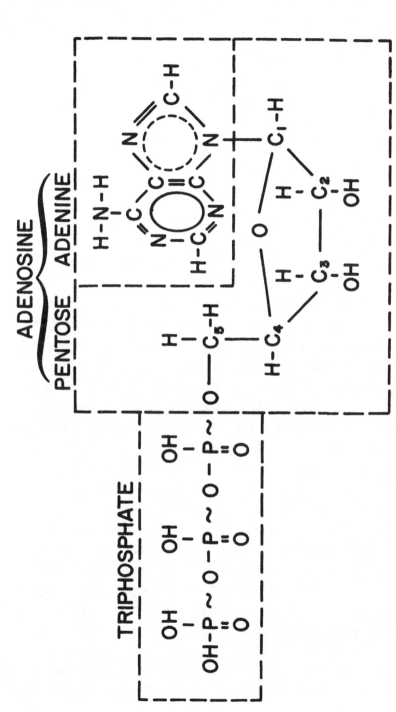

Figure 1-7 The Adenosine Triphosphate (ATP) Complex Composed of Inorganic Phosphate, the Sugar Pentose, and the Base Adenine—the latter two constituting Adenosine. This compound (ATP) contains the high-energy bonds that provide potential energy (Gibbs Free Energy) to drive the biochemical reactions that are involved in muscular contraction.

The muscle action potential (m.a.p.) propagates both longitudinally along the sarcolemma and transversely into the tissue through the previously-described T-system. It also spreads through the SR-system to activate the myofibrils that lie deep in the fiber. Of equal importance, however, these impulses (4 Hz seems to be a necessary minimum) also act to make the membrane of the terminal cisternae of the sarcoplasmic reticulum completely permeable to Ca^{2+}, allowing the cisterns to release and discharge the tightly-sequestered ion into the myofibrillar fluid. For $f_\alpha \sim 4$ Hz, such discharge raises the calcium concentration from a scant $10^{-9} - 10^{-8}$ molar to a very dilute "threshold mechanical response level" of anywhere from 4×10^{-7}M to 8×10^{-7}M, providing the equivalent of one to two calcium ions per cross-bridge, per single muscle "twitch".

This hundred-fold increase in calcium concentration is sufficient both to allow some of these ions to combine with myosin molecules to form the activated myosin catalyst mentioned earlier (ATP-ase), and, to allow others to bind tightly to the afore-mentioned TnC binding sites on the Troponin-Tropomyosin complex. The former allows the hydrolysis of ATP to be catalyzed as follows: it is believed that the myosin cross-bridge is a flexible polypeptide chain which is kept in an extended con-figuration as a result of the mutual electrostatic repulsion between fixed negative charges on the LMM portion of the molecule and the negative phosphate groups of ATP located at the end of the HMM-S-1 portion of the cross-bridge. When positively-charged calcium appears on the scene, it neutralizes some of this negativity, thereby reducing the electrostatic repulsion between the negative charges of the myosin cross-bridge and leading to a shortening of the polypeptide chain. As the mol-ecule thus shortens, it brings the bound ATP into the region of the activated myosin molecule which contains the ATP-ase. The ATP-ase is now in a position to catalyze the hydrolysis of ATP, which releases the energy required for contraction *and* offsets the "Relaxation Role" of ATP mentioned earlier.

When calcium binds to the weakly-connected Troponin-Tropomyosin complex, it strengthens the intermolecular bonding among the subunits, pulling them together. This "distorts" the chain configuration in such a way that the strands are pulled in towards the center of the "groove" between the Actin and Myosin filaments, thus freeing-up (or exposing) the cross-bridge binding sites on the Actin molecules (Cohen, 1975). This having occurred, the Actin monomers are now released from the pre-existing inhibitory influence of the Troponin-Tropomyosin complex and the way is cleared for the cross-bridges to establish the Actomyosin configuration that allows the contraction process to proceed.

Because of the important role that calcium plays in orchestrating the establishment of a contractile milieu within the myofibrillar architecture, the *active state* of a muscle fiber is defined to be the relative amount of Ca^{2+} bound to Troponin (specifically, to Troponin-TnC which apparently contains the calcium binding sites). That is to say, as reflected by the calcium concentration, the active state of a fiber relates to the number of potential interactive sites on the Actin filament that have been exposed by the action of calcium. Based on this definition, the active state is 100% -- that is, *tetanic* -- if the *maximum* number of potential interactive sites on the Actin filament have been exposed, which generally requires a myofibrillar calcium concentration on the order of 40 to 50 thousand times resting value -- or, some 2×10^{-4} molar. The resting state of the fiber thus corresponds to a myofibrillar Ca^{2+} concentration on the order of 5×10^{-9} (zero-percent active state); the threshold state (for a single twitch) of the fiber corresponds to a calcium concentration of around $6 \times 10^{-7}M$ (0.3% active state); and the tetanic state of the fiber corresponds to $[Ca^{2+}] \approx 2 \times 10^{-4}M$ (100% active state) -- with all other contractions involved in the so-called *staircase effect* lying somewhere inbetween. Furthermore, because of the role played by the two regulatory proteins, troponin and tropomyosin, in "turning on" the contractile machinery of muscle, they are sometimes referred to collectively as the *Protein Switch* for the active state.

To summarize, then, a muscle in the active state has four characteristic features:

1) an end-plate-potential-induced *depolarized* Sarcolemma, Sarco-plasmic Reticulum and Transverse Tubular Network that results from stimulation by an α-moto-neuron;

2) a depolarization-induced *release* of significant amounts of calcium ions into the myofibrillar fluid from the now-permeable terminal cisternae of the Sarcoplasmic Reticulum, triggering the *protein switch* that allows (3) and (4) below to take place;

3) a protein-switch-activated *continuous* actomyosin complex formed by the establishment of cross-bridge connections between the HMM-S-1 segments of myosin and the corresponding binding sites on actin; and,

4) a *hydrolyzed* Adenosine Triphosphate Complex that results from a calcium activated, ATP-ase catalyzed reaction that releases the energy required for contraction.

Up to this point, the initial sequence of events that have transpired after the α-moto-neuron generated the end plate potential (i.e., membrane depolarization, calcium release, hydrolysis of ATP, establishment of the actomyosin configuration, and so on) have consumed about 10 milliseconds (0.010 seconds) of time, but, there has been no perceptible alteration in muscle tension or length. One therefore observes a short *latent period* following stimulation during which time the muscle fibers, in a sense, are "preparing" to contract. Also contributing to this latent period are the viscoelastic properties of muscle tissue, a factor that we mention here only in passing, but which we shall get back to in later chapters.

Excitation-Contraction Coupling

The time course of the propagation of a single action potential is nearly complete by the end of the latent period, with the peak of the m.a.p. occurring about 40% into the latent period, i.e., at around 4 milliseconds following stimulation. What happens following the latent period is further summarized in Figures 1-8 and 1-9 for a typical single isotonic twitch.

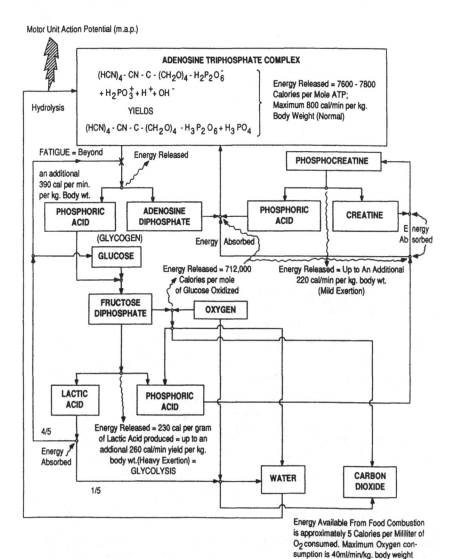

Figure 1-8 Major Biochemical Pathways and Primary Sources of Energy Responsible for Generating a Muscular Contraction.

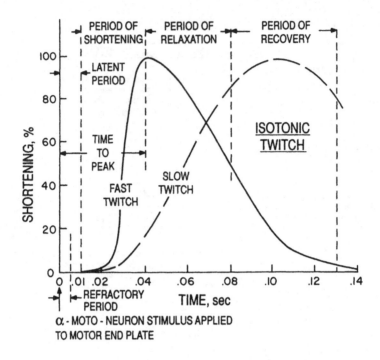

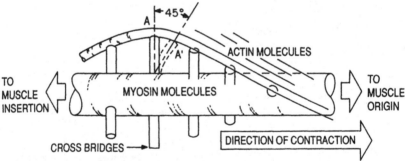

Figure 1-9 The Various Phases of the Contractile Process, Together With The Corresponding Physiologic Events Taking Place At The Time: (i) Cross-Bridge Attaches Itself via an ATP-Driven Endergonic Reaction To Actin Molecule At Point A; (ii) ATP-Driven Electromagnetic and/or Thermal Agitation provide the energy of activation which allows the cross-bridge to reorient itself to a more stable energy level—during which configurational change it moves forward, pulling the Actin molecule to which it is attached forward to new Point A′; (iii) Cross-Bridge releases from Actin molecule at point A′ and oscillates backward again to recycle the entire process.

When a phosphate group splits off of the ATP complex, the energy released drives the endergonic reaction by which the cross-bridge configuration is established between myosin and actin. At the same time, a resulting charge redistribution is believed to produce a prevailing potential difference that sets up an oscillating magnetic field (Hatze, 1981). The potential difference creates both an electromagnetic field and a corresponding flow of charge. Such flow of charge in a magnetic field generates a corresponding mechanical force that tends to separate the two globular subunits comprising the cross-bridge. However, since the mobile HMM-S-1 is now tightly linked (dissociation constant $= 2.9 \times 10^{-4}M$) to actin, a relative movement between the filaments ensues, the former "dragging" the latter.

As the magnetic field increases (and with it, the associated mechanical driving force), an instant occurs when the bond between myosin and actin breaks and the mobile HMM-S-1 subunit, under the influence of elastic restoring intermolecular forces, returns to its original equilibrium position, ready to commence a new cycle with a period of about 3.7×10^{-12} seconds. In the meantime, a new ATP molecule has replaced the one hydrolyzed following excitation, further enhancing the dissociation of actin from myosin, helping to "straighten-up" the cross-bridge again, and allowing the process to recycle as long as there is sufficient calcium present.

The insert to Figure 1-9 summarizes the above, to wit: following the establishment of an "active state", the microscopic cross-bridges begin to undergo electromagnetically-and-thermally-induced mechanical vibrations, such that they start to oscillate back and forth at a frequency of around 0.27 Terahertz, which, in the corresponding electromagnetic spectrum, is equivalent to radiation in the upper micro-wave or lower infra-red range. This helps to explain the noticeable rise in local temperature that accompanies the contractile process. Whereas the cross-bridges remain attached at their base to the myosin molecule (which does not yet move), their connection to the actin molecule is alternately made (by electrostatic forces and biochemical reactions driven by the calcium-activated hydrolysis of ATP) and broken (by mechanical stress and the intervention of new ATP molecules) with each oscillation, as described earlier. Thus, by a kind of "ratchet" action -- collapsing from the metastable position perpendicular to the myosin axis to the stable position at around 45° to the axis -- the bridges drag the thin myofilaments along, causing them to slide in a unidirectional fashion past the thick myofilaments from muscle insertion towards muscle origin. This slipping action causes the contracting fibers to "coil up", decreasing their own length as well as the length of the entire muscle.

Thus, the contraction process closes the H-zones (see Figure 1-3) as the thin filaments slide past the thick ones. Then, the thin filaments overlap until the insertion-end Z-line membranes contact the thick filaments; and finally, the I-bands all close as the thick filaments are pulled by the Z-line membranes towards the muscle origin. This whole process takes anywhere from 5 to 40 msec (most of the time averaging closer to 0.030 sec) for isolated fast twitch fibers, and 50 to 150 msec (most of the time averaging between 110 and 140 msec) for isolated preparations of slow twitch muscle fibers. This time interval is called the *Period of Shortening*, or Contraction, and the events described following the *excitation-contraction coupling* phase represent the *Sliding Filament Model* for contraction, proposed in 1954 by two independent groups of investigators: H. E. Huxley and J. Hanson, and A. F. Huxley and R. Niedergerke. It is important to recognize that, to date, this is *still* only a hypothetical model for muscular contraction -- but, it has so far survived the test of time and is currently able to explain very nicely all of the phenomena observed during the contractile process, both biochemically and physically. It is thus the *prevailing* theory, although not entirely definitive (remember, the "Galenic Tradition" describing the human cardiovascular system survived nearly 1500 years from around 166 A.D., when the "Ebb and Flow" Theory was first introduced, to the year 1628, when William Harvey finally proved this theory to be completely wrong!).

It is also interesting to note that ATP *also* catalyzes the release of the myosin cross-bridges from the Actin molecules. Thus, when death

occurs, the disintegration of the ATP complex causes the bridges to
"freeze up" and firmly bond themselves to the actin chains -- leading to
the condition known as "Rigor Mortis."

The cyclic cross-bridge activity -- attachment, contraction, detach-
ment, return to the equilibrium (metastable) position, reattachment -- and
so on, continues until the stored electrical energy is virtually used up, the
all-or-none law has been satisfied, the available calcium runs out, and/or
the supply of immediately available ATP has been depleted. If a second
or third α-moto-neuron impulse has not in the meantime been delivered
to the muscle, there is a brief interval of time -- on the order of 30 to 50
milliseconds -- following the period of shortening, during which the
bridges stop oscillating and the muscle ceases to contract. This is called
the *Period of Relaxation.*

Relaxation and Recovery Following a Single Twitch

One significant event that takes place during the relaxation
period is that ATP causes dissociation of Troponin from Ca^{2+} and
calcium is *actively* (i.e., via an energy-consuming "pumping" action such
as is described in Schneck, D. J., 1990, for example) transported back
across the new semipermeable-again sarcoplasmic reticulum membrane,
and into the cisternae, where it is again sequestered. This causes the
Actomyosin filaments to become discontinuous as the Troponin-
Tropomyosin complexes "spring back" again to their original configuration, and thus act to block the formation of Actin-Myosin cross-bridges.
Such relaxation occurs as the Ca^{2+} concentration in the myofibrillar fluid
drops back through the range from about 10^{-5} to 10^{-7} Molar.

If the external load against which the muscle was working is still
present, that load now begins to pull the muscle passively back to its original length. Otherwise, the muscle is returned to its original orientation
by a passive gradual relaxation of its own (e.g., flexor) fibers taking place
in conjunction with the activation of the extensor fibers of the corresponding antagonist muscle in the opposing motor unit group. In either

case, the muscle fibers have completed contracting and are now getting ready to "reload" in anticipation of having to fire again.

Another significant event that takes place during the period of relaxation is that ATP is resynthesized via the so-called Lohman Reaction, wherein ADP picks up a phosphate group from the breakdown of Phosphocreatine into Creatine and Phosphoric Acid (see Figure 1-8). In this manner, the primary energy source for muscular contraction is continuously being resupplied (or, the battery is continuing to be recharged), thus allowing the muscle fibers to be ready to react repeatedly to a steady stimulus of reasonable frequency (see later discussion). Moreover, the breakdown of Phosphocreatine is *also* an exergonic reaction, yielding up to an additional 220 calories per minute, per kilogram of body weight. Thus, this second series of reactions (the breakdown of ATP being the first) provides a convenient source of additional energy, when required, for activities that call for mild levels of exertion above those that can be handled by the breakdown of ATP alone.

It is important to realize that the two predominant energy sources for muscular contraction are derived from the breakdown of high-energy phosphate compounds, and that such breakdowns occur in the *absence* of oxygen, i.e., *anaerobically*. In fact, some 80 to 90 percent of the *initial* metabolism of muscles is anaerobic in the sense that it proceeds from stored chemicals that are utilized without oxidation. This turns out to be rather fortuitous, since there is no convenient way of *getting* oxygen *to* the active motor units *while* they are contracting. That is to say, muscles do not receive very much blood (hence oxygen) as they contract because of a phenomenon known as *extravascular compression*. This has to do with the fact that muscle fibers "bulge" as they contract (see Chapter 2), and this bulging action "squeezes" up against the capillary beds that course through the tissue, normally perfusing it with blood. Since the capillary beds are thus "pinched-off" (or occluded) by extravascular compression during contraction, the muscle operates essentially anaerobically during the Period of Shortening of a single twitch. This phenomenon may further explain why a given motor unit has fibers dispersed throughout the muscle, rather than concentrated in one place; and, why motor units are designed to fire in a round-robin, tandem sense as they are recruited, as opposed to uniformly and simultaneously.

Oxygen is, however, an important ingredient in the series of *aerobic* reactions that *replenish* the fuel cell or "re-charge" the battery. Thus, after relaxing, the muscle normally goes through a *Period of Recovery*. During this time interval of from 30 to 50 msec to as much as several minutes, any phosphoric acid which was not immediately used to regenerate ATP combines with the sugar Glucose to form Fructose Diphosphate. The latter may undergo one of two possible fates. It can either be completely *oxidized* to carbon dioxide and water in the mitochondria of the muscle cells (see discussion of Krebs Cycle in, for example, Schneck, D. J., 1990), or, it can be *reduced* to form the products lactic acid and phosphoric acid.

Which of the above two pathways is actually traversed by Fructose Diphosphate depends upon the availability of oxygen during physical exertion and the immediate need for additional energy. That is, if sufficient oxygen is available and the level of physical exertion is no more than "mild", then the glucose is completely oxidized, yielding on the order of 712,000 (range, 675,000 to 738,000) calories per mole, which is sufficient to regenerate 38 moles of ATP (*net* 34 because 4 are re-used to drive some of the biochemical processes involved in the Krebs Cycle) per mole of Glucose metabolized. However, for sustained heavy exercise that lasts beyond four minutes or so, the muscle tissue possesses a means for obtaining from glucose a more limited, but more immediate source of energy without a requirement for molecular oxygen. In this process of *Anaerobic Glycolysis*, the fructose diphosphate is reduced almost instantaneously to form Lactic and Phosphoric Acids. This reaction is again exergonic, and capable of supplying still a third source of energy (up to 20%, or an additional 260 calories per minute per kilogram of body weight) when needed during periods of heavy exertion. The breakdown of Fructose Diphosphate through anaerobic glycolysis also makes available a phosphate group and enough energy for the ultimate resynthesis of only 2 moles of ATP per mole of Glucose reduced. However, about 80% of the Lactic Acid produced during glycolysis is reconverted into the stored sugar, Glycogen, with much of the energy for this process coming from oxidation of the remaining 20% to the waste products Carbon Dioxide and Water. The resynthesized glycogen is then available, again, to generate more ATP at such time as more oxygen becomes available.

Note that during the period of recovery, the metabolism of muscle is aerobic, with oxygen playing a vital role. Note further that if there is enough oxygen available -- both immediately, from quantities bound to the protein *Myoglobin*, and continuously, from heavy breathing (including panting) and a large capillary network to supply the muscle fibers with huge quantities of blood -- then there will be no significant build-up of Lactic Acid in the tissue under normal circumstances. Under these aerobic conditions, Glucose and stored Glycogen are directly and completely oxidized for the regeneration of ATP and Phosphocreatine. However, should muscular effort reach the point where energy demands go some 390 or more cal/min/kg-body weight *beyond* the amounts already made available through the three pathways discussed above, i.e., breakdown of ATP, Phosphocreatine, and Anaerobic Glycolysis, then more lactic acid will be formed per minute than the muscle can handle. That is, the maximum rate of oxygen consumption (some 40 mℓ/min per kg of body weight) will not be sufficient to oxidize all of the lactic acid being formed through anaerobic glycolysis (and hence also to convert a significant amount of it into glycogen). The muscle will therefore experience an *oxygen debt* which will soon (after approximately one to ten minutes of steady state exercise at this level) cause it to become fatigued, or even totally exhausted.

Taking this state of affairs still one step further, when blood flow through a contracting muscle is interrupted as a result of the previously-mentioned extravascular compression, (which shuts off the perfusion of fluid through the tissue), not *only* is the tissue deprived of its crucial supply of oxygen and nutrients, but, perhaps even more importantly, such vascular occlusion *also* impedes the removal of carbon dioxide and waste products from the muscle fibers, allowing these to accumulate at their site of production. This can lead to complete muscle fatigue in as short a time as one minute during a sustained tetanic contraction. This anaerobic state is characterized by a build-up of so much lactic acid that the breakdown of ATP is actually blocked, shutting off the fuel cell and effectively "choking" the engine. Under these extreme conditions, the muscle quickly loses its ability to function (indeed, it may even "cramp", which is an event analogous to rigor mortis) and it must rest long enough to deplete both the lactic acid build-up and the oxygen debt before it can once again become functional.

To summarize, then, the *typical* muscle contraction, or single *twitch* consists of:

1) a *latent period*, during which the *active state* is being established (see previous section);

2) a *period of shortening*, during which *excitation-contraction coupling* elicits a measurable change in the length and/or lengthwise tension of any given motor unit;

3) a *period of relaxation*, during which calcium is actively sequestered again, the active actomyosin complex becomes dissociated, ATP is re-synthesized from Phosphocreatine, and the Sarcolemma, T-and-SR-systems become repolarized; and,

4) a *period of recovery*, during which the state of affairs described for the muscle at rest at the end of the earlier section dealing with the macrostructure of the striated skeletal muscle is essentially completely re-established.

The single muscle twitch (including recovery) is basically completed in anywhere from 75 (in some cases as little as 5) to 220 (in some cases as much as 350) milliseconds, depending on the type and size of the fibers involved. The ratio of the time period of contraction to the time of relaxation plus recovery is called the *duty cycle* of the contractile process. It is an important parameter related to the generation of power when the tissue is subjected to repetitive contraction cycles. For the most part, contraction is under voluntary control because the conscious mind can affect the activation of α-motoneurons. However, if a second neural stimulus attempts to activate a muscle fiber *too soon* after a first one has already elicited a response, this second stimulus will not be effective in generating a contraction. This is because there is a *refractory period* of some 5 milliseconds following its response to one stimulus, during which time the muscle will *not* respond to any other stimulus.

The refractory period accounts for the fact that the sarcolemma and the T-and-SR systems must return to their semipermeable state and become repolarized before they can propagate another end-plate potential. This is accomplished primarily by the afore-mentioned sodium pump mechanism, which actively transports sodium ions to the outside of the muscle fiber membrane, and which takes time to bring the membrane back to its threshold potential.

Summation of Contractions, the Staircase Effect, Tetanus

If several stimuli of adequate and equal threshold intensity, spaced more than 0.005 seconds apart (i.e., at a maximum frequency of no more than 200 per second) are delivered to a muscle in a rapid sequence, each successive stimulus elicits a progressively more intense response -- i.e., there is a summation of contractions -- up to a certain point, called tetanus, which comes from the Greek word for sustained contractions. This phenomenon is called *treppe,* or, the *staircase effect,* and it is attributed to the fact that chemical changes which take place in the muscle as a result of the first contraction make it more irritable to the second, and so on.

That is to say, the amount of *force* that a motor unit can develop depends on the *number* of cross-bridge attachments that are manifest at any given time. The more cross-bridge attachments -- akin to having more "hands" (myosin cross-bridges) pulling on a rope (the Actin molecules) in a tug-of-war -- the higher the *force* that can be developed, even though, in each case, the total *amount* of contraction (change in length) remains the same (the all-or-none response). Now, since the formation of the cross-bridge attachments depends on the concentration of calcium in the myofibrillar fluid (i.e., the *active state* of the motor unit), the more calcium that is released from its sequestered state in the terminal cisternae of the sarcoplasmic reticulum, the more troponin-tropomyosin that is distorted, the more cross-bridge attachments that become possible, the higher the degree of filamentary overlap, the greater the active state of the motor unit, and, finally, the higher the force developed in the subsequent contraction.

Thus, if successive stimuli come in spaced relatively close together, the amount of calcium released by the first stimulus will *add* to the amount released by each successive stimulation, because the timing involved will not allow complete relaxation and recovery after each stimulation. The number of overlapping bridges, and hence, the active state of the motor unit will therefore progressively increase, as will the ability of the motor unit to generate a larger and larger force for the *same* change in length. This is what is behind the concepts of the staircase effect and tetanus, both of which are "rate-coded" into the excitation signal, up to a frequency of 200/sec, maximum, and both of which allow the motor unit to respond more intensely, or to generate a larger force of contraction when a second stimulus arrives soon enough after the first. If the stimuli are delivered at a faster and faster rate, or at a consistent rate continuously, a summation of contractions occurs until *all* of the available calcium has been released, this limit bringing the myofibrillar concentration of calcium up to around 2×10^{-4} Molar (some 40,000 times its resting value). At this point, the contraction is said to be *tetanic*. Note, in particular, that *tetanus* -- describing the *intensity* of *force* developed -- is different from *contraction* -- which relates to the amount of *length* change manifest.

The staircase effect explains why a second stimulus coming in to the muscle *while* it is still contracting in response to a preceding one evokes a total muscular contraction that is more intense than either stimulus alone could have elicited. At low stimulation frequencies, i.e., for impulses arriving at frequencies on the order of around 10 or so per second, the activity of the muscle will show cyclic behavior, with each contraction being followed by a partial relaxation and even recovery before the beginning of the next contraction. *Sustained* stimuli that follow closely enough together to allow the force of adjacent twitches to overlap, but still give the tissue time to at least *partially* recover between twitches, are said to produce an *unfused tetanus.*

In the practical limit, when a series of stimuli are delivered rapidly enough -- usually 25 to 40 per second for slow fibers and around 100 stimuli per second for fast fibers -- the contractions fuse into a maximum continuous tetanus. At these higher frequencies, the effects of summation reach a maximum, with the muscle being maintained in a maximally contracted state with no evidence of, or measurable relaxation between stimuli. Due to changes in the chemical active state of the muscle as a result of its activity, plus the summing effect of successive, superimposed contractions, a tetanic response is greater and more intense -- up to 5 times more intense -- than a corresponding simple twitch, even though, in both cases, the muscle fibers contract (shorten) all the way.

However, as has already been noted, continuous physical exertion and tetanic muscular activity are limited by muscle fatigue (lactic acid build-up) and fuel cell stores (ATP, Phosphocreatine, Glycogen). In general, one cannot voluntarily contract more than about 2/3 of all muscle fibers of a muscle at once. But contraction of all fibers at the same time can occur as a result of proprioceptor reflexes (see later chapters). This can strain the muscle to its total structural tensile capacity, and might even tear it in the eventual limit.

One last point should be made regarding the transmitter substance, Acetylcholine. Following its release into the myoneural junction, ACh is hydrolyzed (destroyed) at the rate of 0.2×10^{-14} moles per millisecond by the enzyme *Acetylcholinesterase* (or, simply, Cholinesterase) located in the subneural clefts of the synaptic region (Marnay and Nachmansohn, 1938). This hydrolysis rate is some 200,000 times faster than the liberation rate of 10^{-17} moles of ACh per action potential (Fleming, 1969). That is to say, f_α would have to *exceed* 200,000 Hz before Cholinesterase would fail to hydrolyze *all* of the ACh released with *each* impulse, before the next one came in. Thus, for all intents and purposes, there is no summation effect for ACh in the myoneural junction; *all* of it is *gone* before the next impulse even arrives; and so, regardless of the frequency f_α, each stimulation of the sarcolemma may be considered to be independent of the last one as far as the generation of an action potential is concerned.

Moreover, *each* impulse that arrives at the neuromuscular junction normally creates an end-plate potential sufficient to depolarize the sarcolemma to threshold -- in fact, each impulse probably causes the release of *three-to-four times* the amount of ACh actually required to stimulate the muscle fiber to threshold. In reality, however, innervation in any motor unit usually produces *volleys* of stimuli or nervous impulses, ranging from several (rarely less than 4 Hz to bring the *calcium* concentration to threshold) to many (rarely more than 80 to 90 Hz); and despite the rapidity with which ACh is eliminated at the myoneural junction, in almost all cases it has sufficient time to excite the muscle fiber to threshold. This it does by binding to special protein molecule "Acetylcholine Receptors" lying in the muscle membrane. The binding process produces a conformational change, or geometric reorientation, if you will, that increases the sarcolemma permeability sufficiently (i.e., some 5000-fold) to open large 6 to 7 Angstrom pores in the membrane. This brief, momentary increase in membrane permeability is what starts the action potential propagating down the membrane.

The Metabolic Equivalent, or "MET" Measure of Exertion

Energy for the resynthesis of Adenosine Triphosphate, Adenosine Diphosphate, Phosphocreatine and Glycogen all comes from the air we breathe and the food we eat, which eventually finds its way into the *mitochondria* of the muscle cells (Schneck, D. J., 1990). These tiny processing plants can convert food into a stored form of chemical potential energy, which can subsequently be retrieved to yield up to 5 thermodynamic calories per milliliter of oxygen consumed (i.e., 5000 calories, or 5 dietary Calories per liter of O_2; ibid.). Obviously, this rate of

energy production by direct oxidation, which amounts to:
$5 \dfrac{cal}{m\ell\ O_2} \times 40 \dfrac{m\ell\ O_2}{min\text{-}kg} = 200$ calories per minute (maximum), per kilogram of body weight, is much slower than the rate of energy consumption in the muscle during contraction (on the order of 800 cal/min, maximum, per kg of body weight). Thus, the ATP, Phosphocreatine and Glycogen *stores* of muscle tissue are key factors in determining one's endurance limit during physical exertion. That is to say, muscles cannot "recharge" themselves as fast as they can potentially "discharge" during contraction. Their ability to work continuously and strenuously depends, therefore, upon how "charged-up" their "batteries" are when they begin to perform. This may vary from individual to individual, and also helps to explain why some are more suited for certain types of physical or athletic activities than are others.

A convenient measure of physical exertion is the *Metabolic Equivalent,* or the MET. One MET is defined to be the rate of energy expenditure requiring an oxygen consumption of 3.5 $m\ell$/kg body weight, per minute -- which corresponds approximately to the basal metabolic rate associated with sitting quietly in a chair. One MET is thus this "basal" rate; two METS is twice the energy expenditure of resting; three METS corresponds to three times the resting energy expenditure, and so on, so that the metabolic "cost" of various activities can be expressed as multiples of the basal energy cost. Some examples are illustrated in Table 1-I, reproduced by permission from Erb, B. D., "Applying Work Physiology to Occupational Medicine," *Occupational Health and Safety 81,* Vol. 50, No. 6, pp. 20-25, June, 1981. This table lists the MET-equivalents for a variety of common activities.

Taking one MET as the basal energy cost while sitting, and ten METS as a reasonable maximum (almost 40 $m\ell$ O_2/min-kg body weight) gives one a useful scale of 1 to 10 for measuring physical activity. For example, sedentary work may be defined as 2.1 METS, light work as 2.4 to 4.15 METS, medium work as 4.2 to 6.4 METS, heavy work as 6.4 METS, and very heavy work as above 6.4 METS (ibid.). Empirical ob-

TABLE 1–I
Metabolic Costs of Activities

ACTIVITY	METS	VO_2 ml/kg/min
Sitting at Desk, Writing, Calculating, Etc.	1.5	5.25
Standing Quietly, Assembling Light Machine Parts, Working at Own Pace	2.5	8.75
Kneeling or Squatting Doing Light Work	3.0	10.50
Walking 2.0 mph	2.5	8.75
3.0 mph	3.0	10.50
3.5 mph	4.0	14.00
Lifting and Carrying Objects		
20 − 44 lbs. (09 • 20 kg.)	4.5	15.75
45 − 64 lbs. (20 • 29 kg.)	6.0	21.00
65 − 84 lbs. (30 • 38 kg.)	7.5	26.25
85 − 100 lbs. (39 • 45 kg.)	8.5	29.75
Cycling (9.4 mph), Fishing, Hiking, Hunting, Mowing Lawn, Softball Game, Square Dancing, Water Skiing, Water Volleyball	6.0	21.00
Swimming		
Backstroke 40 yd./min.	8.0	28.00
Breaststroke 40 yd./min.	9.0	31.50
Crawl 45 yd./min.	9.5	33.25
Cycling (13 mph)	9.0	31.50
Shoveling (10/min. − 23 lbs.)	15.0	52.50

Table 1–I: Metabolic Costs Of A Variety Of Physical Activities, measured in "MET" Units: 1 MET = 3.5 mℓ 0_2 ($\dot{V}O_2$) per minute, per kilogram of body weight. Table reproduced by permission from Erb, B. D., "Applying Work Physiology to Occupational Medicine," Occupational Health And Safety, Volume 50, Number 6, Pages 20–24, June, 1981.

servations suggest that an individual can function at 25 to 40 percent of his or her maximum capacity for an eight-hour shift. This increases to nearly 67% if the activity period is reduced to only one hour.

Rarely do muscles in the body undergo simple twitches. Nor are they ever completely relaxed. More often than not, they are maintained in a state of partial tetanic contraction by volleys of nervous impulses that represent an individual's desire to maintain some body posture or move in some prescribed fashion. The mechanics of such behavior is a function of the anatomy and physiology of the striated skeletal muscles from which it is generated, and of their corresponding stress-strain and/or stress-strain-rate characteristics. The latter constitutes much of the material covered in the following three chapters.

****

Problem 1-1: Based on the anatomical and physiological description of muscular contraction presented in this chapter, construct a *flow chart* detailing the cascading series of events that occur from initial alpha-motoneuron excitation at the motor end plate to the final generation of a single motor unit "twitch".

****

Problem 1-2: As a first approximation, let the rate-of-change of Calcium concentration in the sarcoplasm, with respect to α-motoneuron excitation frequency, f_α, i.e., let the "staircase" effect be defined by the so-called *Logistic Equation,*

$$\frac{d[Ca^{++}]}{df_\alpha} = k_o[Ca^{++}](M_\infty - [Ca^{++}]) \qquad [1\text{-}1]$$

which accounts for the observed facts that this rate-of-change depends *both* on the *actual* amount of Ca^{++} present in the sarcoplasm at any given time (a diffusion-type asymptotic effect), and, on the *difference* between this actual amount and some upper limiting value, $M_\infty = 2 \times 10^{-4}$ (the tetanic state of the tissue).

Using the method of separation of variables, solve equation [1-1] to obtain the *Sigmoidal Function*,

$$[Ca^{++}] = \frac{[Ca^{++}]_o M_\infty}{[Ca^{++}]_o + (M_\infty - [Ca^{++}]_o)e^{-M_\infty k_o f_\alpha}} \qquad [1-2]$$

where: For $f_\alpha = 0$, i.e., the "resting state" of the muscle, $[Ca^{++}]_o = 5 \times 10^{-9}$; for $f_\alpha \to \infty$ (realistically, about 200 Hertz), $[Ca^{++}] \to M_\infty$; and, use the "threshold state" boundary condition that $[Ca^{++}] = 6 \times 10^{-7}$ when $f_\alpha = 4$ Hz to solve for k_o. The latter is approximately the threshold excitation frequency required to elicit a single twitch of the earliest and smallest motor units of a muscle.

Then, with appropriate values for $[Ca^{++}]_o$, M_∞, and k_o obtained from the boundary conditions, *plot* the S-shaped curve defined by equation [1-2] for $[Ca^{++}]$ vs. f_α. This curve approximates the *active state* of the motor unit, as defined in the text.

****

Problem 1-3: A second equation which is sometimes used to define the active state of a motor unit is the so-called *Hill Equation*:

$$\frac{[Ca^{++}] - [Ca^{++}]_o}{[Ca^{++}]_\infty} = \frac{\left(\dfrac{f_\alpha}{f_{1/2}}\right)^\psi}{1 + \left(\dfrac{f_\alpha}{f_{1/2}}\right)^\psi} \qquad [1-3]$$

where $[Ca^{++}]_o = 5 \times 10^{-9}$; $[Ca^{++}]_\infty = 2 \times 10^{-4}$; $f_{1/2}$ is the alpha-motoneuron firing frequency at which $[Ca^{++}] \approx \frac{1}{2} [Ca^{++}]_\infty$, which, for illustrative purposes, we may take equal to 50 cycles per second; and ψ is an exponent whose value may be determined from the requirement that $[Ca^{++}] = 6 \times 10^{-7}$ (threshold) when $f_\alpha = 4$ Hz.

Using the above constraint, calculate the appropriate value of ψ and plot equation [1-3] with f_α as the abscissa and $[Ca^{++}]$ as the ordinate. Compare your results with those of equation [1-2] and discuss which of

these you believe to be the better model for frequencies in the range from
0 to 200 Hz.

****

Problem 1-4: "Fault-tree" analysis is an organizational chart from which
one can deduce the failures that can contribute to an undesired event.
The "top" of the tree represents the single most undesired event; all of the
potential "failures" constitute the "branches" of the tree and are organized
as a flow of information from the tips of the branches in toward the trunk
and up towards the top. Let failure of the motor unit to contract represent the single most undesired event and construct a fault-tree to define
the process of muscular contraction.

****

References for Chapter 1

1. Bourne, S. H., (Editor), *The Structure and Function of Muscle*, New
   York, Academic Press, Second Edition, 1972.

2. Cohen, C., "The Protein Switch of Muscle Contraction," *Scientific
   American*, Vol. 233, No. 5, pp. 36-45, November, 1975.

3. DeVries, H. A., *Physiology of Exercise for Physical Education and
   Athletics*, Dubuque, Iowa, William C. Brown Company, Third
   Edition, 1980.

4. Elftman, H., "Skeletal and Muscular Systems: Structure and Function," in: Glasser, O., (Editor), *Medical Physics*, Volume 1,
   Chicago, The Year Book Publishers, Inc., pp. 1420-1430, 1944.

5. Erb, B. D., Fletcher, G. F., and Sheffield, T. L., "Standards for
   Cardiovascular Exercise Treatment Programs," *Circulation*, Vol.
   59, Page 1084A, 1979.

6. Erb, B. D., "Applying Work Physiology to Occupational Medicine,"
   Occupational Health and Safety 81, Vol. 50, No. 6, pp. 20-24,
   June, 1981.

7. Fleming, D. G., "Physiology of Nerve and Muscle," in: Plonsey, R.,
   Bioelectric Phenomena, New York, McGraw Hill, 1969, pp. 1-22.

8. Fung, Y. C., Perrone, N., and Anliker, M., (Editors), *Biomechanics --
   Its Foundations and Objectives*, Englewood Cliffs, New Jersey,
   Prentice-Hall, Inc., 1972.

9. Guyton, A. C., *Textbook of Medical Physiology*, Philadelphia, Pennsylvania, W. B. Saunders Company, Sixth Edition, 1981.

10. Harper, H. A., *Review of Physiological Chemistry*, Los Altos, California, Lange Medical Publications, 11th Edition, 1967.

11. Hoyle, G., "How is Muscle Turned On and Off?" *Scientific American*, Vol. 222, No. 4, pp. 84-93, April, 1970.

12. Huddart, H., *The Comparative Structure and Function of Muscle*, Oxford, The Pergamon Press, 1975.

13. Huxley, H. E., "Electron Microscope Studies of the Organization of the Filaments in Striated Muscle," *Biochem. Biophys. Acta*, Vol. 12, pg. 387, 1953.

14. Huxley, H. E., "The Double Array of Filaments in Cross-Striated Muscle," *J. Biophys. Biochem. Cyt.*, Vol. 3, pg. 631, 1957.

15. Huxley, H. E., "The Contraction of Muscle," *Scientific American*, Vol. 199, No. 5, pp. 66-82, November, 1958.

16. Huxley, H. E., "The Mechanism of Muscular Contraction," *Science*, Vol. 164, pp. 1356-1366, 1969.

17. Ingels, N. B., (Editor), *The Molecular Basis of Force Development in Muscle*, Palo Alto, California, The Palo Alto Medical Research Foundation, 1979.

18. Jacob, S. W., Francone, C. A., and Lossow, W. J., *Structure and Function in Man*, Philadelphia, W. B. Saunders Company, Fifth Edition, 1982.

19. Junge, D., *Nerve and Muscle Excitation*, Sunderland, Mass., Sinauer Associates, Inc., Second Edition, 1981.

20. Karpovich, P. W., *Physiology of Muscular Activity*, Philadelphia, W. B. Saunders Company, 1959.

21. Katz, B., *Nerve, Muscle and Synapse*, New York, McGraw-Hill Book Company, 1966.

22. Loeb, E. G., and Gans, C., *Electromyography for Experimentalists*, Chicago, The University of Chicago Press, 1986.

23. Margaria, R., "The Sources of Muscular Energy," *Scientific American*, Vol. 226, No. 3, pp. 84-91, March, 1972.

24. Marnay, A. and Nachmansohn, D., "Choline Esterase in Voluntary Muscle," *J. Physiology, London*, Vol. 92, pp. 37-47, 1938.

25. Mommaerts, W. F. H. M., *Muscular Contraction*, New York, Interscience Publishers, 1950.

26. Podolsky, R. J., (Editor), *Contractility of Muscle Cells and Related Processes,* Englewood Cliffs, New Jersey, Prentice-Hall, Inc., 1972.

27. Ralston, H. J., "Special Review: Recent Advances in Neuromuscular Physiology," *American J. Physical Med.,* Vol. 36, No. 2, pp. 94-120, April, 1957.

28. Rasch, P. J., and Burke, R. K., *Kinesiology and Applied Anatomy,* Philadelphia, Lea and Febiger, 1959.

29. Ruch, T. C., and Patton, H. D., *Physiology and Biophysics,* Philadelphia, W. B. Saunders Company, 1979.

30. Schneck, D. J., *Engineering Principles of Physiologic Function,* New York, The New York University Press, 1990.

31. Selim, R. D., *Muscles: The Magic of Motion,* Washington, D. C., U. S. News Books Series on the Human Body, 1982.

32. Sienko, M. J., and Plane, R. A., *Chemistry,* New York, McGraw-Hill Book Company, Inc., 1957.

33. Squire, J., *The Structural Basis of Muscular Contraction,* New York, Plenum Press, 1981.

34. Stacy, R. W., Williams, D. T., Worden, R. E., and Morris, R. O., *Essentials of Biological and Medical Physics,* New York, McGraw-Hill Book Company, Inc., 1955.

35. Stein, R. B., *Nerve and Muscle: Membranes, Cells, and Systems,* New York, Plenum Press, 1980.

36. Szent-Gyorgyi, A., *Chemistry of Muscular Contraction,* New York, Academic Press, Inc., Second Edition, 1951.

37. Szent-Gyorgyi, A., *Chemical Physiology of Contraction in Body and Heart Muscle,* New York, Academic Press, Inc., 1953.

38. Tokay, E., *Fundamentals of Physiology,* New York, Barnes and Noble, 1959.

39. Wilkie, D. R., *Muscle,* London, Edward Arnold Publishers, Second Edition, 1976.

40. Wilson, L. G., "William Croone's Theory of Muscular Contraction," *Notes and Records of the Royal Society of London,* Vol. 16, pg. 158, 1961.

Chapter 2

A Nonlinear, Elastic, Continuum Constitutive Model for Striated Skeletal Muscle

Introduction

As an engineering material, muscles fall into the category of substances that exhibit time-dependent, nonlinear viscoelastic behavior. They are *viscous* in the sense that their behavior depends not only on the *amount* by which they are deformed, but also on the *rate* at which they are deformed. Their behavior is *time-dependent* in the sense that the loading-response (stress-strain or stress-strain-rate) curves for this type of physiologic tissue all exhibit *hysteresis*. That is, starting with the tissue at rest, if one subjects it to cyclic loading and unloading, one does not travel up (loading) and down (unloading) the *same* stress-strain or stress-strain-rate curve, such that the material response at any *given* time depends upon its *history of deformation* up *to* that time.

Muscle tissue is *elastic* in the sense that following deformation (stretching, twisting, squeezing, contracting, and so on) the material returns to its original length and shape. Although individual muscle fibers may or may not be approximately *linearly* elastic, the whole muscle, which contains significant amounts of connective tissue and other materials that exhibit a wide range of mechanical properties, definitely deviates from showing any reasonable degree of linear behavior. Moreover, because of its anatomical configuration and chemical composition (which includes polarized protein molecules that exhibit complicated patterns of electric charge distribution), the typical striated skeletal muscle is a non-homogeneous, anisotropic, discontinuous mass of complex consistency, that develops intricate secondary microstructural configurations.

From an engineering point of view these characteristics are disturbing in that they make it difficult to develop a comprehensive mathematical model to describe muscle behavior. Nevertheless, several more simplified approaches have yielded meaningful and relevant results. In particular, the nonlinear elastic theory postulated by Nubar (1962), the linear viscoelastic model developed by Bahler (1968) and Soechting, et al. (1971), and the nonlinear viscoelastic formulations of Decraemer, et al. (1980) and Hatze (1981), are worthy of careful study in that they predict quite accurately the major features of muscular performance. All three types of models shall therefore be presented and discussed in this and subsequent chapters, beginning here with Nubar's nonlinear-elastic *continuum* model for muscular contraction.

Analysis of Strain

Figure 2-1a shows an isolated (i.e., free of external attachments and constraints) muscle of length, L, and assumed circular cross section of maximum diameter, D, in a resting state. Under this no-load condition, simultaneous stimulation of all of its fibers will cause it to contract to its smallest length, with maximum average velocity and without the development of any tension (Atonic contraction). Furthermore, because its volume will remain essentially unchanged, the muscle will also experience a correspondingly large increase in diameter. Figure 2-1b shows the more realistic situation, in which the muscle has first been stretched passively between two supports before being stimulated to contract against an external load. The supports, of course, are the origin and insertion of the muscle tendons into the bones on either side of the joint spanned by the muscle. Stretching the muscle *passively* between these two boundaries will produce a *decrease* in diameter due to a generalized Poisson effect.

This is in contrast to what happens when the muscle is stimulated to contract *actively*, at which time its diameter tends to *increase* as tension is developed in the fibers.

Even as it contracts, the muscle is kept *passively* in a state of tension by the resistance of the external constraints (bones) against which it is pulling. This *tensile* resistance (force) on the *contracting* fiber leads to a generalized Poisson effect that tends to *thin* the fibers. On the other hand, the nearly isovolumetric *active* contraction process *itself* tends to *thicken* the fibers as they shorten. Therefore, a muscle stimulated to contract under *loaded* conditions may be considered to respond in some *net* fashion that results from both active and passive effects taking place simultaneously. That is, it will have a tendency to thicken as a result of the contraction mechanism, but this tendency will be modified by a general Poisson effect due to the tensile load imposed by the external restraints against which the muscle acts. Assuming that the muscle cross section still remains circular following contraction, it is now considered to have some deformed length, $L + \Delta L$, and some new maximum diameter, D'.

To develop an equation for muscle strain, attention is focussed first on a single circular muscle fiber which starts out at some original radial location, x, measured outward from the longitudinal axis of the muscle. This fiber has a length, ℓ, and thickness, dx, when the muscle is in a resting state (or, in some initially stressed reference state). Following stretching and contraction, the fiber length becomes $\ell + \Delta\ell$ and its thickness changes to dx'. Finally, the fiber now finds itself at a new radial location, x', relative to the longitudinal axis of the muscle, which is considered to have remained colinear with its position prior to deformation. In accordance with the previous discussion, one may write the following equation to describe the lateral deformation:

$$dx' = dx(1 + q)(1 - p) \qquad \text{[2-1]}$$

where: q represents the *active* increase in thickness (lateral strain) due to stimulation (contraction), and

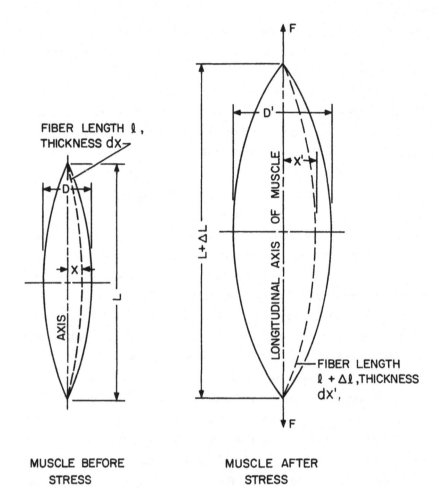

MUSCLE BEFORE   MUSCLE AFTER
    STRESS   STRESS

Figure 2-1 Schematic Continuum Representation of a Striated Skeletal Muscle: (a) *Before* being subjected to a Contraction Under Load, F; and, (b) *After* being Stressed Under This Loading.

p represents the *passive* retarding Poisson effect (lateral strain) due to tensile external loading.

Assume, now, that the effects q and p are nonlinear functions of longitudinal fiber engineering strain, which is defined to be the change in fiber length, $\Delta\ell$, divided by the *original* fiber length, ℓ. Assume further that these nonlinear functions may be expressed in power series of the form:

$$q = q_0 + q_1\left(\frac{\Delta\ell}{\ell}\right) + q_2\left(\frac{\Delta\ell}{\ell}\right)^2 + q_3\left(\frac{\Delta\ell}{\ell}\right)^3 + \cdots \qquad [2\text{-}2]$$

$$p = p_1\left(\frac{\Delta\ell}{\ell}\right) + p_2\left(\frac{\Delta\ell}{\ell}\right)^2 + p_3\left(\frac{\Delta\ell}{\ell}\right)^3 + \cdots \qquad [2\text{-}3]$$

In equation [2-2], q_0, q_1, q_2, q_3, ... , are experimentally determined non-dimensional coefficients assumed to be dependent on stimulation and vanishing with it. They are thus related in some sense to the excitation dynamics of the contractile element of a single muscle fiber (Hatze, 1981), as determined by its active state, and hence the concentration of calcium in the sarcoplasm (c.f., Chapter 1, pgs. 25 to 30). The coefficients q_i, $i = 0, 1, 2, 3, \ldots$, are called *stimulation coefficients.* They are maximized as the action of calcium gradually exposes all of the potential cross-bridge interactive sites on the Actin filaments, i.e., as a result of the staircase effect up to a tetanic contraction, c.f. Problems 1-2 and 1-3.

Hatze (1981) defines a parameter p^* as the rate-of-change of the stimulation coefficient q with respect to the active state of the fiber, $[Ca^{++}]$:

$$p^* = \frac{dq}{d[Ca^{++}]} \qquad [2\text{-}4]$$

where $[Ca^{++}]$ is given by an equation similar to [1-1]. He then goes on to propose that p^* satisfies a second-order differential equation of the form:

$$\frac{d^2q}{d[Ca^{++}]^2} = \frac{dp^*}{d[Ca^{++}]} = g_1\left(\frac{\Delta\ell}{\ell}\right)(1-q) - g_2\left(\frac{\Delta\ell}{\ell}\right)p^*,$$

or,

$$\frac{d^2q}{d[Ca^{++}]^2} + g_2\left(\frac{\Delta\ell}{\ell}\right)\frac{dq}{d[Ca^{++}]} - g_1\left(\frac{\Delta\ell}{\ell}\right)(1-q) = 0 \qquad \textbf{[2-5]}$$

where the coefficients $g_1\left(\frac{\Delta\ell}{\ell}\right)$ and $g_2\left(\frac{\Delta\ell}{\ell}\right)$ are both functions of engineering strain, which depends also on $[Ca^{++}]$. Details of the solution
to equation [2-5] are not immediately relevant to the subject matter of this
chapter, and may be found elsewhere (Hatze, 1981). Suffice it to say here
that for an isometric fiber contraction, $\Delta\ell = 0$ and q reduces to q_0, which
is a function of the isometric active state of the fiber. Hatze's formulation
is developed further in Chapter 4.

In equation [2-3] the coefficients p_1, p_2, p_3, ... , are experimentally
determined parameters which represent *generalized Poisson ratios*. Note
that for an isometric fiber contraction, $p = 0$, since there will be no
Poisson effect if there is no longitudinal change in fiber length, $\Delta\ell$. Thus,
for an *isometric fiber* contraction,

$$dx' = dx(1 + q_0) \qquad \textbf{[2-6]}$$

****

Problem 2-1: Consider the *passive* behavior of muscle ($q = 0$). For this
case, show that the leading term in the expansion of p (i.e., p_1 in equation
[2-3]) is the classical Poisson ratio (i.e., $\dfrac{\text{lateral strain}}{\text{longitudinal strain}}$) considered in
the *linear* mechanics of deformable bodies.

****

Problem 2-2: Show that if an elastic continuum is incompressible, it must
have a Poisson ratio equal to 1/2, which is equivalent to saying that the
continuum undergoes *isovolumetric* expansions or contractions. Is the
converse of this statement necessarily true? That is, *if $p_1 = 1/2$, must* the

continuum be incompressible? Explain and mathematically verify your answer.

****

Substituting equations [2-2] and [2-3] into equation [2-1], expanding and neglecting terms of order $\left(\frac{\Delta \ell}{\ell} \right)^4$ and higher (the longitudinal fiber strains are considered to be small enough for this to be justified) yields, after simplification,

$$dx' = dx[1 + r_1 \varepsilon_z + r_2 \varepsilon_z^2 + r_3 \varepsilon_z^3 + q_0] \qquad [2\text{-}7]$$

where: $r_1 = q_1 - p_1(1 + q_0),$

$r_2 = q_2 - p_2(1 + q_0) - p_1 q_1,$

$r_3 = q_3 - p_3(1 + q_0) - p_2 q_1 - p_1 q_2,$ and,

$\varepsilon_z = \dfrac{\Delta \ell}{\ell}$

The corresponding relation between cross-sectional areas (stressed vs. unstressed) is:

$$dA' = dA[1 + q_0 + r_1 \varepsilon_z + r_2 \varepsilon_z^2 + r_3 \varepsilon_z^3]^2 \qquad [2\text{-}8]$$

In order to integrate equation [2-7], one must develop an equation for ε_z in terms of x and x'. This can be done by noting that, for a simple convex curve that is flat enough to allow the fourth and higher powers of $\frac{x}{L}$ to be neglected, the length, ℓ, of the curve may be very closely approximated by the equation:

$$\ell \approx L\left[1 + \frac{8}{3} \left(\frac{x}{L} \right)^2 \right] \qquad [2\text{-}9]$$

where L is the distance spanned by the entire curve. Similarly, one can write further for the corresponding stressed muscle fiber case:

$$\ell + \Delta \ell \approx (L + \Delta L)\left[1 + \frac{8}{3} \left(\frac{x'}{L + \Delta L} \right)^2 \right] \qquad [2\text{-}10]$$

****

Problem 2-3: In order to gain some confidence in the limiting approximation given by equation [2-9], consider a symmetric curve spanning a distance L through some maximum height x. To order $\left(\frac{x}{L}\right)^4$, find the approximate length of the curve if it is assumed to have the following functional forms:

a) Two simple straight-line segments: $X = mz + b$ for $0 \leq z \leq \frac{L}{2}$, $0 \leq X \leq x$ (i.e., half the curve), and the mirror image of this function for $\frac{L}{2} \leq z \leq L$;

b) A polynomial of the form: $X = b_0 + b_1 z + b_2 z^3 + b_3 z^5$;

c) A sine curve of the form: $X = x \sin \frac{z\pi}{L}$;

d) An Exponential of the form: $X = x[1 - e^{-(16/3)(z/L)}]$ for $0 \leq z \leq \frac{L}{2}$, $0 \leq X \leq 0.93x$ (slightly flatter than the height x), and the mirror image of this function for $\frac{L}{2} \leq z \leq L$.

****

For convenience, introduce the following dimensionless variables:

$$\beta = \frac{x}{L} \qquad \text{and} \qquad \beta' = \frac{x'}{L + \Delta L}, \quad \text{and}$$

substitute into equations [2-9] and [2-10]. Then, substitute equation [2-9] for ℓ into equation [2-10] for $\Delta\ell$, and divide the result by equation [2-9] to get, after some algebraic manipulation and the neglect of terms of order $\beta'^2\beta^2$ and β^4:

$$\varepsilon_z = \alpha + (1 + \alpha)\left[\frac{8}{3}\left(\beta'^2 - \beta^2\right)\right] = \text{Muscle Fiber Strain} \qquad \textbf{[2-11]}$$

where: $\alpha = \frac{\Delta L}{L} = $ Total Muscle Strain.

From the definition of β and β', note further that:

$$\frac{dx'}{dx} = (1 + \alpha)\frac{d\beta'}{d\beta} \qquad \textbf{[2-12]}$$

Equations [2-11] and [2-12] can now be substituted back into equation [2-7] to yield, after expanding and again neglecting terms of order $(\beta'^2 - \beta^2)^2$ and $(\beta'^2 - \beta^2)^3$:

$$\frac{d\beta'}{d\beta} = N + \frac{8}{3}\left(\beta'^2 - \beta^2\right)\left[r_1 + 2r_2\alpha + 3r_3\alpha^2\right] \qquad [2\text{-}13]$$

where: $N = \dfrac{1 + q_0 + r_1\alpha + r_2\alpha^2 + r_3\alpha^3}{1 + \alpha}$.

Equation [2-13] is a differential equation with β' acting as the dependent variable and β serving as the independent variable. The most convenient means for solving such an equation is to seek a series solution of the form:

$$\beta' = \sum_{i=0}^{\infty} A_i \beta^i \qquad [2\text{-}14]$$

and applying appropriate boundary conditions.

****

Problem 2-4: Assuming $\beta' = 0$ when $\beta = 0$, which is to say, the longitudinal axis $(x = 0)$ of the muscle remains fixed $(x' = 0)$ as the muscle undergoes deformation, and, neglecting higher order terms involving those from β^4 up, substitute the series expansion [2-14] into the differential equation [2-13] and equate respective coefficients of the various powers of β to show that the solution to the differential equation may be written as:

$$\beta' = A_1\beta + A_3\beta^3 \qquad [2\text{-}15]$$

where: $A_1 = N$, and
$$A_3 = \frac{8}{9}\left(r_1 + 2r_2\alpha + 3r_3\alpha^2\right)(N^2 - 1)$$

****

Finally, substitute equation [2-15] back into equation [2-11], and drop the terms of order β^4 and β^6 to get the resulting equation for muscle fiber strain:

$$\varepsilon_z = \frac{\Delta \ell}{\ell} = \alpha + Q\beta^2 \qquad [2\text{-}16]$$

where: $Q = \frac{8}{3}(1 + \alpha)(N^2 - 1)$.

Equation [2-16] represents the engineering strain in a muscle fiber located an arbitrary distance x from the longitudinal axis of the entire muscle. Note that it is the resultant of both the passive cumulative longitudinal engineering strain, $\alpha = \frac{\Delta L}{L}$, of the entire muscle, (i.e., *all* fibers) plus an additional effect, $Q\beta^2$, which accounts for the *individual* changes that take place in the thickness of all fibers located at the radial location, x, owing to the combination of active stimulation and generalized Poisson effects. Relative changes in muscle thickness and cross-sectional area can now be determined by integrating equation [2-15].

****

Problem 2-5: From equation [2-15] and the definitions of β and β', show that the relative change in muscle thickness, $\frac{D'}{D}$, is given by:

$$\frac{D'}{D} = (1 + \alpha)\left[N + \frac{A_3 D^2}{4L^2} \right] \qquad [2\text{-}17]$$

****

Problem 2-6: To order $\left(\frac{D}{L}\right)^2$, what is the corresponding relative change in cross-sectional area, $\frac{A'}{A}$?

****

Analysis of Stress

As was mentioned previously, muscle as a whole deviates from a linear form of Hooke's Law for perfectly elastic solids due to the lack of homogeneity, simplicity and isotropy of the structure. However, one can assume that the longitudinal strain, $\frac{\Delta \ell}{\ell}$, of the fiber and its unit tension or stress are related to each other through a generalized nonlinear form of Hooke's law, written as:

$$\frac{f}{a} = E_1\left(\frac{\Delta \ell}{\ell}\right) + E_2\left(\frac{\Delta \ell}{\ell}\right)^2 + E_3\left(\frac{\Delta \ell}{\ell}\right)^3 \qquad \text{[2-18]}$$

to the order of approximation in this analysis. In equation [2-18], f is tensile force in the fiber, a is its original cross-sectional area, $\dfrac{\pi(dx)^2}{4}$, before stimulation, and E_1, E_2 and E_3 are generalized Young's moduli characteristic of the fiber. By analogy with the earlier definition of engineering strain, and to remain consistent with it, equation [2-18] defines *engineering* stress and so relates f to the unstressed cross-sectional area as a reference. If one preferred to define true stress, the "instantaneous" cross-sectional area could be used since equation [2-1] or the solution to Problem 2-6 are available to relate the two areas.

Substituting equation [2-16] into equation [2-18], expanding and neglecting higher order terms yields, after simplification,

$$\frac{f}{a} = Q\beta^2\left[E_1 + 2E_2\alpha + 3E_3\alpha^2\right] + \alpha\left[E_1 + E_2\alpha + E_3\alpha^2\right] \qquad \text{[2-19]}$$

Equation [2-19] gives the tensile engineering stress in a *single,* circular muscle fiber located an arbitrary distance x from the longitudinal axis of the muscle at any given time. The tensile *force* in the fiber is then simply $(f/a) \cdot a$. To get the total force in an *annulus* of fibers located at the radial location x, each having a diameter dx, one can define some "average" fiber force per unit circumferential length as $a \cdot (f/a) \div dx$. Then, the force, f_x, in the ring of fibers located a distance x from the axis would be given by:

$$f_x = \frac{f}{a}\frac{a}{dx}2\pi x = \frac{f}{a}\frac{\pi(dx)^2}{4}\frac{2\pi x}{dx} = \frac{\pi^2 x\,dx\,f}{2a} \qquad \text{[2-20]}$$

Substituting for x, $L\beta$ and for dx, $L\,d\beta$, equation [2-20] becomes:

$$f_x = \frac{\pi^2 L^2 \beta\,d\beta\,f}{2a}. \qquad \text{[2-21]}$$

Thus, to get the *total* force (or tension), F, in the *muscle,* one substitutes equation [2-19] into equation [2-21] and performs the appropriate integration on the independent variable, β, which has limits from $\beta = \frac{x}{L} = 0$ (the longitudinal axis of the muscle) to $\beta = \frac{x}{L} = \frac{D}{2L}$ (where D is the actual original diameter of the muscle, since β corresponds to the original x). Finally, if this result is divided by the cross-sectional area, A, of the muscle, one gets the total force per unit area, or stress in the muscle as a whole, which is:

$$\sigma = \frac{F}{A} = \frac{\pi}{4}\left[E_1\alpha + E_2\alpha^2 + E_3\alpha^3 + \frac{QD^2}{8L^2}\left(E_1 + 2E_2\alpha + 3E_3\alpha^2\right)\right] \quad \text{[2-22]}$$

Kuhn, (1936, 1939; see also King and Lawton, 1950) attempted to calculate E_1 from statistical mechanics theory. He examined the case of randomly oriented rigid rods connected end to end by flexible links and embedded in an isotropic fluid matrix. If one takes this to be an approximate model for myofilaments, the modulus of elasticity obtained for such a system at zero extension is:

$$E_1 = \frac{9}{5}\frac{RTW}{M} \quad \text{[2-23]}$$

where: R is the universal gas constant, $8.37 \times 10^7 \frac{\text{ergs}(=\text{ dyne-cm})}{\text{°K-gm-mole}}$,

$\quad\quad W$ is the nondimensional weight fraction (weight of elastic material, in grams, per unit gram weight of total material) per cubic centimeter,

$\quad\quad T$ is the absolute temperature, $310°K$ for a normal body temperature of $37°C$, and,

$\quad\quad M$ is the molecular weight per gram mole of each element of the chain.

Recall that muscle consists by weight of about 20% protein, of which 62% - 85% are the Actomyosin filaments that comprise the elastic material of the tissue. Thus, using the mean of this range, one observes that these filaments account for some 14.7% (0.735×0.20) of the total muscle weight, or, stated another way, the weight fraction of elastic material in muscle is 0.147. This weight fraction is distributed fairly uniformly throughout the tissue, so that W can be taken to be 0.147 grams of elastic material per gram of muscle tissue in each cubic centimeter of same.

Going one step further, recall that myosin has a molecular weight up to about 490,000 (some texts quote this even as high as 500,000) and actin has a molecular weight up to about 76,000 (some texts quote a range from 40,000 to 85,000). Now, the estimated myosin-to-actin *mass* ratio is about 2.1:1. Hence, for every 490,000 grams or mole of Myosin there are some 233,333 grams of Actin, or $\dfrac{233,333}{76,000} = 3.07$ moles. The Actin/Myosin *Molar* Ratio is thus around 3:1, so that the molecular weight, M, of an element of Actomyosin is approximately 490,000 + 3(76,000) = 718,000. Again, some literature references quote the Actin/Myosin molar ratio in striated skeletal muscle to be as high as 3.5-4.0:1.0, depending on the values assigned to the molecular weights of Myosin and Actin.

In any event, putting all of this information together, one can calculate E_1 approximately from equation [2-23]:

$$E_1 = \left(\frac{9}{5} \right) \frac{8.37 \times 10^7}{718,000/\text{gm-mole}} \frac{\text{dyne-cm}}{°\text{K-gm-mole}} \, 310°\text{K}(0.147) \frac{\text{gm}}{\text{gm-cm}^3}$$

$$= 0.9562 \times 10^4 \text{ dyne/cm}^2 \approx 10^4 \text{ dynes/cm}^2$$

The problem with Kuhn's statistical theory is that it assumes the total material is made up simply of elastic elements embedded in a fluid matrix. Thus, it does not take into account all of the collagenous connective tissue that is an integral part of the muscle fiber. Recall that the elastic elements (Actomyosin filaments) are supported by dense membranes (Z-lines) and are packed tightly into myofibril bundles covered by endomysium. Recall further that fibrils are also packed together into bundles wrapped by more fibrous tissue (fascia), and that the muscle fiber itself is ultimately covered by the semipermeable sarcolemma.

Now, the Young's Modulus for collagen is about 5×10^9 dynes/cm^2. Thus, if the value $E_1 \approx 10^4$ calculated from statistical theory is compared with the Young's modulus for collagen, one can conclude that a complicated geometrical arrangement of elastic and fibrous tissue should exhibit strength properties that lie somewhere between 10^4 and 10^9 dynes/cm^2. It is not surprising to learn, therefore, that the modulus of elasticity, E_1, for extracted muscle *fibers* at their natural length has been found experimentally to be, on the average, 6.2×10^7 dynes/cm^2. This is more than 30 times larger than that for rubber and about 10^5 smaller than the elastic modulus for mild steel.

Considering the simplicity of the statistical theory, it reasonably predicts the characteristics of the *elastic* elements of muscle tissue. Moreover, if one accepts that the modulus E_1 for myofilaments is theoretically of order 10^4, and that this modulus increases to the experimentally determined value between 10^7 and 10^8 for muscle *fibers* because of the effects of fibrous connective tissue, then one would expect still a further increase in E_1 for the entire muscle -- since the latter contains still *more* collagenous material than do the individual fibers of which it is composed. In fact, one would expect the modulus E_1 for *total* muscle to lie somewhere between 10^7 (for muscle fibers) and 10^9 (for pure collagen). It is interesting to note, therefore, that the elastic modulus for muscle *tendons* has been measured to be some 1×10^8 dynes/cm^2. Based on these observations and the logical reasoning behind them, the modulus E_1 for muscle is taken to be equal to 10^8 dynes per square centimeter in the work which follows. This appears to be a reasonable estimate, as we shall see further in the next chapter.

A convenient means for determining the stimulation coefficient q_0 is to examine an isometric contraction, described in equation [2-22] by letting $\alpha = 0$. For this case, $N = 1 + q_0$, $Q = \dfrac{8}{3} q_0(2 + q_0)$ and,

$$\sigma = \frac{\pi}{4} \ \frac{q_0}{3} (2 + q_0) \ \frac{D^2}{L^2} \ E_1 \qquad\qquad \text{[2-24]}$$

Note that equation [2-24] is of the *linear* Hookean form, $\sigma = \varepsilon E_1$ where:

$$\varepsilon = \frac{\pi q_0}{12} (2 + q_0) \ \frac{D^2}{L^2} = \text{"Isometric Strain"} \qquad\qquad \text{[2-25]}$$

Isometric strain refers to the fact that *myofilaments* undergo a change in length during an isometric contraction, even though the total length of the *muscle* (from origin to insertion) remains constant. Thus, by measuring ε, together with muscle length, L, and diameter, D, during an isometric contraction, one can compute q_0 from equation [2-25]. This has been done, with the empirical result that $\varepsilon = .1152 \ \frac{D^2}{L^2}$. Substituting this into equation [2-25] yields:

$$\pi q_0^2 + 2\pi q_0 - 1.3824 = 0,$$

from which the positive fractional root $q_0 = 0.20$ is obtained (the negative root, -2.2, is not physically meaningful).

It should be pointed out again that for isometric contractions or passive deformations that involve small muscular strains, the behavior of muscle tissue is essentially linearly elastic in the Hookean sense. On the other hand, to examine what happens at larger passive deformations, or, in cases involving isotonic or isokinetic contractions, one must utilize the entire nonlinear form of equation [2-22]. Thus, values of p_i, q_i, and E_i which are required in order to use equation [2-22] as a stress-strain relationship for striated skeletal muscle have been determined from available experimental data (e.g., that of Ramsey and Street, 1940, Buchthal, 1942, Ramsey, 1944, Bull, 1945, Ramsey, 1947, Buchthal and Rosenfalck, 1957, and others). Comparison of this data with the nonlinear equation derived earlier gives a good regression fit for the following range of values:

$$0.30 \leq p_1 \leq 0.50 \qquad 0.40 \leq q_1 \leq 0.50$$

$$0.20 \leq p_2 \leq 0.30 \qquad -0.30 \leq q_2 \leq -0.20$$

$$p_3 = 0.10 \qquad -0.20 \leq q_3 \leq -0.10$$

$$\frac{E_2}{E_1} = 0.20$$

$$\frac{E_3}{E_1} = 0.60$$

Nonlinear Passive Behavior of Striated Skeletal Muscle

With the information above, let us describe first the *passive* behavior of muscle, i.e., the behavior of the tissue as a nonlinear engineering material in an unstimulated state. this can be done by *nulling* the stimulation coefficients q_0, q_1, q_2, and q_3 so that:

$$r_1 = -p_1 \qquad N_{(q_i = 0)} = \frac{1 - p_1\alpha - p_2\alpha^2 - p_3\alpha^3}{1 + \alpha} = N_0$$

$$r_2 = -p_2$$

$$r_3 = -p_3 \qquad Q_{(q_i = 0)} = \frac{8}{3}(1 + \alpha)(N_0^2 - 1) = Q_0$$

Values of p_1, p_2, p_3, E_1, E_2 and E_3 will be taken to be average quantities from the ranges quoted earlier. Recall that p_1 is the classical Poisson ratio considered in the linear mechanics of deformable bodies (Problem 2-1), and that $p_1 = 0.50$ for a material that undergoes isovolumetric expansions or contractions (Problem 2-2). One therefore makes the interesting observation that muscle tissue may deviate from showing isovolumetric behavior under certain circumstances, since p_1 may vary from the isovolumetric value of 0.50 down to as low as 0.30. This is simply a manifestation of the "compressibility" of the long chain Actomyosin, helically-coiled filaments and the nonlinear and viscoelastic properties of the material, which come more into evidence the greater it is deformed (see below). Do realize, however, that $p_1 = 0.5$ for isovolumetric deformations of *linearly elastic* materials. Deviations from linearity, and the introduction of additional coefficients p_2, p_3, ... , may allow p_1 to take on other values while still preserving the isovolumetric behavior of the material. Indeed, many investigators (see, for example, Hatze, 1981) still insist that muscular contraction *is* isovolumetric, under *any* circumstances, but *this* author is not necessarily convinced that this is unequivocally the case.

To examine a representative case illustrating the passive characteristics of muscle tissue, let:

$$p_1 = 0.40 = -r_1 \qquad E_1 = 1.00 \times 10^8 \text{ dynes/cm}^2$$
$$p_2 = 0.25 = -r_2 \qquad E_2 = 0.20 \times 10^8 \text{ dynes/cm}^2$$
$$p_3 = 0.10 = -r_3 \qquad E_3 = 0.60 \times 10^8 \text{ dynes/cm}^2$$

$$\left(\frac{D}{L} \right) = 0.20$$

and solve equation [2-22] for $\sigma_o = \dfrac{F_o}{A_o}$ as a function of α. The subscripts "o" are being used here to designate passive, unstimulated behavior, and the corresponding stress-strain diagram for muscle is illustrated in Figure 2-2. Note, first of all, the nonlinear nature of the curve compared with a linear Hookean material. This, of course, was to be anticipated because of the nonlinear form of equation [2-22]. Of interest, however, is the suggestion in Figure 2-2 that muscles appear to get *stiffer* the more they are deformed. That is, the shape of the curve shows clearly that to achieve a given deformation, ΔL, requires a progressively larger force increment, ΔF, the more the muscle is passively stretched from its resting length. The slope of the muscle curve in Figure 2-2 increases with α, illustrating a phenomenon similar to what is known as *strain hardening* or *work hardening* in deformable crystals. The latter is characterized by the fact that the shear stress required to produce crystal slip continuously increases with increasing shear strain.

Strain hardening in crystals is caused by dislocations interacting with each other and with barriers that impede their motion through the crystal lattice. Strain hardening in *muscle tissue* can be attributed to the stretching out of progressively stiffer elements as the deformation con-

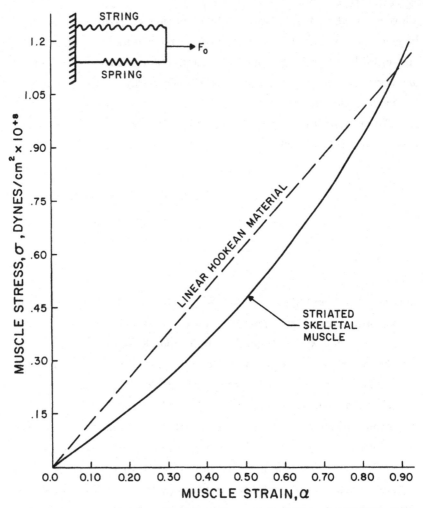

Figure 2-2   Nonlinear Passive Stress-Strain Characteristics Of Striated Skeletal Muscle.

tinues from resting length to maximum extension. That is, consider the hypothetical model depicted by the insert in the upper left hand corner of Figure 2-2. Here, the spring element may represent the more elastic myofilament portions of muscle tissue, and the parallel string element could correspond to the stiffer collagenous matrix of the tissue. At rest, the collagen fibers and membranes are in a relatively loose, or "slack" state. As deformation ensues, however, the string gets pulled taut, and soon the force F_o must stretch a tight string, rather than an elastic spring in order to generate a further deformation. Since the string is less elastic than the spring, the composite material appears to get stiffer as it undergoes a tensile deformation -- and vice versa as the string slackens during compression. Now, if one imagines a complicated continuous network of highly elastic tissue, covered with and permeated throughout by a stiffer but looser collagenous matrix, which, indeed, describes the anatomical configuration of the striated skeletal muscle, then the strain hardening nonlinear behavior described by equation [2-22] and shown in Figure 2-2 can certainly be explained physically (i.e., as the result of a composite material which is composed of elements having different elastic properties).

Active Nonlinear Behavior of Striated Skeletal Muscle

Bearing the above in mind, we turn our attention now to the active characteristics of stimulated muscle tissue. To examine this case, values of the stimulation coefficients, q_1, q_2, and q_3 are taken to be:

$$q_1 = 0.45$$
$$q_2 = -0.25$$
$$q_3 = -0.15$$

and the other quantities needed to solve the full equation [2-22] are as previously defined.

****

Problem 2-7: To examine the pure effects of stimulation on the development of active muscle tension, one can solve the *full* equation [2-22] and subtract off the passive behavior obtained by nulling the stimulation coefficients. Show first, that:

$$Q - Q_o = \frac{8}{3}(1 + \alpha)(N^2 - N_o^2)$$

$$= \frac{8}{3}\frac{B_1 + B_2\alpha + B_3\alpha^2 + B_4\alpha^3}{1 + \alpha} \qquad \text{[2-26]}$$

where: $B_1 = q_o(2 + q_o)$

$B_2 = 2[r_1(1 + q_o) + p_1]$

$B_3 = r_1{}^2 + 2r_2(1 + q_o) - p_1{}^2 + 2p_2$, and,

$B_4 = 2[r_1r_2 + r_3(1 + q_o) - p_1p_2 + p_3]$

Then define the nondimensional active tension, Φ, as:

$$\Phi = \left\{ \frac{F_{\text{total}} - F_{\text{passive}}}{F_{\text{isometric}}} \right\} B_1$$

and show that:

$$\Phi = \frac{B_1 + B_2\alpha + B_3\alpha^2 + B_4\alpha^3}{1 + \alpha}\left[1 + 2\frac{E_2}{E_1}\alpha + 3\frac{E_3}{E_1}\alpha^2\right] \qquad \text{[2-27]}$$

****

Equation [2-27] is plotted in Figure 2-3, where it is observed that the active tension which a striated skeletal muscle can develop in a single twitch depends on its state of elongation at the time. More specifically, the active tension increases with length up to a maximum at $\alpha = 0.2678$, and then begins to fall off rapidly to zero at $\alpha = 0.7182$. As was true for the passive behavior discussed earlier, so, too, can the active behavior of muscle be explained by anatomical considerations based on the sliding filament theory of contraction (see Chapter 1). Thus, Figure 2-3 suggests that when a muscle is at its resting length ($\alpha = 0$) there is probably some compression of the sarcomeres, leading to a slight crowding of the cross-bridges that link the Myosin molecules to the Actin molecules. This crowding interferes with the ability of the bridges to oscillate or otherwise move freely relative to one another when they are activated. Thus, if the muscle is stimulated in this condition, it can only develop about 88% of a full contractile force.

Carrying this line of reasoning one step further, one can surmise that if the muscle is compressed below its resting length (i.e., for negative α) the cross-bridge interference will get still worse and so, too, will the ability of the fibers to generate a force. Indeed, the curve in Figure 2-3 does confirm such logic. In the limit, therefore, one might expect the situation to continue to worsen until the I-bands are effectively closed up and there is virtually a complete overlap of Actin molecules, so that the cross-bridges are completely squeezed together and not free to move at all (insert A in Figure 2-3). In this case (see Figure 1-3) $\frac{\Delta L}{L} \equiv \alpha \approx \frac{-0.8}{2} = -0.40$. Looking again to Figure 2-3 for confirmation, one finds the interesting result that Φ, indeed, approaches zero as α goes to -0.3763. While such findings show the self-consistency of the physics and the mathematics, it should be pointed out that in real life the tension developed by muscle tissue does not actually go all the way to zero when it is stimulated from a severely compressed state. However, it *is* true that the tension developed by a muscle in this condition is *drastically* reduced because of the interference imposed by crowding of the vibrating cross-bridges.

Going now in the other direction, one finds that if a muscle is stretched to about 27% more than its resting length (insert B in Figure 2-3), then there are a maximum number of unobstructed cross-bridges making contact between the muscle filaments, and these cross-bridges are completely free to oscillate unimpeded. Therefore, maximum twitch tension is possible and can be achieved. It is interesting to note, in this respect, that unstimulated skeletal muscle at rest in the body is *normally* under slight tension -- a fact borne out by the observation that the tissue *shortens* about 20% if the tendons are cut from their respective attach-

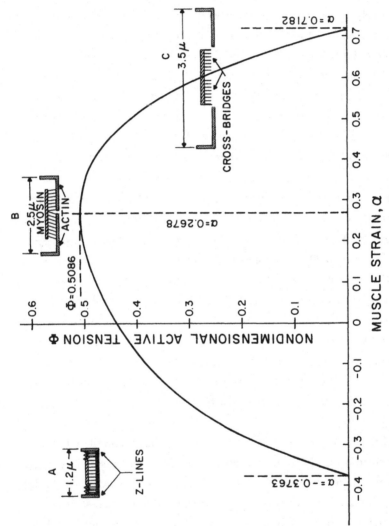

Figure 2-3 Nondimensionalized Active Tension Developed By Striated Skeletal Muscle As A Function Of Its Length (Active Stress-Strain or Length-Tension Behavior).

ments to bone with the muscle in a relaxed state. Because active tension *increases* with muscle length for $-0.3763 \leq \alpha \leq +0.2678$ in Figure 2-3, this portion of the curve is sometimes called the *compensation phase* of the length-tension diagram for striated skeletal muscle.

The Parameter Φ/B_1 essentially gives the ratio of an active *isotonic* contraction to an active *isometric* contraction ($\Phi = B_1$ for $\alpha = 0$) and, with $B_1 = 0.44$ ($q_o = 0.20$) and $\Phi_{max} = 0.5086$, we see that this ratio is of unit order when the muscle is experiencing a maximum isotonic contraction. That is to say, a complete isometric contraction represents the largest force that any single muscle can *actively* generate (per stimulation, or for a *given* frequency of stimulation) from a given starting length.

To illustrate this, consider what happens when a person attempts to flex the elbow while holding a weight in one hand. If the weight is very light, an adequate isotonic contraction can be generated in the Biceps Brachii muscle (see Figure 1-6) and elbow flexion can be accomplished with little effort. As the weight is gradually increased, the isotonic force necessary to accomplish elbow flexion will also increase. However, there is an upper limit to the isotonic force that the muscle can actively generate, and this limit will be reached when a weight of sufficient magnitude is placed in the hand such that the person can no longer flex the elbow regardless of how hard he or she tries. At this point, since the joint does not flex, the contraction of the Biceps Brachii is, by definition, an isometric contraction and, again, since the person cannot get the weight to move, this isometric contraction represents the upper limit of the force that can be generated by an isotonic contraction of the muscle.

The obvious extension of this reasoning to the case where the weight placed in the hand is so heavy that it causes the elbow joint to *passively extend, despite* the efforts of the Biceps Brachii to produce an *active* elbow *flexion,* shall be considered in Chapter 5 (when the force-velocity characteristics of muscle are discussed in some detail). Suffice it to say at this point that this situation tends to *inhibit* the Biceps from generating an active contraction at all (by, for example, the inverse myotatic reflex -- see Chapter 6 later); that the force generated in the muscle is now determined more by its *passive* behavior (Figure 2-2) than by its active behavior; and that this milieu defines an *eccentric* contraction. Thus, one observes that the *total* tension in the tissue *can* exceed the isometric value, but not due to an active contractile mechanism.

In general, isotonic contractions tend to generate smaller forces than do isometric contractions because their intent is less to *favor* force than it is to produce motion of parts or all of the animal body (i.e., to generate kinetic energy). However, if the maximum weight against which the person above is trying to produce an elbow flexion, should be suddenly removed, it is obvious that the isometric tension generated by the muscle would be quickly converted into an isotonic contraction, and that the potential energy stored in an "isometric" form would soon appear as kinetic energy of high-speed limb movement. Thus, one may think of isometric contractions as generating potential energy and isotonic contractions as generating kinetic energy, with the two being able to be transformed into one another, and with the former being the upper limit of the latter. This limit, in turn, is a function of muscle length in accordance with the behavior illustrated in Figures 2-2 and 2-3.

The relatively horizontal plateau which occurs around $\alpha = 0.2678$ in Figure 2-3 is due to the fact that the 0.15-micron-H-Zones in the muscle filaments are devoid of cross-bridge attachments between Myosin and Actin molecules (see Figure 1-3 in Chapter 1). Thus, *increasing* filament overlap (contraction) which occurs in this anatomical region, and resulting cross-bridge crowding, is essentially without consequence until α drops below around 0.20. Similarly, *decreasing* filament overlap (extension) with the resulting breakdown of cross-bridge binding to Actin does not seriously impede muscular performance until α exceeds roughly 0.30. Due to the cross-bridge-free H-zone region, therefore, the force curve essentially reaches a plateau for $0.20 \leq \alpha \leq 0.30$.

To conclude our discussion of Figure 2-3 and equation [2-27], we note that as the muscle is stretched beyond $1.27L$ the filaments are pulled apart to the point where the cross-bridges attached to the Myosin molecules begin to lose contact with the Actin chains. This reduction in the number of cross-bridge attachments progressively diminishes the capability of the muscle fibers to generate a tension actively. By the time the filaments have been pulled out a total of about 1.5 microns, there are *no* cross-bridges able to make contact with the Actin molecules (insert C, Figure 2-3) and the muscle, indeed, even in real life, completely loses its ability to generate a contractile force. Observe, again, that this deformation of 1.5 microns corresponds to a muscle strain of 0.750, which is remarkably close to the value 0.7182 predicted by the nonlinear theory.

Note again, also, that, while such a strain impedes the muscle from having the ability to generate a *contractile* force, it does not alter the *passive* characteristics of the muscle, as indicated in Figure 2-2. Thus, to reiterate what was previously mentioned, the *total* force in muscle continues to increase as it is stretched, but the component that is due to *active* contraction is no longer a factor in determining this force. In fact, active muscular contraction is *inhibited* from occurring under these circumstances by a variety of reflex mechanisms that are described in more detail in Chapter 6.

Because active tension *decreases* with muscle length for $0.2678 \leq \alpha \leq 0.7182$ in Figure 2-3, this portion of the curve is sometimes called the *Decompensation Phase* of the length-tension diagram for striated skeletal muscle. The compensation/decompensation characteristics that result from the anatomical structure of this tissue give rise to the famous *Starling's Law of the Heart* that governs intrinsically the cardiac output of this organ -- i.e., as inflow (venous return) to the heart increases (*lengthening* the myocardial muscle fibers just prior to cardiac contraction), the subsequent strength of contraction (development of muscle fiber *tension*) increases with it, thereby insuring that as much blood gets pumped *out* of the heart as comes *in*, on the average, over a period of time.

In addition to its state of elongation at the time of stimulation, the amount of force that any one muscle in the body can develop depends also on such factors as the active state of its fibers; the number of cross-bridges that are *active*, or *activated* with each stimulation; the total number of motor units contained in the muscle; the strength of individual motor units; the degree of filamentary overlap; the velocity of shortening; certain intermolecular secondary forces; and the geometric arrangement of motor units in the muscle. For example, a muscle with its fibers inserted obliquely into the muscle tendon (Penniform) cannot exert as much tension on the tendon as can a muscle of the same size and individual unit strength with its fibers inserted parallel (Fusiform) to the axis of the tendon.

Moreover, the fact that all cross-bridges may be in an *optimal* configuration to form a bond with Actin, and to oscillate back and forth unimpeded, does not necessarily insure that they *will*. Indeed, an isometric contraction represents the largest force that a muscle can develop for a *given* stimulation frequency and state of activation of its actomyosin complex -- not the largest force that the tissue can develop in an *absolute* sense (e.g., a tetanic contraction). The active tension could be increased, for example, by factors such as the staircase effect discussed in Chapter 1 (to which we shall return in Chapter 5). Various other "extrinsic" mechanisms that affect membrane permeability, calcium metabolism, enzyme systems, ATP-utilization, and so on, can also produce so-called *Inotropic effects* on striated skeletal and cardiac muscle. The word, inotropic, derives from the Greek prefix, "ino-," meaning, "fiber," and suffix, "-tropic," meaning, "a turning toward." Within this context, it refers, generally, to the activity of endocrine hormones and/or autonomic nervous system stimulation that influences the contractility (length-tension and force-velocity characteristics) of muscular tissue by mechanisms such as are mentioned above (and described in somewhat more detail in Chapter 6).

Furthermore, the variation in total strength of specific muscles is great -- the Sartorius muscle that flexes and laterally rotates the thigh to cross the legs in a "tailor's position" is one of the strongest muscles in the body; the Rectus Femoris Gastrocnemius muscle of the thigh is one of the weaker ones; and flexor muscles tend to be *actively* stronger than extensors (although, interestingly enough, the latter have a higher ultimate strength in *passive* tests) -- and the variation in *passive* strength of individual motor units in different muscles is also great -- and depends as well on the *age* of the individual.

Up to age 20, muscle tissue matures (or is *capable* of maturing) to 100% of its potential material strength (e.g., Figure 2-2). Within the next ten years, to age 30 or so, the strength drops off to about 80% of its maximum value. This continues to decrease over the next 20 years (to age 50) by about another 20% of maximum (roughly 10% per decade) before tapering off as one enters into "senior citizenhood". Past age 60, on up to age 80, passive muscle strength asymptotically stabilizes at around 47% to 50% of its age 20 value so that, barring any serious musculoskeletal diseases, one should still be able to function at about half of his or her "youthful vigor" through to the individual's demise (Yamada, H., 1973).

By contrast, *active* muscle strength (e.g., Figure 2-3) peaks, for most muscle groups, between the ages of 25 and 30 (Fisher and Birren, 1947), and decreases very slowly during maturity up through at least the fifth decade. Beyond that point, the active strength decrease accelerates (perhaps due more to disuse than to aging, per se); but even into the sixties the loss does not generally exceed 10 to 20 percent of maximum, and rarely does it drop much below that value, until sizable decrements in strength *do occur* in old age for legitimate reasons that are independent of use patterns.

All of the above factors are taken into account by the total of ten experimental coefficients that are used in this analysis -- four stimulation factors (q_0, q_1, q_2, q_3, which may also include inotropic effects), three generalized Poisson ratios (p_1, p_2, p_3), and three generalized Young's Moduli (E_1, E_2, E_3). Depending on the values of these ten parameters, one thus gets a *family* of length-tension diagrams for striated skeletal muscles. However, as good as the nonlinear theory may be in modelling the stress-strain behavior of striated skeletal muscle, it does *not* account for some of the more significant strain-*rate*-dependent characteristics of the tissue. For this reason, the chapter that follows shall address a phenomenological, linear viscoelastic model that does, indeed, describe the time-dependent nature of this complicated material.

****

Problem 2-8: For values of the relevant parameters given in the text, plot the *full* equation [2-22] for $-0.40 \leq \alpha \leq +1.50$, in order to get a complete stress-strain diagram for muscle.

****

Problem 2-9: a) Nubar's nonlinear theory for muscular contraction contains no time-dependent or viscous behavior. At what point in the formulation of his theory might visco-elastic behavior have been introduced?

b) Write an equation that Nubar might have used to formulate a *nonlinear, viscoelastic* theory for muscular contraction.

****

References for Chapter 2

See at end of Chapter 4.

Chapter 3

A Linear, Viscoelastic, Phenomenological Constitutive Model
for Striated Skeletal Muscle

Introduction and Mathematical Formulation

Since muscle tissue consists of 75% water by weight, and much of what remains is Amorphous, long-chain polymer, composite material, it is not surprising to learn that it exhibits quite a bit of viscous behavior. In order to account for the time-dependence resulting from such behavior, the four-element viscoelastic model depicted in Figure 3-1 is one that has been proposed. In this model, the contractile elements (Actomyosin cross-bridge configuration) of the muscle are assumed to generate some force, P, (perhaps calculated from the nonlinear analysis of the previous chapter) and this force is considered to be modulated by the spring-dashpot system shown before appearing in the tendons as the tensile force, F. Thus, c represents the dashpot constant (force per unit velocity of deformation), k_s is the series spring constant (force per unit length of deformation), k_p is the parallel spring constant, and the other dimensions of the model are as shown.

The series spring corresponds physically to secondary elastic configurations within the cross-bridge structure, to the passive elasticity of the actomyosin architecture, to the sarcomere Z-discs, and to the passive activity of muscle tendons (see later). The parallel spring corresponds physically to elastic structures that lie passively parallel to the force-

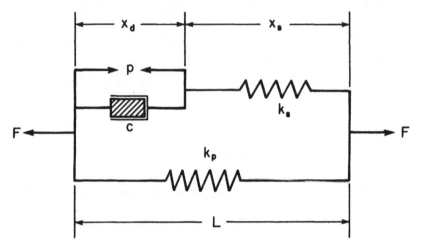

Figure 3-1   Four-Element Viscoelastic Model For Striated Skeletal Muscle

producing sarcomeres -- such as connective tissue sheaths, the various fasciae, and coverings that include the endomysium, sarcolemma, epimysium, and perimysium (see also later). The viscous element, of course, again accounts for the enormous fluid content of muscle tissue, as well as for "delayed elasticity" due to secondary electrochemical structures (more on this later). Note the conspicuous absence of *mass* in this model, making it respond as a first-order, rather than a second-order physical system (i.e., no inertia). It can be shown that, within certain limits, the choice of the value of the sarcomere mass is not critical or even significant as regards the model response. It appears, therefore, permissible to neglect this mass altogether, or, to locate the *total* sarcomere mass right at the Z-disc if one wishes to include it in the analysis (see Problem 3-7).

It should be emphasized that complicated spring-dashpot models such as that shown in Figure 3-1 are *phenomenological* rather than *physical*. That is to say, the *behavior* of the material is well represented and predicted by the differential equations and parameters that govern the *model*, even though the *real* material is not actually composed of tiny elastic springs and viscous dampers. Some attempt will be made to relate the model to the physics of muscle as we examine the behavior of the spring-dashpot system (sometimes called a Kelvin Model) illustrated in Figure 3-1. To develop the governing equation for this system, consider first the loop containing the contractile elements and the viscous damper. Contracting against an external tensile resistance, F, pulling on the muscle tendons, the force generated by the dashpot will be equal to $c\dot{x}_d$ (where the dot over a symbol indicates differentiation with respect to time) and the force generated by the contractile elements of the muscle will be equal to P, as previously defined. Thus, because the dashpot and the contractile unit are connected in parallel, one component of the tensile forces generated by the muscle in order to overcome the resistance F can be written as:

$$f_1 = P + c\dot{x}_d \qquad\qquad \text{[3-1]}$$

from which:

$$\dot{x}_d = \frac{f_1 - P}{c}$$ [3-2]

Since the spring with constant k_s is in *series* with the dashpot-contractile-element-loop, one can write further,

$$f_1 = k_s(x_s - x_{os})$$ [3-3]

where x_{os} represents the (constant) undeflected resting length of the series spring and x_s, its actual length at any time, t. Differentiation of equation [3-3] with respect to time yields:

$$\dot{x}_s = \frac{\dot{f}_1}{k_s}$$ [3-4]

Now, $L = x_d + x_s$, so, $\dot{L} = \dot{x}_d + \dot{x}_s$. Substituting into this last expression equation [3-2] for $\dot{x}_d$ and equation [3-4] for $\dot{x}_s$, and solving for $\dot{f}_1$ gives the following result:

$$\dot{f}_1 = k_s \dot{L} - \frac{k_s}{c} f_1 + \frac{k_s}{c} P$$ [3-5]

Turning our attention now to the branch of the model that contains the parallel spring element, we can write *its* response to the pull F as:

$$f_2 = k_p(L - L_{op})$$ [3-6]

where L_{op} represents the (constant) undeflected resting length of the parallel spring, and, from which:

$$\dot{f}_2 = k_p \dot{L}$$ [3-7]

Equations [3-5], [3-6], and [3-7] can now be used to derive the governing differential equation for total tensile force F as a function of total muscle length L. That is, because the branches generating forces f_1 and f_2 are arranged in parallel, one can write:

$$F = f_1 + f_2 \qquad [3\text{-}8]$$

Substitute equation [3-6] for f_2 into equation [3-8] and multiply the result by $\dfrac{k_s}{c}$ to get:

$$\frac{k_s}{c} F = \frac{k_s}{c} f_1 + \frac{k_s}{c} k_p (L - L_{op}) \qquad [3\text{-}9]$$

Now differentiate equation [3-8] with respect to time:

$$\dot{F} = \dot{f_1} + \dot{f_2} \qquad [3\text{-}10]$$

Substitute equation [3-5] for $\dot{f_1}$ and equation [3-7] for $\dot{f_2}$ into equation [3-10] to get:

$$\dot{F} = k_s \dot{L} - \frac{k_s}{c} f_1 + \frac{k_s}{c} P + k_p \dot{L} \qquad [3\text{-}11]$$

The term $\left[\dfrac{k_s}{c} f_1 \right]$ can be eliminated from equation [3-11] by adding it to equation [3-9] to get:

$$\frac{k_s}{c} F + \dot{F} = k_s \dot{L} + \frac{k_s}{c} k_p (L - L_{op}) + \frac{k_s}{c} P + k_p \dot{L} \qquad [3\text{-}12]$$

Finally, introduce the new variable $\xi = L - L_{op} =$ the total deformation of the muscle relative to its resting state, and note that $\dot{\xi} = \dot{L}$ (since L_{op} is just some reference constant) so that equation [3-12] becomes:

$$\dot{F} + \frac{k_s}{c} F = (k_s + k_p)\dot{\xi} + \frac{k_s k_p}{c} \xi + \frac{k_s}{c} P \qquad [3\text{-}13]$$

Passive Rheologic Behavior of Muscle

Equation [3-13] defines the Force-Deformation relationship for the viscoelastic model depicted in Figure 3-1, just as equation [2-22] does for the nonlinear model developed from Figure 2-1. Thus, as was done in the nonlinear case, let us examine first the *passive* behavior of muscle as predicted by equation [3-13]. This requires that we null the effects of neural stimulation, i.e., set P equal to zero, and consider the equation:

$$\dot{F} + \frac{k_s}{c} F = (k_s + k_p)\dot{\xi} + \frac{k_s k_p}{c} \xi \qquad [3\text{-}14]$$

Several specific cases of equation [3-14] may be considered. The simplest involves looking at steady-state events which are time-independent. For this situation, $\dot{F} = \dot{\xi} = 0$, and

$$F = k_p \xi \qquad [3\text{-}15]$$

Note the linear form of equation [3-15], which represents the steady-state elastic response, F, of muscle tissue to passive displacements, ξ. This equation, therefore, provides a convenient means for calculating k_p based on laboratory experiments of the force-deformation characteristics of muscle. As expected, such experiments reveal that k_p is not constant, but rather varies widely (at least by an order of magnitude) depending on animal species, individual experimental subjects, muscle geometry, type, and so on. One conclusion that *can* be drawn, however, is that k_p is frequently an order of magnitude smaller than the other parameters in the viscoelastic model (see later). In general, the parallel spring constant can take on values that range from 8.75×10^5 dynes/cm to a maximum of around 9.5×10^6 dynes/cm (875-9500 Newtons/meter).

It is interesting to compare the passive behavior predicted by equation [3-15] with the corresponding behavior predicted by the nonlinear theory for the unstimulated muscle, i.e., Figure 2-2. Observe from the definition of $\xi = L - L_{op} = \Delta L$ that ξ also equals αL (c.f., equation [2-11]. Moreover, if equation [3-15] is divided on both sides by $A = \frac{\pi D^2}{4}$, the cross-sectional area of the muscle, then one obtains:

$$\frac{F}{A} = \sigma = \frac{4k_p}{\pi D^2} \alpha L = E\alpha \qquad [3\text{-}16]$$

where E represents the Young's Modulus in a Hookean Elastic sense for a given muscle, i.e., a given L, D and k_p. Thus,

$$E = 4 \frac{k_p}{\pi L} \left(\frac{L}{D} \right)^2 \qquad [3\text{-}17]$$

Equation [3-17] can be generalized into some generic form, $V_m = G_n V_n$ (Gottlieb, Agarwal and Stark, 1969), where V_m is some mechanical or structural parameter (such as the parallel spring constant, k_p, the series spring constant, k_s, or the viscous damper, c) measured from an intact muscle; V_n is a normalized parameter (such as the Young's Modulus, $E = \frac{\sigma}{\alpha}$, or the Viscous Modulus, $\eta = \frac{\sigma}{\alpha}$) characteristic of the basic properties of the biological muscle tissue; and G_n defines a geometric ratio or characteristic length, which in this case is the ratio of muscle cross-sectional area to muscle length. The physical significance of the latter is that both the elasticity and viscosity of the total muscle will be directly proportional to the number of fibers in *parallel*, as manifest by the muscle cross-sectional area, and *inversely* proportional to the number of elements in series, as reflected in muscle length (ibid.). Thus, G_n relates a muscle's structural parameters, which characterize the muscle as a whole, to its normalized parameters, which are basic properties of the biological materials, i.e.,

$$G_n = \frac{V_m}{V_n} = \frac{\pi D^2}{4L} = \frac{k_p}{E}, \qquad [3\text{-}18]$$

for example, as derived from equation [3-17].

Moreover, Gottlieb, et al., (1969) suggest that the muscle model as depicted in Figure 3-1 is actually representative of a *single* sarcomere, with each muscle fiber being composed of many (say n_o) sarcomers linked in series, and each muscle, itself, being made up of many fibers linked both in series and in parallel. For this more complicated arrangement, Decraemer, Maes, and Vanhuyse (1980) define an "Effective" Young's Modulus, for a fiber, i.e.,

$$E_{eff} = \sum_{i=1}^{n_o} \frac{k_i \ell_i}{A_i} \simeq n_o \frac{k_p L}{A} \qquad [3\text{-}19]$$

in terms of equation [3-17], and assuming the k_i's, ℓ_i's and A_i's are approximately equal and uniform for the entire fiber. Note from equations [3-17] or [3-19] that there is a *difference* between saying that k_i is constant, and saying that E_i is constant. The latter may vary even if the former does not (and vice versa), depending on the corresponding values of L (or ℓ_i) and A (or A_i). We shall have much more to say about the work of Decraemer, et al., in Chapter 4, so, for now, we return to the more simple analysis of Figure 3-1 and examine again the case for $\frac{L}{D} = \frac{1}{0.20} = 5$.

Taking $8.75 \times 10^5 \leq k_p \leq 9.5 \times 10^6$, equations [3-16] or [3-17] yield:

$$\frac{1}{L}(2.79 \times 10^7) \leq E \leq \frac{1}{L}(3.02 \times 10^8) \text{ dynes/cm}^2$$

Depending on the length of any given muscle, which in most cases would be (in centimeters) of the same order as the mantissa in the above relationship, the steady-state value of E predicted by the viscoelastic theory is thus in the range $10^7 - 10^8$ dynes/cm^2 ($10^6 - 10^7$ Newtons/m^2). Turning now to the secant modulus of the stress-strain curve illustrated in Figure 2-2 -- i.e., the slope of the dashed line labelled, "Linear Hookean Material," one finds that $E_{secant} = \frac{1.12 \times 10^8}{0.90} = 1.25 \times 10^8$ dynes/cm^2. Moreover, near $\alpha = 0$, the tangent modulus of the striated skeletal muscle curve has a value of about 7.65×10^7 dynes/cm^2 and near $\alpha = 0.9$, the tangent modulus increases to 2.03×10^8 dynes/cm^2 due to the strain hardening effect discussed earlier.

Therefore, it is clear that the linear, viscoelastic theory and the nonlinear elastic theory give results so far that are self-consistent, quite compatible and reconcilable. They also agree with published data in the literature. Let us, then, take a closer look at what equation [3-14] tells us about the *time-dependent* behavior of muscle. To do so, two simple cases shall first be examined -- one involving a step-strain input and one involving a step-stress input.

Step-Strain Input: Stress Relaxation

Suppose a muscle is at rest when, at some reference time, $t = 0$, it is suddenly stretched a finite amount, ξ_o, and held that way for a long period of time thereafter. What happens? The answer to this question may be obtained by solving equation [3-14] with $\xi = \xi_o =$ constant for $t \geq 0$ and $\dot{\xi} = 0$ for all time. Thus, for a step-strain input:

$$\dot{F} + \frac{k_s}{c} F = \frac{k_s k_p}{c} \xi_o = \text{constant} \qquad \text{[3-20]}$$

Equation [3-20] is a linear, first order, nonhomogeneous, ordinary differential equation with assumed constant coefficients. It can be solved rather easily by multiplying the equation through by the integrating factor $e^{(k_s/c)t}$, to get:

$$e^{(k_s/c)t}\dot{F} + e^{(k_s/c)t}\left(\frac{k_s}{c}\right)F = \frac{d}{dt}\left\{Fe^{(k_s/c)t}\right\}$$

$$= e^{(k_s/c)t}\left(\frac{k_s}{c}\right)k_p\xi_o = \frac{d}{dt}\left\{k_p\xi_o e^{(k_s/c)t}\right\}$$

from which,

$$e^{(k_s/c)t}F = k_p\xi_o e^{(k_s/c)t} + \text{constant} \qquad \text{[3-21]}$$

The constant in equation [3-21] can be determined by observing that at $t = 0$, the instant the muscle contracts or is stretched, it reacts right at that moment with a purely elastic response. As is true of most good "shock absorbers", they are relatively unresponsive to sudden impact loading, of which the case being examined here is an example. In fact, that is *why* such dampers are called "shock" absorbers! Therefore, for $t = 0$ one may impose the physical constraint that:

$$f_1 = k_s \xi_o \quad \text{and} \quad f_2 = k_p \xi_o$$

so that, from equations [3-8] and [3-21] (with $t = 0$),

$$k_s \xi_o + k_p \xi_o - k_p \xi_o = \text{constant} = k_s \xi_o.$$

Equation [3-21] may now be solved for F, to get:

$$F = k_p \xi_o + k_s \xi_o e^{(-k_s/c)t} \qquad \qquad \text{[3-22]}$$

Note that for $t = 0$, the initial condition $(F)_{t=0} = \xi_o(k_p + k_s)$ is recovered. In fact, this condition provides a convenient means for calculating k_s, the series spring constant. That is, with k_p already known, one can measure $(F)_{t=0}$ at the muscle tendons for any given sudden stretch, ξ_o, and then simply use equation [3-22] applied at $t = 0$ to calculate the corresponding value of k_s. This has been done in a series of "quick release", abrupt acceleration tests, with the result that

$$3.25 \times 10^7 \le k_s \le 2.50 \times 10^8 \ \text{dynes/cm}$$

As already mentioned, observe that k_s, the series spring constant, is generally in a range an order of magnitude above the parallel spring constant, k_p, where:

$$8.75 \times 10^5 \le k_p \le 9.5 \times 10^6 \ \text{dynes/cm}.$$

Some physical reasoning to explain this situation shall be presented a bit later on. For now, note further in equation [3-22] that as $t \to \infty$, F approaches the value $k_p \xi_o$ exponentially; which means that eventually, the parallel spring winds up carrying the entire deformation load, while the force in the series spring is gradually "relaxed". This corresponds to the steady-state case considered earlier and defined by equation [3-15]. Taking the ratio of $(F)_{t=0}$ to $(F)_{t\to\infty}$, one finds that:

$$\frac{(F)_{t=0}}{(F)_{t\to\infty}} = \frac{\xi_o(k_p + k_s)}{k_p\xi_o} = 1 + \frac{k_s}{k_p} > 1,$$

since both spring constants are positive-valued. Thus, we conclude that $(F)_{t=0} > (F)_{t=\infty}$, or, that the total tensile force in the muscle *decreases* exponentially with time to some asymptotic value, if the deformation is maintained constant.

This behavior is called *stress-relaxation* and is related to the chemical kinetics associated with long chain polarized macro-molecules (such as Actomyosin filaments) that are embedded in a viscous fluid medium. At rest, these long molecules equilibrate into a complicated overlapping structure that is held together not only by several types of strong primary covalent and chemical ionic bonds, but also by weaker Van der Waals' electrostatic forces and physical dipole-dipole interactions caused by the polarized charges on the filament chains. When subjected to a sudden pull or stretch (or to an instantaneous contraction), this structure deforms, but it does so against intermolecular restoring forces that do not give way easily or quickly. Thus, if the muscle is released from its deformed state within a reasonably short period of time, the viscoelastic material shows a purely elastic compliance that returns it almost at once to its original molecular configuration. Initially, strong intermolecular and intramolecular restoring forces thus allow the muscle to show a purely elastic response early in its deformation history.

However, if the tensile strain is held constant for a longer period of time, the weakest electrostatic and *physical* molecular bonds (Van der Waals and dipole-dipole) will eventually "break" under the load and molecules will start to "unwind" and "slip" past one another. As the bonds come apart and reform, and as the material "yields" to its deformed shape, and as the molecular configuration restructures itself to conform to its new environmental constraints, there results a relaxation of stress because the restoring forces gradually diminish (but not to zero) and it becomes progressively less difficult to hold the tissue at its new length. Such behavior is often referred to as *retarded elasticity* associated with the molecular process of *configurational* change under stress.

It also helps to explain why, phenomenologically, k_p is much smaller than k_s. That is, the *series* spring, since its effect damps out with time, represents conceptually the stronger component of initial elastic restoring forces that dominate the early deformation history of the material. This situation prevails when there is much molecular overlapping in evidence and where many, many inter- and intra-molecular bonds are acting to hold the muscle in its resting configuration. On the other hand, the parallel spring, since it eventually picks up the entire load, represents conceptually the lesser component of forces that are primarily responsible for holding the structure together in its deformed state -- when entire polymer chains have unwound and slipped past one another and where significantly less molecular overlapping, and hence molecular interactions are occurring. In reality, of course, these "initial" and "delayed" effects are not individually identifiable specific "elements" of the muscle; but they can be *modelled* as such by considering a stronger spring in parallel with a weaker one, where the effects of the stronger one are gradually damped out with time. The restoring forces generated by the weaker spring (or the lesser molecular interactions taking place in the deformed muscle) *do* start the recovery process when the muscle tissue is eventually released at some later point in time. Thus, given enough time, the *original* equilibrium configuration of the tissue is restored once the deforming strain is released.

A measure of the *rate* at which stress-relaxation (i.e., the making and breaking of intermolecular bonds, together with the slipping diffusional motion that takes place between long chains) occurs is called the Relaxation Constant, $\frac{k_s}{c}$, or, in its inverted form, the Relaxation Time Constant,

$$\tau_\varepsilon = \frac{c}{k_s}$$

The nondimensionalized form of equation [3-22] can thus be written:

$$\frac{F(t)}{F_{t \to \infty}} = 1 + \frac{k_s}{k_p} e^{-t/\tau_\varepsilon} = F^*(t) \qquad \text{[3-23]}$$

Figure 3-2A is a plot of equation [3-23] for $\frac{k_s}{k_p} = 10$, and the exponential stress relaxation or decay is immediately obvious. Furthermore, since the equation is intrinsically linear, it can be used in a simplified form to calculate τ_ε. Thus, writing:

$$-\ell n \left[\frac{k_p}{k_s} (F^* - 1) \right] = \frac{1}{\tau_\varepsilon} t, \qquad \text{[3-24]}$$

which follows directly from equation [3-23], one is left with a linear equation having slope $\frac{1}{\tau_\varepsilon}$. Plotting the left side of equation [3-24], then, as a function of time, one can easily measure the slope of the regression line to obtain $\frac{1}{\tau_\varepsilon} = \frac{k_s}{c}$, which turns out to be in the range: $2 \leq \frac{k_s}{c} \leq 26$ sec^{-1} for muscles *in vivo*, under loaded conditions (Stewart, et al., 1971). Substituting in, now, the range quoted earlier for k_s, we conclude that the dashpot constant, c, is in the approximate range:

$$1.25 \times 10^6 \leq c \leq 1.25 \times 10^8 \ \frac{\text{dynes}}{\text{cm/sec}} .$$

This range was calculated based on the *smallest* value of k_s (3.25×10^7) coupled with the *largest* value of $\left(\frac{k_s}{c} \right)$, 26, giving the lower limit for $c = \frac{3.25}{26} \times 10^7 = 1.25 \times 10^6$; and, the *largest* value of k_s (2.5×10^8) coupled with the *smallest* value of $\frac{k_s}{c}$, 2, giving the upper limit for $c = \frac{2.5}{2} \times 10^8 = 1.25 \times 10^8$.

Some investigators have found the damping component of the series element to be very much smaller than these values. Bahler (1967), for

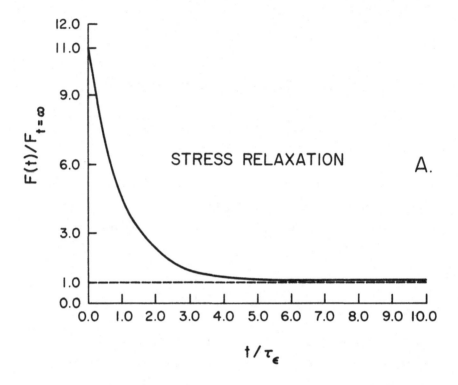

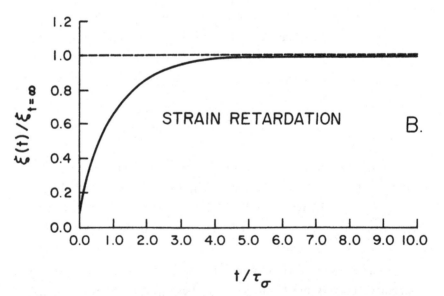

Figure 3-2   Response of Four-Element Viscoelastic Model for Striated Skeletal Muscle to: (A) Step-Strain Input (illustrating the phenomenon of Stress Relaxation), and (B) Step-Stress Input (illustrating the phenomenon of Creep). Both are for the Passive Case Corresponding to $P = 0$ in Figure 3-1.

example, reports c to be about 300 dynes/cm/sec for the Gracilis Anticus muscle of the rat, while Woledge (1961) found the viscous coefficient for the frog sartorius muscle to be in the range from 200 to 500 dynes/cm/sec (0.2 to 0.5 Newtons/m/sec). Gottlieb, et al., (1969), however, find c to be one to two orders of magnitude *larger* than this range, i.e., 8100-67,000 dynes/cm/sec for the musculature of the *human* arm, although this range is *still* much smaller (by at least one or two orders of magnitude) than that quoted earlier based on Stewart's, et al. (1971) results.

Suffice it to say, that these model parameters are very much species-dependent; their numerical value seems to be very much investigator-and-experiment-dependent (in vitro, in situ, in vivo, isolated muscle preparations vs. intact experimentation on entire systems, and so on); and the numbers will vary depending on the complexity of the actual phenomenological model chosen to simulate the tissue. Thus, at best, we can only state that the range $10^6 \leq c \leq 10^8$ dynes/cm/sec derives from the *reasonable* values quoted earlier for k_s, and from the results of at least one group of investigators for the range of (k_s/c). Certainly, c will be no *larger* than these values. Anything said further must await additional information and more laboratory results.

Observe that the dashpot constant has units of $\dfrac{\text{dynes - sec}}{\text{cm}}$ which, if divided by the length, L, of the material, converts to units of $\dfrac{\text{dynes - sec}}{\text{cm}^2}$ which are units of dynamic viscosity. Thus, one may think of the viscous behavior of muscle *in vivo* as being expressed in the range:

$$\frac{1}{L}(1.25 \times 10^6) \leq \mu_d \leq \frac{1}{L}(1.25 \times 10^8) \quad \text{Poise.}$$

Once again we note that the length (in centimeters) of many muscles of the human body is of the same order of magnitude as the mantissa of the above relationship, so we conclude that muscle contracting under loaded conditions shows viscous properties that are analogous to fluids having viscosities in the range $10^6 - 10^8$ Poise. For purposes of comparison, Table 2-I gives the approximate viscosity, in Poises, of some familiar materials. Muscle, then, *in vivo* is seen to show viscous behavior somewhere between that of Molten Lava at 1100°C and Pitch at 20°C, which also is in the range just below soft glass in its workable or gel-like state.

Note from the table that *isolated* muscle (upon which most of Bahler's, Woledge's, and Gottlieb's results are based) *does* exhibit viscous behavior several orders of magnitude below that of muscle tissue *in vivo*. We shall have more to say about *isolated* muscle tissue in a later section of this chapter, but observe that its viscous behavior is closer to Confectioner's Glucose ($10^4 - 10^5$ Poise).

****

Problem 3-1: For the case of a step stretch of finite amount, ξ_o, one can define a *Relaxation Modulus, $\mathscr{R}$,* as the subsequent ratio of muscle stress to muscle strain. Show that the Relaxation Modulus for the passive behavior of the model depicted in Figure 3-1 is given by:

$$\mathscr{R}(t) = F^*(t)\, E$$

Where: $F^*(t)$ is defined by equation [3-23], and

E is defined by equation [3-17].

****

Step-Stress Input: Creep

Let us turn our attention, now, to the solution of equation [3-14] for the case of a step-*stress* input. Suppose a muscle is at rest when, at some reference time, $t = 0$, a finite tensile force, F_1, is suddenly applied to the tendons and held there for a long period of time thereafter. The response of the muscle to this situation may be analyzed by solving equation [3-14] with $F = F_1 = $ constant for $t \geq 0$ and $\dot{F} = 0$ for all time. Thus, for a step-stress input:

$$\dot{\xi} + K\xi = \frac{K}{k_p} F_1 = \text{Constant} \qquad [3\text{-}25]$$

where: $K = \dfrac{k_s k_p}{c(k_s + k_p)}$

TABLE 3–I		
Viscosity of Some Familar Materials		
MATERIAL	TEMPERATURE	APPROXIMATE VISCOSITY, POISES
Ether	68° F (20° C)	10^{-3}
Water	68° F	10^{-2}
Kerosene	68° F	10^{-1}
S.A.E. 10 Motor Oil	68° F	$10^0 = 1$
Glycerin or Caster Oil	68° F	10^1
Karo corn syrup, Honey	68° F	10^2
Molasses	68° F	10^3
Confectioner's Glucose	68° F	10^4
Striated Skeletal Muscle, Isolated	37° C	$10^4 - 10^5$
Molten Lava	1100° C	10^5
Striated Skeletal Muscle, In Vivo	37° C	$10^6 - 10^8$
Pitch	68° F	10^8
Sodium Silicate Glass	650° F (near the annealing point)	10^8
	600° C	10^9
	550° C (glass can hold its shape)	10^{10}

****

Problem 3-2: Using the integration factor e^{Kt} and appropriate elastic initial conditions for $t = 0$, solve equation [3-25] to show that:

$$\xi = \frac{F_1}{k_p} - \frac{k_s}{k_p(k_s + k_p)} F_1 e^{-Kt} \qquad \text{[3-26]}$$

****

In equation [3-26] note again the purely elastic response for $t = 0$, and the result that $F_1 = k_p\xi$ as $t \to \infty$. Thus, one recovers once more the fact that the parallel spring eventually picks up the entire load as the situation approaches a steady state. In the limit, we find that:

$$\frac{(\xi)_{t=0}}{(\xi)_{t \to \infty}} = \frac{F_1 k_p}{(k_s + k_p)F_1} = \frac{1}{1 + k_s/k_p} < 1,$$

or, $(\xi)_{t=\infty} > (\xi)_{t=0}$. Thus, when subjected to a constant loading, the deformation of muscle will *increase* exponentially with time to some asymptotic value. This type of behavior is called *strain retardation,* or *creep* and is caused by the same chemical kinetics that are associated with stress relaxation or retarded elasticity. That is, the bent, convoluted, secondary overlapping equilibrium structure of the muscle molecules at rest is altered by the application of a tensile stress. The stress tends to "straighten out" and stretch the macro-molecules while orienting them in the direction of pull. The result, again, is that the weak Van der Waals and electrostatic molecular bonds break apart, allowing the molecules to elongate and slide past one another. This process will continue to some limiting value as long as the disturbing force is maintained, and so the tissue gradually deforms at a continuous rate (or "creeps") with time until the load is removed or until the entire secondary structure has completely unraveled, whichever comes first. A recovery process then ensues.

A measure of the *rate* at which the muscle creeps is called the strain retardation constant, K, or, in its inverted form, the Retardation Time Constant,

$$\tau_\sigma = \frac{1}{K}.$$

The nondimensionalized form of equation [3-26] can thus be written:

$$\frac{\xi(t)}{\xi_{t \to \infty}} = 1 - \frac{1}{1 + k_p/k_s} \, e^{-(t/\tau_\sigma)} = \xi^*(t) \qquad [3\text{-}27]$$

Figure 3-2B shows a plot of equation [3-27] for $k_p/k_s = 0.10$, and the exponential strain retardation or creep is immediately obvious. Note from the definition of K, that all the parameters needed to compute its range of values are known quantities from previous calculations. Thus, for any given value of k_s, k_p and c, K can be readily determined. It is of greater interest, however, to look at the ratio of the two time constants, τ_σ and τ_ε, i.e.,

$$\frac{\tau_\sigma}{\tau_\varepsilon} = \frac{c(k_s + k_p)}{k_s k_p} \frac{k_s}{c} = 1 + \frac{k_s}{k_p} >> 1,$$

since k_s is generally an order of magnitude larger than k_p for reasons given earlier. Therefore, the time constant for creep is much larger than the time constant for stress relaxation. This is related to the fact that in the case of stress-relaxation the deformation is *imposed* upon the molecular configuration of the material, whereas, in the case of creep the material is allowed to deform at its own rate -- which is inherently much slower. Thus, as opposed to the Relaxation Modulus, $\mathscr{R}$, which was defined for the case of a step-stretch disturbance (stress-relaxation), one can define

for the case of a step-force disturbance a *Creep Compliance*, $\mathfrak{C}$, which is the ratio of subsequent strain (creep) to the applied stress.

****

Problem 3-3: Show that the Creep Compliance, $\mathfrak{C}$, can be written as:

$$\mathfrak{C}(t) = \frac{1}{E} \; \xi^*(t)$$

Where: $\xi^*(t)$ is defined by equation [3-27] and

        E is defined by equation [3-17].

****

Problem 3-4: Using the definition of the Laplace Transform,

$$\bar{g}(s) = \int_o^\infty g(t)e^{-st}dt$$

derive the fact that the relaxation modulus of Problem 3-1 and the Creep Compliance of Problem 3-3 are related by the simple equation:

$$\overline{\mathfrak{C}}(s) \, \overline{\mathscr{R}}(s) = \frac{1}{s^2}$$

This equation can actually be generalized for the product of the Laplace Transform of *any* corresponding pairs of Creep Compliance and Relaxation Modulus -- i.e., the product of their respective Laplace Transforms is always equal to $\frac{1}{s^2}$.

****

The same physical phenomena that give rise to stress-relaxation and creep also cause the tissue to exhibit a characteristic known as *hysteresis* (see Figure 3-3). That is to say, if one loads muscle tissue (by stressing or deforming it), then unloads it (Loading-Unloading Cycle 1), then loads it again, then unloads it again (Loading-Unloading Cycle 2), and so on -- one finds that he or she does not travel along the same stress-strain curve with each loading cycle. On the contrary, because of stress-relaxation and strain-retardation effects, the tissue appears to be easier to deform (i.e.; the same stress generates a larger strain) if it is disturbed relatively soon after just having been deformed. Thus, with each loading cycle, a somewhat different form is obtained for the loading of the speci-

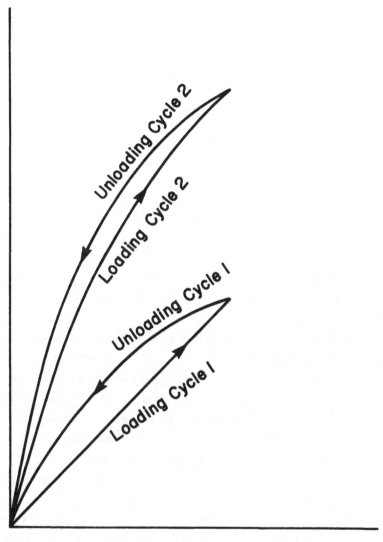

Figure 3-3 Passive Hysteresis Loops

men from that recorded for its unloading. This, of course, assumes that the tissue has not been allowed to recover fully from having been deformed before the next loading is applied.

Because hysteresis results from the breaking of weak, polar bonds in the material, it obviously has an upper limit. Indeed, it has been observed that the shape and characteristics of the stress-strain behavior of muscle tissue tends to become fixed (i.e., the area between the curves in Figure 3-3 tends to zero) as the number of loading-unloading cycles increases. Thus, the tissue will first go through a *transient stage* as it is stressed cyclicly, and then it will reach some equilibrium configuration which can be determined as seen in the next section. Hysteresis is a way of saying that the behavior of muscle at any given time depends on its loading-history, sometimes referred to as an "after-effect" or "preload" or "pre-stress" condition. After a number of loading and unloading cycles, the hysteresis effects approach a steady-state situation, which is described more fully below.

An interesting extension of this reasoning suggests that hysteresis, while governing the response of the tissue to a sinusoidal input, *also* plays a role in the staircase effect, wherein successive contractions can be summed to yield a tetanus. Each incoming stimulus excites the tissue from a pre-stressed condition (caused by the previous stimulus), so that the resulting force which can be generated by a succession of stimuli is much larger (because the *internal* passive resisting stresses are *smaller*) than that which would result from each stimulus applied separately over isolated periods of time.

The ratio $\frac{\tau_\sigma}{\tau_\varepsilon} = 1 + \frac{k_s}{k_p}$ given earlier is of significant interest because it is a measure of the dynamic behavior of muscle tissue as compared to its static behavior. This will become clearer when we examine the dynamic behavior of the tissue in the section that follows.

****

Problem 3-5: Show that the steady-state solution ($t \to \infty$) of the viscoelastic model described by equation [3-14] to a *sinusoidal* forcing function of the form $\xi = \xi_m \sin \omega t$ is:

$$F = Ck_p\xi_m \sin(\omega t + \phi) \qquad [3\text{-}28]$$

where:

$$C = \sqrt{\frac{\left(\dfrac{k_s}{c\omega}\right)^2 + \left[1 + \dfrac{k_s}{k_p}\right]^2}{1 + \left(\dfrac{k_s}{c\omega}\right)^2}} \quad = \text{ Magnification Factor, and,}$$

$$\tan\phi = \frac{(k_s/c\omega)}{[(k_s^2/c^2\omega^2) + (1 + k_s/k_p)]k_p/k_s} = \text{ Phase Angle}$$

****

Sinusoidal Input: Phase and Amplitude Relationships

Equation [3-28] reveals that when a muscle is subjected to a dynamic (in this case, simple periodic) loading, there is a phase difference, ϕ, between the applied deformation, ξ, and the resulting stress distribution represented by F (or, vice versa if the applied load is a force instead of a displacement). This phase difference is positive (lead) or negative (lag) depending on how the output of the tissue (force or displacement) is related to the input disturbance (strain or stress). That is to say, if the output of a system is a function of the *derivative* (or derivatives) of the input, then the output *leads* the input, since derivatives always lead their respective function. For example, you experience a resting *force* in a viscous damper *before* it starts to move, because the force is proportional to the *derivative* of displacement and thus *leads* the displacement, itself. On the other hand, if the output of a system is a function of the *integral* (or integrals) of the input, then the output always *lags* the input. And finally, if the output of a system is proportional *directly* to the input, or powers thereof, then the two will generally be perfectly *in phase*.

A convenient way to relate to these concepts is to recall that one must have an acceleration (*derivative* of velocity) *before* one can have a velocity, and one must have a velocity (*derivative* of displacement) *before* one can have a displacement. Thus, velocity (output) *lags* acceleration (input) because the output (velocity) is the time *integral* of the input (acceleration); and displacement (output) lags velocity (input) for the same reason. Conversely, acceleration leads velocity, which leads displacement. Applying this reasoning to the problem at hand, we note that the force (stress) in a viscoelastic system is proportional to both the *gradient* (visco-) *and* the magnitude (-elastic) of displacement, and thus force *output* (*F*) will *lead* displacement *input* (ξ). On the other hand, if the driving *input* were force (proportional to $\dfrac{d\xi}{dt}$) then the displacement *output* (ξ) would *lag* the input.

In addition to *leading* the strain input by a phase angle ϕ, the amplitude of the response *F* is also frequency-dependent due to the existence of the Magnification Factor, *C*, defined above. Both of these effects can be attributed directly to the time-dependent, series elastoviscous elements of the model shown in Figure 3-1 (see discussion that follows). The tangent of ϕ, or ϕ (which generally lines between 0 and $\dfrac{\pi}{2}$), either of which may be considered to be a direct measure of the internal friction of the material, and the magnification factor, *C*, are frequency-dependent for physical reasons that will be discussed more fully below.

Phase angle ϕ can easily be shown to lie somewhere between zero and $\dfrac{\pi}{2}$. If we let $c \to \infty$ and null *P* in Figure 3-1, then the system reduces to a *purely* elastic one. Force *F* thus becomes proportional directly to ξ through k_s and k_p, and we may write $F = (k_p + k_s)\xi = (k_p + k_s)\xi_m \sin \omega t$; $\phi = 0$. On the other hand, if we let $k_p = 0$ and null the effects of k_s by letting $k_s \to \infty$, then the system reduces to a *purely* viscous one. Force *F* thus becomes proportional to $\dfrac{d\xi}{dt}$ through *c*, and we may write:

$$F = c \frac{d\xi}{dt}$$

$$= c\xi_m \omega \, \cos \omega t$$

$$= c\xi_m \omega \, \sin \left(\omega t + \frac{\pi}{2} \right),$$

and immediately see that $\phi = \frac{\pi}{2}$. Note, mathematically, that these two extremes also agree with the definition of $\tan \phi$ given under equation [3-28]. For the more complex arrangement depicted in Figure 3-1, then, we would expect something between a *purely* elastic response ($\phi = 0$) and a *purely* viscous response ($\phi = \frac{\pi}{2}$).

In Figure 3-4, the phase angle, ϕ, and the magnification factor, C, have been plotted as a function of linear frequency, f_ω, (where *angular* frequency, ω, is equal to $2\pi f_\omega$) for $k_s/c = 15$, and $k_s/k_p = 10$. Observe, first, that ϕ increases with frequency from zero when $f_\omega = 0$, to a maximum value of about 56.5° for f_ω equal to nearly 0.75 cycles per second (45 cycles per minute), but then decreases to zero again for very high oscillation frequencies on the order of $10^3 - 10^4$ cycles/sec. This behavior can be explained physically on the basis of the fact that events such as stress-relaxation and strain retardation (i.e., secondary structures breaking, re-forming, and so on), discussed earlier take *time* to occur and to develop. Similarly, it also takes time to *reverse* these effects when the disturbance causing them changes direction. Thus, if the time scale of the oscillations is significantly shorter than a representative time scale of the retardation phenomena, then one will see a phase-shift between the disturbing input and the responding output. On the other hand, if the time scale of the oscillations is much larger than a representative time scale of the retardation phenomena, then the two will appear to be in phase because the response of the tissue will occur at a much faster rate than that at which the disturbance is changing (i.e., the disturbance is changing slow enough to let the physical response "catch up" to it prior to the start of the next cycle). In other words, time of disturbance is "short" or "long" when

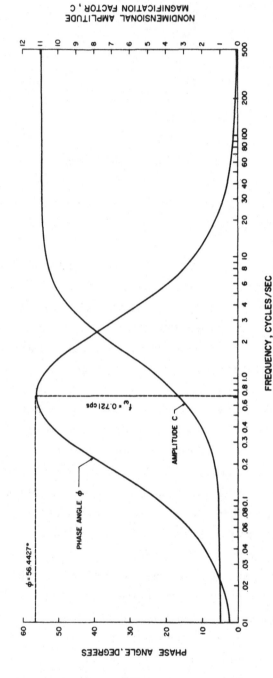

Figure 3-4 Dynamic Viscoelastic Behavior of Unstimulated (Passive) Striated Skeletal Muscle Subjected to Cyclic (Sinusoidal) Loading. Shown are the Phase Angle and Amplitude Response of the Tissue as a Function of the Disturbance Frequency.

compared to some mean relaxation time of the tissue. If not enough time has elapsed for there to be any measurable stress-relaxation, we call the response purely elastic. Otherwise, we must take into account viscous behavior as well.

For example, in Figure 3-2A, or from equation [3-23], we see that theoretically, it takes an infinitely long period of time for the stress-relaxation process to have been completed in response to a step-strain input. Therefore, hypothetically, if in a "dynamic" experiment, the muscle could be stretched *gradually* and *slowly* from $\xi = 0$ to $\xi = \xi_m$ over an infinite period of time, and then back again to $- \xi_m$ over an equally infinite period of time, and then forward again, ... , ad infinitum, -- then F would be theoretically defined by the steady state equation [3-15] at each instant of time, it (F) would be exactly in phase with ξ and ϕ would be identically equal to zero -- as indeed it is when the period of oscillation is infinite and $\omega \rightarrow 0$ in the expression for tan ϕ.

For this limiting case of an oscillation with an infinite time period, the effects of the *series* spring element in Figure 3-1 would always be essentially damped out completely and instantaneously ($x_s - x_{os} = 0$ in equation [3-3]), so k_s could be taken to be effectively infinite in equation [3-28]. This means that the series spring undergoes virtually no *change* in length (deformation) when it is "stretched" by ξ ($x_s - x_{os} = 0$), but, rather, simply gets displaced as an entire unit (i.e., undergoes pure translation), without deforming. In other words, a slight, slow movement of its right end (see Figure 3-1) is countered almost immediately (compared to the time scale of the oscillatory motion) by a corresponding movement of its left end, so the spring gets entirely *displaced*, but not *stretched* or deformed per se. It therefore offers no significant resistance to the motion (i.e., $f_1 \simeq 0$).

Neither does the dashpot, since *its* resistance to motion depends on the *rate of change* of the motion ($\dot{x}_d$), which is basically zero when the period of oscillation is infinite. The net effect of all of this, since k_s is the *stronger* of the two springs in the model, is that eliminating it from the response equation reduces the magnification factor to unity and effectively makes the force response to the displacement ξ a function only of the *smaller* spring constant, k_p. Thus, with $C = 1$ and $\phi = 0$, equation [3-28] would reduce to:

$$F = k_p \xi_m \sin \omega t, \qquad\qquad\qquad [3\text{-}29]$$

which is the same as equation [3-15] with $\xi = \xi_m \sin \omega t$, and which says, effectively, that the purely elastic tissue response is in phase with the disturbance, and oscillating around its limiting mean value. One could then conclude that muscle shows a *purely elastic*, "flat" response at near-zero disturbance frequencies because it has a *great deal of time* to adjust to $F_{t \to \infty}$ in the sense of equation [3-23] as the disturbance changes with very small increments of displacement over very long periods of time.

In a more realistic sense, one can now envision that if the disturbing displacements (or forces) are fluctuating with a very *low*, but finite frequency, events can be changing so slowly with time that the tissue is able to adjust very quickly (relative to the period of the disturbance) to any given loading -- almost as if each specific loading were, in fact, held constant for long periods of time, and the disturbance was not oscillating at all. In such cases, the response of the muscle will *tend* to be essentially in phase (timewise) with the disturbance, which is to say, a change in the disturbance will result virtually instantaneously in a corresponding change in the muscle, with no significant time lead or lag. But, how *low* is low frequency in order for this to hold true? The answer can be obtained mathematically by noting that, for ω very small, but finite, one can write, approximately:

$$C = 1$$

$$\phi = \frac{c\omega}{k_p} = \frac{c}{k_s} \frac{k_s}{k_p} \omega, \text{ and}$$

$$F = k_p \xi_m \sin (\omega t + \phi) \qquad\qquad\qquad [3\text{-}30]$$

Recall that the relaxation time constant, τ_ε, is given by (c/k_s), so that the phase angle for small oscillation frequencies can also be written as:

$$\phi = 2\pi \, \frac{\tau_\varepsilon}{T_\omega} \, \frac{k_s}{k_p} \qquad\qquad [3\text{-}31]$$

where $T_\omega = \dfrac{1}{f_\omega} = $ the time period of the oscillation. With $(k_s/k_p) = 10$, equation [3-31] reduces to $\phi = 62.8(\tau_\varepsilon/T_\omega)$ radians, or, $3600 \, (\tau_\varepsilon/T_\omega)$ degrees. Thus, we see that the phase angle will be small when the period of the oscillation is very much bigger than the relaxation time constant, or, when:

$$\frac{\tau_\varepsilon}{T_\omega} \leq 0(10^{-3}),$$

which gives phase angles on the order of $3.6°$ or less. Observe from Figure [3-4] that these are, indeed, very small phase leads. In fact, for $\tau_\varepsilon = \dfrac{c}{k_s} = \dfrac{1}{15}$, $\phi = 240f_\omega$ degrees, and so the phase angle increases approximately linearly from $0°$ to $3.6°$ as f_ω increases from zero to 0.015 cycles/sec (around one cycle per minute). In this range, the amplitude response, C, is also nearly flat and equal to unity. The tissue behaves essentially linearly elastically and its material properties are defined quite appropriately by a *static* modulus of elasticity, E, in the sense given by equations [3-17] and [3-18].

As the oscillation frequency of the disturbance goes up, or, as T_ω comes down from its "large" value of $1000\tau_\varepsilon$, viscous time-dependent effects cause the phase lead between displacement input and force output to go up as well, such that ϕ now becomes more prominent. For the situation being considered here, the maximum is reached at a frequency of 0.721 cycles per second, which corresponds to a period of 1.387 seconds. At this point, T_ω has been reduced to almost 21 times the relaxation time constant of $(1/15) = 0.0667$ seconds, which is a decrease of almost two orders of magnitude. Let us take a closer look at what this implies.

If the disturbance is oscillating with a period of 1.387 seconds, this means that ξ goes from its minimum value to its maximum value in one-half that time, or, 0.6935 seconds, which translates into just 10 relaxation time constants. Now, note from Figure 3-2A that by the time 10 relaxation time constants have gone by, most of the relaxation process has been completed for a given sudden muscle stretch ($F^*(t) = 1.0005$ when $t = 10\tau_\varepsilon$). Thus, we conclude that this "critical" oscillation frequency of 0.721 cycles per second is "just" slow enough to allow the tissue to respond with almost a complete stress relaxation during (and "between") each cycle, but fast enough to cause that response to lead the disturbance by a maximum phase angle of some 56.5°. Again, the phase lead is due to the fact that the system response (F) becomes more a function of $\dot{\xi}$ than of ξ as f_ω increases and the dashpot assumes progressively more prominence. In other words, a resisting *force* develops in the tissue (due to $\dot{\xi}$) *before* a tissue displacement (due to ξ) becomes manifest. But, what happens if the oscillation frequency *continues* to rise above this critical value?

For still higher oscillation frequencies, the phase lead begins to decrease because now events are starting to change so fast with time that the tissue *cannot* respond fully with each cycle. By the time $T_\omega = \tau_\varepsilon$, for example, which corresponds to a frequency of 15 cycles per second, ϕ is already down to only 8.2°, and equation [3-23] indicates that for $t = (0.50)\tau_\varepsilon$, $F^*(t) = 7.0653$ -- which is still nearly two-thirds of its initial value at $t = 0$. Thus, what is happening in this case is that the role of the *dashpot* is being minimized (c is effectively becoming infinite in equation [3-28]), just as that of the series spring ($k_s \to \infty$) was for low frequencies, and more and more of the total response is becoming purely elastic again. Furthermore, the elastic response is starting to be governed progressively more by ($k_s + k_p$), rather than by just k_p as it was earlier, so the material appears to be getting stiffer and stiffer -- as evidenced by the sudden rapid rise in the value of C between one and fifteen cycles per second.

In the limit, when the disturbing influences fluctuate *extremely* rapidly with time ($\omega \to \infty$), the phase lead is virtually wiped out and the left end of the series spring in Figure 3-1 might as well be rigidly attached in parallel with the parallel spring. In effect, such rapid fluctuations act like a sequence of sudden, alternating step-strain or step-stress inputs because the rise time of a high-frequency sinusoidal signal is so short that it deviates only slightly from a corresponding square-wave-type signal. The striated skeletal muscle thus finds itself in a constant state of *initial* response to these high-frequency, changing strain inputs. Recall that such an initial response is *strong* and *purely elastic* for reasons already discussed, so there is no, or virtually no time shift between input (ξ) and output (F). In other words, by the time the tissue *would* respond in a viscoelastic sense to whatever state of instantaneous stress or strain is being imposed, that stress or strain has changed abruptly and the muscle starts all over again. In the final limit of $\omega \to \infty$, ϕ, indeed, once again goes to zero as it did for $\omega \to 0$, but F approaches the stiffer limit $(k_p + k_s)\ \xi_m \sin \omega t$ (compared to equation [3-29] for $\omega \to 0$). For ω very large, but finite, one can write, approximately:

$$C = 1 + \frac{k_s}{k_p}$$

$$\phi = \frac{k_s}{k_p} \frac{k_s}{c} \frac{1}{\omega\left(1 + \frac{k_s}{k_p}\right)} = \frac{k_s}{k_p} \frac{T_\omega}{\tau_\varepsilon} \frac{1}{2\pi\left(1 + \frac{k_s}{k_p}\right)}, \text{ and,}$$

$$F = (k_p + k_s)\xi_m \sin (\omega t + \phi) \qquad\qquad \text{[3-32]}$$

which says, effectively, that the tissue response is virtually in phase (elastic) with the disturbance (ϕ is nearly equal to zero), and oscillating around its initial value, i.e., the elastic boundary conditions on equations [3-20] or [3-25] for $t = 0$. Once again, putting in parametric values that are being used in the sample problem under consideration, the phase angle for large oscillation frequencies can be written: $\phi = 0.1447(T_\omega/\tau_\varepsilon)$ radians, or, 8.29 $(T_\omega/\tau_\varepsilon)$ degrees. Thus, we see that the phase angle in this case varies *inversely* with f_ω, and that it will be small again when the period of the oscillation is of the same order as the relaxation time constant, or, when:

$$\frac{T_\omega}{\tau_\varepsilon} \leq 0(1),$$

which gives phase angles of the order of 8.3° or less.

Frequently, the elastic constants of viscoelastic materials are determined by high-frequency methods *because* no relaxation effects will occur ($c \rightarrow$ negligible effect) under these conditions and the strain in the material will be a rapidly alternating function of time. The elastic modulus which one measures in this high frequency "flat response" range is then termed the "unrelaxed elastic modulus", or the *dynamic modulus of elasticity*, E_{dyn}, defined by the equation:

$$E_{dyn} = \frac{\sigma_{max} - \sigma_{min}}{\alpha_{max} - \alpha_{min}} = \frac{\text{Stress Range}}{\text{Strain Range}} \qquad [3\text{-}33]$$

As was done before, the force F defined by equation [3-28] can be referred to the cross-sectional area, $A = \frac{\pi D^2}{4}$ to convert it into an engineering stress, and the deformation, ξ can be set equal to αL to express it as an engineering strain. Furthermore, since both stress and strain are considered here to vary as pure sine waves, the difference between their maximum and minimum values (i.e., their range) will simply be equal to twice their respective amplitudes. Thus, the dynamic modulus of elasticity becomes:

$$E_{dyn} = \frac{2Ck_p\xi_m}{\pi D^2}\ 4\ \frac{L}{2\xi_m} = 4\left(\frac{L}{D}\right)^2 \frac{Ck_p}{\pi L} = E_{static}(C) \qquad [3\text{-}34]$$

where E_{static} is the so-called "relaxed elastic modulus" defined earlier by equation [3-17]. Since the dynamic elastic modulus defined above is determined by high-frequency methods, one can write as before, for ω very large, $C = 1 + \dfrac{k_s}{k_p}$. Therefore, we conclude that the quantity, $1 + \dfrac{k_s}{k_p} = \dfrac{E_{\text{dynamic}}}{E_{\text{static}}}$, also provides a measure of the dynamic behavior of muscle tissue as compared to its static behavior, and that muscle appears to be stronger under dynamic loading than under static loading; this, due to the fact that more work has to be done against stronger inter- and intra-molecular bond configurations in dynamic, high-frequency situations where stress-relaxation has been effectively nulled, than in lower-frequency, viscoelastic, quasi-steady situations. With $\dfrac{k_s}{k_p} = 10$, E_{dynamic} is about an order of magnitude larger than E_{static}, which would put it in the range $10^8 - 10^9$ dynes/cm^2.

One may therefore conclude that the behavior of muscle tissue is basically elastically-dominated by k_p and E_{static} for very low (< 1 cycle per minute) frequencies; that it is essentially elastically-dominated by $k_s + k_p$ and E_{dynamic} for very high (> 15 cycles per second) frequencies; and that muscle shows viscoelastic behavior in between these two extremes -- which we might call the "Response Range", or *Bandwidth* of the viscous damper, c. That is to say, the tissue is elastic at low frequencies because it has a *great deal* of time to adjust to external disturbances; it is elastic at high frequencies for exactly the opposite reason, i.e., it has *not enough* time to adjust in a viscous sense to external disturbances.

Moreover, the low-frequency response is governed primarily by the weaker parallel spring, k_p (E_{static}), whereas, the high-frequency response is governed primarily by the stronger combination of the parallel and series springs, $k_s + k_p$ (E_{dynamic}). Taking the ratio of equation [3-32] to equation [3-29], one obtains still again (with ϕ negligibly small):

$$\frac{F_{\text{very high frequency}}}{F_{\text{very low frequency}}} = 1 + \frac{k_s}{k_p} ,$$

which is identical to the ratio given earlier for the two time constants, τ_σ and τ_ε, and, for the two elastic moduli, E_{dynamic} and E_{static}. Thus, as has already been stated twice, this ratio provides a measure of the dynamic behavior of muscle tissue as compared to its static behavior. A similar relationship may be obtained by taking the ratio of equation [3-32] to equation [3-30].

Letting $k = 1 + \dfrac{k_s}{k_p}$, one can write the magnification factor, C, as:

$$C = \sqrt{\frac{1 + (\omega\tau_\varepsilon k)^2}{1 + (\omega\tau_\varepsilon)^2}}$$

and,

$$\tan\phi = \frac{\omega\tau_\varepsilon}{1 + k(\omega\tau_\varepsilon)^2}\frac{k_s}{k_p}$$

The circular frequency for which $\omega\tau_\varepsilon = \dfrac{1}{k}$ is defined to be the *lower breakpoint*, or *lower corner* frequency of the amplitude response curve. At this frequency,

$$C = \sqrt{\frac{2k^2}{k^2 + 1}} \quad \text{and,}$$

$$\phi = \text{Arc Tan } \frac{1}{k+1}\frac{k_s}{k_p}$$

If $\dfrac{k_s}{k_p} = 10$, then $k = 11$, for which value $C = 1.4084$ and $\phi = 39.8056°$. Moreover, with $\dfrac{k_s}{c} = 15 = \dfrac{1}{\tau_\varepsilon}$, $\omega = (15/11) = 1.3636$ radians/second $= 2\pi f_\omega$, so, $f_\omega = 0.2170$ cycles/sec $= 13$ cycles per minute. Note from Figure 3-4 that the system *amplitude* response is essentially "flat" (i.e., C remains very nearly constant with decreasing frequency) for f_ω below the lower breakpoint frequency of 0.2170 cps. Thus, *this* characteristic frequency is a convenient demarcation to define the *beginning* of the major frequency-response range for the *magnification factor*. (Recall that $f_\omega = 0.015$ cps was the corresponding prominent feature of the phase angle response curve.) Defining further the *decibel*, db, as 20 times the log of C, we observe that:

(a) for ω small $(T_\omega \geq 1000\tau_t)$, $C \simeq 1$, $\phi \simeq 0°$ and 20 log C
    $= 20 \log 1 = 0$ db; and,

(b) for $\omega = 1.3636$ rad/sec, $C = 1.4084$, $\phi = 39.8°$ and $20 \log C$
$= 2.9746 \simeq 3$ db.

Thus the lower breakpoint frequency (0.2170 cps) which defines the beginning of the response range for the magnification factor, corresponds to a point where C is some 3 decibels above the value it has at the beginning of the response range for ϕ, where *phase* relationships begin to be important (i.e., when $C \simeq 1$ and $T_\omega \geq \dfrac{1000}{15} = 66\ 2/3$ seconds/cycle; $f_\omega = 0.015$ cps). In other words, the amplitude-frequency-response of the system continues to remain essentially "flat" for some three decibels past where the phase-angle-frequency-response of the system ceased to be "flat".

On the other end of the spectrum, the amplitude-frequency-response of the system becomes nearly flat again some three decibels past where the phase angle is again equal to 39.8056°. This phase angle thus defines the *upper breakpoint* frequency, which corresponds to $\omega \tau_t = 1$. That is to say, when $\omega \tau_t = 1$,

$$C = \sqrt{\frac{1 + k^2}{2}} = 7.8102$$

$20 \log C = 17.8533$ db

$$\phi = \text{Arc Tan } \frac{1}{k+1} \frac{k_s}{k_p} = 39.8056°, \text{ and}$$

$$f_\omega = 2.3873 \text{ cps}$$

and, when $C = 11$, $20 \log C = 20.8279$, so the difference between 20.8279 and 17.8533 is again 2.9746 decibels; and furthermore, for $C \simeq 11$, and $T_\omega \simeq \tau_\varepsilon = 0.067$ seconds/cycle, $f_\omega = 15$ cycles/sec, and phase angle ϕ is once more becoming negligibly small. The magnification factor and phase angle thus both have a flat frequency response from 3 decibels below the lower breakpoint frequency on down to zero cycles per second and from 3 decibels about the upper breakpoint frequency on up to an infinite number of cycles per second. This frequency *range* (from 3 db *below* 0.2170 cps to 3 db *above* 2.3873 cps) is sometimes called the *band width* of the frequency response characteristics of the system. In the case of striated skeletal muscle, the band width spans a frequency range of three decades from around 0.015 cps to about 15 cycles/sec, or 3 orders of magnitude, within which the tissue response is viscoelastic.

Finally, the *maximum* phase lead occurs when $\omega\tau_\varepsilon = \dfrac{1}{\sqrt{k}}$, at which point,

$$C = \sqrt{k} = 3.3166$$

$$\phi = \text{Arc Tan } \frac{k_s}{k_p} \frac{1}{2\sqrt{k}} = \text{Arc Sin } \frac{k-1}{k+1} = 56.4427°$$

and $f_\omega = 0.72$ cps.

****

Problem 3-6: For $k_p = 0$, show that equation [3-28] reduces to the governing response equation that describes a spring (constant k_s) and a dashpot (constant c) in series. This is a so-called Maxwell Body. What are the corresponding relationships for $Ck_p\xi_m$ and tan ϕ for a Maxwell body?

Problem 3-7: For k_s infinite (almost like a rigid body) show that equation [3-28] describes the behavior of a spring (constant k_p) and a dashpot (constant c) in parallel. This is a so-called Voigt Body. What are the corresponding relationships for $Ck_p\xi_m$ and tan ϕ for a Voigt Body?

****

Just as the low-frequency response of the model in Figure 3-1 can be characterized by the elastic modulus, E_{static}, and the high-frequency response can be defined by the elastic modulus, E_{dynamic}, the response of the system in its *band-width range* has associated with it *several* parameters that characterize viscoelastic behavior. The first of these is a quantity called the *complex elastic modulus*, E_{complex}, which, unlike the previous two, *is* a function of circular frequency, ω. The complex elastic modulus is obtained by defining the stress-strain equations for muscle in more general terms utilizing complex notation. Thus, for example, one can write, from Problem 3-5:

$$\frac{F}{A} = \sigma = \frac{4Ck_p\xi_m}{\pi D^2} e^{i(\omega t + \phi)}$$

$$\frac{\xi}{L} = \alpha = \frac{\xi_m}{L} e^{i\omega t},$$

and then define:

$$E_{complex} = \frac{\sigma}{\alpha} = \frac{4Ck_p}{\pi L} \left(\frac{L}{D}\right)^2 e^{i\phi}$$

where ϕ, the phase angle is, of course, frequency dependent, as is C. Observe that the dynamic modulus, as defined by equation [3-34] represents, the *magnitude* of the complex elastic modulus. The reciprocal of the complex elastic modulus is called the *complex compliance, J*, of the muscle tissue, so that:

$$\sigma = E_{complex}\alpha,$$
$$\alpha = J\sigma, \text{ and,} \qquad \text{[3-35]}$$
$$JE_{complex} = 1$$

The complex compliance can actually be determined from the Creep Compliance defined earlier using what is known in viscoelastic theory as a "hereditary" integral. The reader is referred to the literature for more details. Writing,

$$E_{complex} = \frac{4Ck_p}{\pi L} \left(\frac{L}{D}\right)^2 [\cos\phi + i\sin\phi] \qquad \text{[3-36]}$$

we comment further that, sometimes, the real part of equation [3-36] is used as an alternate definition of the dynamic elastic modulus (in this case, however $E_{dynamic}$ *is* frequency-dependent). More often, however, the real part is called the *storage modulus, E$_{storage}$*, and, the imaginary component of equation [3-36] is referred to as the *dynamic loss* or *viscous modulus, $E_{viscous}$*, of the material. The names, storage modulus and loss modulus, imply something to do with energy storage and energy loss. Indeed, writing:

$$\sigma = E_{complex}\alpha = (E_{storage} + iE_{viscous})\alpha,$$

and realizing that $i\alpha = \frac{\alpha}{\omega}$ for $\alpha L = \xi_m e^{i\omega t}$, one finds that the stress can be represented as an elastic (energy-storing) part dependent on strain, α, with modulus $E_{storage}$, plus a viscous (energy-dissipating) part dependent on strain-*rate*, $\dot{\alpha}$, with viscosity $(E_{viscous}/\omega) = \eta$:

$$\sigma = E_{storage}\alpha + \eta\dot{\alpha}$$

Then,

$$\tan \phi = \frac{E_{viscous}}{E_{storage}}$$

represents the ratio of the energy-dissipating characteristics of the tissue to the energy-storing nature of the material.

Note that $E_{viscous} < E_{storage}$ as long as $\phi < 45°$, but that the viscous modulus can become much larger than the storage modulus for larger values of ϕ up to 90°. In the sample case, for $\phi_{max} = 56.4427°$, $E_{viscous}$ climbs to about one and one-half times $E_{storage}$. There is an interesting moral here -- namely, that based on the rheologic and energy-dissipating characteristics of muscle, there may be some optimum frequencies at which cyclic physical exertion should be accomplished in order to maximize performance and minimize energy expenditure. For instance, in the sample case that we have been examining throughout this chapter, it would appear that energy losses for this particular muscle are maximized when it is cycled at a frequency of around 40-45 per minute, but minimized if the oscillation frequency either exceeds 15 cycles per second or is less than about 1 cycle per minute. Thus, one is led to wonder if the "natural" heart rate of around 70 beats per minute, or the "optimum" walking cadence of 80 steps per minute (see Chapter 6), or the inherent periodicities that manifest themselves in other musculoskeletal activities, might, in some sense, reflect a trade-off between energy conservation and energy dissipation, at least within the constitutive framework described above. It is certainly a point worth exploring further.

At the higher frequencies, there may also be some optimum trade-off between the viscoelastic characteristics of the tissue and its fuel-cell fatigue properties as discussed in Chapter 1. We will get back to this point in later chapters, but for now it is important to realize that findings such as these could be of great value to work physiologists, athletes, trainers, rehabilitation engineers, choreographers, dancers, and others who may be concerned with optimizing human performance.

Just as the complex elastic modulus, $E_{complex}$, has a *real* and an *imaginary* part, in the sense of equation [3-36], so, too, has the complex compliance, J, as defined by equation [3-35]. Thus, from [3-35],

$$J = \frac{\pi L}{4 C k_p} \left(\frac{D}{L} \right)^2 e^{-i\phi} = \frac{\pi L}{4 C k_p} \left(\frac{D}{L} \right)^2 [\cos \phi - i \sin \phi] \qquad [3\text{-}37]$$

The reciprocal of the dynamic modulus defined by equation [3-34] is called the *dynamic compliance*. The real part of equation [3-37] is called the *storage compliance* and the imaginary part is called the *viscous compliance*. (Incidentally, one might also define the reciprocal of the low-frequency static Young's modulus as the *static compliance*).

In a manner similar to that developed above, but relating stress to the *rate*-of-strain rather than to the strain, one can define further a *mechanical impedance function*, E_μ, such that:

$$E_\mu = \frac{\sigma}{\dot{\alpha}} = \frac{4 C k_p}{i \pi L \omega} e^{i\phi} \left(\frac{L}{D} \right)^2,$$

and a corresponding *complex viscous modulus*,

$$\omega E_\mu = \frac{4Ck_p}{i\pi L} \left(\frac{L}{D}\right)^2 [\cos\phi + i\sin\phi] \qquad [3\text{-}38]$$

Then, going through the same game of amplitude, real part, imaginary part, and reciprocals of these functions, as before, one could identify at least six, or more (up to 12) *additional* material properties that would serve to describe the mechanical behavior of the tissue. Rather than do that, however, we point out two things: First, from equations [3-36] and [3-38], we conclude that:

$$i\omega E_\mu = E_{complex} \qquad [3\text{-}39]$$

so that a knowledge of *either* the complex elastic modulus *or* the complex viscous modulus, at all frequencies, is sufficient to describe completely the viscoelastic material. And second, that *all* of the quantities, ϕ, E_{static}, $E_{dynamic}$, $E_{storage}$, $E_{viscous}$, $E_{complex}$, η, and so on can be determined from their basic definitions, which revert back to having to know only the values of k_p, k_s, c, L and D, all of which *are* either known, or, can be measured. Thus, having characterized the rheologic properties of muscle in a purely passive, i.e., unstimulated state, let us now examine the response of the tissue to situations in which $P \neq 0$, i.e., we consider now the *active* rheologic behavior of muscle.

Active Rheologic Behavior of Muscle

To examine the active rheologic behavior of muscle, consider, first, an isometric tetanic contraction, which is defined in equation [3-13] by setting $\xi = \dot{\xi} = 0$, to get:

$$\dot{F} + \frac{k_s}{c} F = \frac{k_s}{c} P = \text{constant} \qquad [3\text{-}40]$$

in the simplest case where P is assumed not to vary with time. Again, use the integrating factor $e^{(k_s/c)t}$ to integrate equation [3-40] from some initial time, $t = 0$, at which the isometric contraction is assumed to begin, to some arbitrary time, t, later. This gives the result:

$$F = P[1 - e^{-(k_s/c)t}] \qquad [3\text{-}41]$$

where $F_{t=0}$ is taken to be equal to zero. This initial condition assumes that the isometric contraction begins with the muscle at rest ($F = 0$). Otherwise, the left side of equation [3-41] would read: $F(t) - F(0^-)$, where the superscript ($-$) means, "just at the time the isometric contraction begins." In either case, one notes that at the start of the contraction, the step-force input generated by the contractile elements of the muscle is not manifest initially at the muscle tendons. This is because P must be transmitted through the viscous damping element, c, before it shows up at the tendons, and so at first, the dashpot or "shock absorber" totally dominates (dampens) the muscle response.

This is exactly the *reverse* of what was the situation when a step-input was applied to the *tendons* with $P = 0$. In the latter case, the fact that it takes *time* for the viscous damper to react caused the initial response of the muscle to be purely elastic when the input came from the "spring-side." Now, this same phenomenon causes the initial response of the muscle to be completely damped when the input originates in the dashpot loop. Thus, whereas passive step-inputs at the tendons are associated with such subsequent events as stress-relaxation and strain retardation, active step-inputs originating from the contractile elements are associated with a physical response called *stress retardation*. The latter is characterized by a progressive *increase* in F with time at the muscle tendons, rather than the *decrease* associated with stress relaxation. Thus, as the dashpot "yields" to the persistence of P with time, the contractile force is ultimately transmitted through the series and parallel spring elements to the tendons, and $F \to P$ as $t \to \infty$. This type of behavior is illustrated in Figure 3-5A for an isometric contraction.

Observe that the rate at which the active exponential transfer of load occurs is the same as the rate at which passive stress relaxation takes place. That is, the stress retardation time constant, τ_p is also given by the ratio c/k_s. Observe further, then, that experiments carried out isometrically on stimulated muscle tissue *also* provide a convenient means for determining the ratio c/k_s. In this case, a muscle is suspended between two fixed supports, stimulated to contract isometrically in a tetanic fashion, and $F(t)$ at the tendons is measured as a function of time for a very long period of time. For t large, $F(t) \simeq P$, so the value of P may be taken to be the asymptotic value of $F(t)$ measured at the tendons long after the muscle has equilibrated in its isometric state. With P thus determined and $F(t)$ known as a function of t, a regression analysis on equation [3-41] then yields the value of k_s/c as the only unknown quantity. The analysis may be simplified even further by linearizing equation [3-41], i.e.,

$$\tau_p = -\frac{t}{\ell n\left(1 - \dfrac{F}{P}\right)} \qquad\qquad \text{[3-42]}$$

It might be mentioned parenthetically that viscoelastic events such as stress retardation, and phase lag relationships (displacement lags force), are also contributing factors to the presence of a *latent period* following α-motoneuron stimulation of a motor unit. In other words, the latent period is due not only to the sequence of biochemical events that transpire following stimulation, but also to the viscoelastic physical properties of the muscle tissue itself.

The final case to be examined for the rheologic model of muscle illustrated in Figure 3-1 is that of an isotonic contraction. By definition, this is a contraction that takes place with a constant force being maintained at the muscle tendons. Therefore, one can write in equation [3-13], $\dot{F} = 0$, and $F = $ constant $= F_T$, to get:

$$\dot{\xi} + K\xi = \frac{k_s}{c(k_s + k_p)}(F_T - P) = \text{constant} \qquad\qquad \text{[3-43]}$$

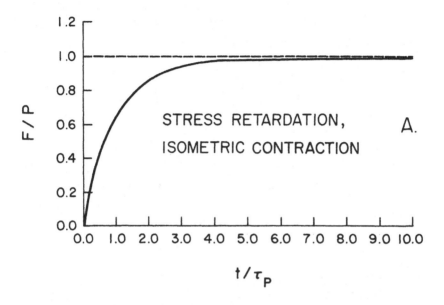

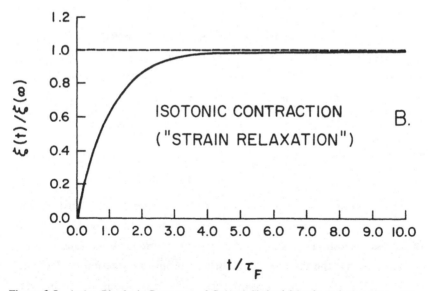

Figure 3-5 Active Rheologic Responses of Striated Skeletal Muscle to both an Isometric (showing Stress Retardation) and an Isotonic (showing Strain Relaxation) Contraction.

if P is assumed again not to vary with time. Multiplying equation [3-43] through by the integrating factor, e^{Kt}, one obtains:

$$e^{Kt}\dot{\xi} + Ke^{Kt}\xi = \frac{d}{dt}\left[\xi e^{Kt}\right] = \frac{1}{k_p}Ke^{Kt}(F_T - P)$$

$$= \frac{F_T - P}{k_p}\frac{d}{dt}\left[e^{Kt}\right]$$

[3-44]

Assuming, as was done in the case of an isometric contraction, that the isotonic contraction begins with the muscle at rest, i.e., taking ξ to be equal to zero, for simplicity, at $t = 0$, equation [3-44] can be integrated to yield:

$$\xi(t)e^{Kt} = \frac{F_T - P}{k_p}\left[e^{Kt} - 1\right],$$

or,

$$\xi(t) = \frac{F_T - P}{k_p}\left[1 - e^{-Kt}\right]$$

[3-45]

Equation [3-45] may be taken to be the mathematical description of the Period of Shortening, illustrated in Figure 1-9 of Chapter 1, for a typical isotonic muscle twitch. As $t \to \infty$, $\xi(t)$ approaches its maximum value, which is to say, the muscle has contracted as far as it will go. In the limit, $\xi(\infty) = \frac{F_T - P}{k_p}$, so,

$$\frac{\xi(t)}{\xi(\infty)} = 1 - e^{-(t/\tau_F)}$$

[3-46]

where τ_F, the isotonic twitch time constant is given by $\frac{1}{K}$. Just as the stress-retardation constant for an isometric contraction was the same as the stress-relaxation constant for a step-strain input at the tendons, so we see here that the time constant for an isotonic contraction is identical to the strain-retardation constant for a step-stress input at the muscle tendons. In keeping with the terminology describing these occurrences, one might classify the behavior defined by equation [3-46] and illustrated in Figure 3-5B as "strain relaxation", since, the muscle length as $t \to \infty$ is considerably less than its length at $t = 0$, which is exactly the opposite of what happens in the case of strain retardation, where the muscle length *increases* with time. Observe, again, that:

i) for $t = 0$, the viscous damper prevails and there is momentarily no immediate contractile response, i.e., $\xi(0) = 0$;

ii) for $t \to \infty$, the parallel spring element picks up the entire load, i.e., $(F_T - P) \to k_p\xi(\infty)$; and,

iii) for $0 < t < \infty$, $F_T < P$ since $\xi(t)$ is a *negative* quantity (i.e., $L < L_{op}$) for an isotonic contraction. This, again, illustrates the point made earlier (pages 73 and 74 in our discussion of Nubar's nonlinear theory), namely, that an *isometric* muscular contraction represents the largest force that any single muscle can actively generate at a given length. That is, equation [3-45] clearly reveals that the force manifest in the tendons, F_T, approaches the contractile force, P, only when $\xi(t) = 0$ for all t, which defines precisely an isometric contraction. In this sense, the viscoelastic theory is again consistent with the nonlinear theory in its prediction of muscular behavior.

****

Problem 3-8: From equations [3-17] and [3-36], we can define a *nondimensional* complex elastic modulus,

$$E^*_{complex} = \frac{E_{complex}}{E} = C \cos\phi + iC \sin\phi \qquad \text{[3-47]}$$

From the results of Problem 3-5, where C and ϕ are defined in terms of k_s, k_p, c, and ω, and, using the fact that $\tau_\varepsilon = \dfrac{c}{k_s}$, *show* that $E^*_{complex}$ as defined by equation [3-47] can be written as:

$$E^*_{complex} = \left\{ \left[1 + v\, \frac{\omega\tau_\varepsilon}{\omega\tau_\varepsilon + \dfrac{1}{\omega\tau_\varepsilon}} \right] + iv\, \frac{1}{\omega\tau_\varepsilon + \dfrac{1}{\omega\tau_\varepsilon}} \right\} \qquad \text{[3-48]}$$

where:

$$v = \frac{k_s}{k_p} = \frac{\tau_\sigma}{\tau_\varepsilon} - 1 = v(\tau_\varepsilon)$$

****

Referring back to Figure 1-9, suppose the period of shortening is defined as the time it takes for the muscle to achieve over 99% of its total contracted length. From equation [3-46] or Figure 3-5B, we see that this can be accomplished in five isotonic time constants, or, when $t = 5\tau_F$, at which point, $\xi(t) = 0.9933\xi(\infty)$. Since $\tau_F = \frac{1}{K}$ and $K = 1.3636$ for $\frac{k_s}{c} = 15$ and $\frac{k_s}{k_p} = 10$, one concludes that the single twitch period of shortening for this sample illustration is $t = 3.6667$ seconds. This value is incredibly high when compared with "time-to-peak" figures of 15-50 milliseconds for fast twitch muscle fibers and 60-120 milliseconds for slow twitch fibers. However, one must realize that the latter time scales are obtained for the most part by stimulating muscles which are not contracting under load, whereas values for $\frac{k_s}{c}$ quoted earlier were obtained on the basis of experiments conducted on muscle *in vivo*, under loaded conditions. (In the animal body, a muscle *never* contracts under zero load.) It may be intuitively clear (although it shall become clearer in Chapter 5) that muscular responses become much more "sluggish" the greater the load that is imposed upon them during contraction. In fact, even under *light* loads, the presence of connective tissue around the muscle, and the surrounding constraints imposed by the tissues within which the muscle is embedded, all act to retard its response time to stimulation.

These effects, of course, have not been *explicitly* identified in the model depicted in Figure 3-1 because, among other things, this model is assumed to be a mass-less system -- such that inertial terms involving $\ddot{\xi}$ do not appear in equation [3-13] -- and, the isotonic behavior of the muscle has been derived to show how a force F_T, is generated at the tendons -- but the subsequent kinematic response has been assumed to take place against *no* external resistance, R_T, or tethering effect that might act to control further the rate constant, K. In general, the mass (or equivalent mass) that a muscle has to move is *large* when compared with its (i.e., the muscle's) *own* mass. Hence, under these conditions, the internal mass of the *muscle* may be neglected relative to the mass of the *resistance*, and the force relationships for the distributed muscle model system may be developed from simple kinematical equilibrium conditions that set the *muscle* mass equal to zero. However, see Problem 3-9 and discussion that follows.

****

Figure 3-6

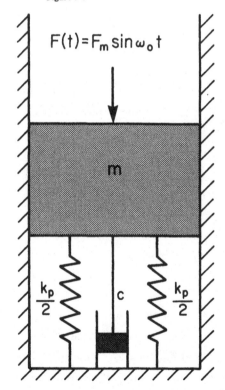

$$F(t) = F_m \sin \omega_o t$$

$$m$$

$$\frac{k_p}{2} \qquad c \qquad \frac{k_p}{2}$$

Note: All surfaces may be
        assumed to be
        frictionless

Problem 3-9: Consider the mass-spring-dashpot system shown to the left here.   If this system is driven by a periodic force of the form: $F(t) = F_m \sin \omega_o t$, derive a differential equation of motion for this system.

Obtain the steady state solution of this equation by assuming ξ to be of the form:

$$\xi = \xi_m \sin (\omega_o t - \phi)$$

and show that:

$$\tan \phi = \frac{c\omega_o}{k_p - m\omega_o^2} \quad \text{and,}$$

$$\xi_m = \frac{F_m}{\sqrt{(k_p - m\omega_o^2)^2 + (c\omega_o)^2}}$$

****

In problem 3-9, note the dependence of the results on the mass, m, of the system. In particular, observe that the phase lag goes to zero *not only* if $c = 0$ (no damping), $\omega_o \to 0$ (very slow oscillations), $\omega_o \to \infty$ (very fast oscillations), or $k_p \to \infty$ (very stiff spring), but, *also if* $m \to \infty$ (very large mass). Moreover, the magnification factor, ξ_m, *also* depends on mass, m, going to zero as $m \to \infty$ (all other variables held constant). This is merely an expression of the *inertial* properties of the system -- namely, that if a system has a great deal of mass, it cannot be easily moved, *especially* at high frequencies which involve rapidly changing its *direction* of motion as well. If we relate this back to Figure 3-4, we would find that for a *real* muscle containing *mass* as well as viscoelastic properties, the plateau reached by the magnification factor, C, at high frequencies would not go on forever, as implied by the simple theory. Rather, at super high frequencies the inertial properties of the tissue would start to predominate, and, for second-order systems, we would find still *another* breakpoint frequency beyond which C would again start declining asymptotically towards zero (as does ϕ). For *isolated* muscle preparations, the mass of the tissue is relatively small and so may be effectively neglected in studying the behavior of the tissue even up to rather high frequencies ($m \to 0$ in problem 3-9, which reduces it to a simple first-order Voigt Model). In other words, the next breakpoint frequency for *isolated* muscle preparations is high enough so that the frequency response characteristics of the magnification factor may be considered to be essentially "flat" for all practical purposes.

This is not true, however, in real life -- where muscles must contract against significant resisting masses and constraining forces. From the equations of problem 3-9, we see that reducing m *increases* the denominator in the expressions for *both* $\tan \phi$ and ξ_m, thereby decreasing their values. This is also accomplished by reducing the value of c in the phase angle relationship, which, in turn, is related to the time-constant associated with the response characteristics of the system (see, for example, equations [3-31] and [3-32]). Thus, take away from a *real* model the effects of mass, external constraints, resisting loads, and so on ... and it has effects similar to reducing the viscous properties of the muscle tissue, thus lowering the corresponding dashpot constant, c, which raises the value of K, thereby decreasing τ_F and allowing the tissue to respond a great deal faster.

How *much* faster? Well, suppose that the period of shortening is, on the average, 20 milliseconds for fast twitch muscle fibers and 80 milliseconds for slow twitch fibers. Then, for fast twitch fibers, $t = 0.020 = 5\tau_F = \dfrac{5}{K}$, $K = 250$; and, for slow twitch fibers, $t = 0.080$, $K = \dfrac{k_s/c}{1 + k_s/k_p} = 62.5$. Thus, with $\dfrac{k_s}{k_p} = 10$, we find that the ratio $\dfrac{k_s}{c}$ jumps from the earlier quoted "loaded" range of 2 to 26 sec^{-1} to the hypothetically-calculated "no-load" range of 688 to 2750 sec^{-1}. With k_s assumed to remain constant, this two-order-of-magnitude increase in $\dfrac{k_s}{c}$ corresponds to a two-order-of-magnitude *decrease* in c, a similar decrease in τ_F (to around 10^{-3} sec), and a concomitant decrease in the "time-to-peak" characteristics of the muscle. The result is that *isolated* muscle preparations show viscous properties that are closer to Confectioner's Glucose (see Table 3-I) than to molten lava or glass, and they show rise times that are correspondingly two or more orders of magnitude faster than those measured in the actual human body.

While inertial and constraint effects are not accounted for explicitly in the model, they can be taken into account *implicitly* by measuring the variables k_s, k_p and c under *in vivo*, real-life loaded conditions, so that the model is "phenomenologically" *forced* to describe actual physical events realistically. In other words, one can choose values for the system parameters such that it is fair to say that in real life, under actual loaded conditions the tissue "acts" as though it were composed of the spring-dashpot-contractile-element systems having representative moduli in the ranges given. In fact, one can go even further, to develop a *network* of Kelvin elements assembled into interconnecting functional blocks that, together, make up the mechanical equivalent of the skeletal muscle (Fung, 1972, Hatze, 1981). Such Kelvin networks introduce the concept of a *Relaxation Time Spectrum.*

The Relaxation Time Spectrum

For the Kelvin model depicted in Figure 3-1, Figure 3-4 reveals a continuous dependence of phase angle ϕ (hence internal damping) on frequency ω (c.f., Problem 3-5). But in real life, some well-known experimental findings (see, for example, Fung, 1972) suggest that internal friction (hysteresis loops such as are shown in Figure 3-3) is *insensitive* to frequency ω -- at least within a certain range of frequency within physiologic limits. That is to say, the well-defined *peak* for ϕ in Figure 3-4 is actually more like a *plateau* in real life. To "spread out" the curve and introduce a range of frequency within which damping "plateaus" with respect to ω, one can superimpose a large number of Kelvin models in series upon one another, and introduce the concept of a *continuous spectrum of relaxation times* into our formulation.

To implement this idea, let us first rewrite equation [3-48] in terms of the *dynamic* elastic modulus defined by equation [3-34], rather than the *static* elastic modulus defined by equation [3-17], i.e., let:

$$E^*_{\text{complex}} = \frac{E_{\text{complex}}}{E} = \frac{E_{\text{complex}}}{E_{\text{dynamic}}} \times \frac{E_{\text{dynamic}}}{E_{\text{static}}} \qquad \text{[3-49]}$$

where, following the reasoning developed for equation [3-32], and the discussion relevant to equation [3-34], we have, for large but finite ω,

$$\frac{E_{\text{dynamic}}}{E_{\text{static}}} = C = 1 + \frac{k_s}{k_p} = 1 + v(\tau_\varepsilon) \qquad \text{[3-50]}$$

Then, substituting equations [3-49] and [3-50] into equation [3-48], we have:

$$\frac{E_{\text{complex}}}{E_{\text{dynamic}}} = \frac{E^*_{\text{complex}}}{1 + v}$$

$$= \frac{1}{1 + v} \left\{ \left[1 + v \frac{\omega\tau_\varepsilon}{\omega\tau_\varepsilon + \frac{1}{\omega\tau_\varepsilon}} \right] + iv \frac{1}{\omega\tau_\varepsilon + \frac{1}{\omega\tau_\varepsilon}} \right\} \qquad \text{[3-51]}$$

In order to extend equation [3-51] to a *network* of Kelvin elements combined in series, we let the *discrete* variable τ_ε be replaced by a *continuous* variable τ^*, and $v(\tau_\varepsilon)$ be a function of τ^*. For such a system with a *continuous relaxation time spectrum*, we may then define the following nondimensionalized complex modulus:

$$\frac{E_{complex}}{E_{dynamic}}(\omega) = \frac{1}{1 + \int_0^\infty v(\tau^*)d\tau^*} \left\{ 1 + \int_0^\infty v(\tau^*) \frac{\omega\tau^*}{\omega\tau^* + \frac{1}{\omega\tau^*}} d\tau^* \right.$$

$$\left. + \int_0^\infty iv(\tau^*) \frac{d\tau^*}{\omega\tau^* + \frac{1}{\omega\tau^*}} \right\}$$

[3-52]

The problem, then, is to find a particular form for the function $v(\tau^*)$ which will make the nondimensional complex modulus defined by equation [3-52] nearly constant for a frequency band within the physiologic range. One such form suggested (Fung, 1972) is:

$$v(\tau^*) = \frac{c^*}{\tau^*} \text{ for } \tau_1^* \le \tau^* \le \tau_2^*$$

$$= 0 \text{ for } \tau^* < \tau_1^* \text{ and}$$

$$\tau^* > \tau_2^*$$

[3-53]

****

Problem 3-10: Substitute equation [3-53] into equation [3-52] and integrate to verify that:

$$\frac{E_{complex}}{E_{dynamic}}(\omega) = \frac{1}{1 + c^* \ell n \frac{\tau_2^*}{\tau_1^*}} \left\{ 1 + \frac{c^*}{2} \left[\ell n \frac{1 + \omega^2\tau_2^{*2}}{1 + \omega^2\tau_1^{*2}} \right] \right.$$

$$\left. + ic^* [\tan^{-1}(\omega\tau_2^*) - \tan^{-1}(\omega\tau_1^*)] \right\}$$

[3-54]

We are left, then, with three parameters, c^*, τ_1^*, and τ_2^*, to determine from experimental data. For *arbitrary* $c^* = 1$, $\tau_1^* = 10^{-2}$ and $\tau_2^* = 10^2$, plot separately the *stiffness* (real part of equation [3-54]) and the *damping* (imaginary part of equation [3-54]) as functions of the common logarithm of the circular frequency ω, for $10^{-3} \leq \omega \leq 10^3$ (i.e., six decades) -- and note the rather constant damping for $\dfrac{1}{\tau_2{}^*} \leq \omega \leq \dfrac{1}{\tau_1{}^*}$.

****

The form of equation [3-53] is by no means unique, and several others have been suggested (Fung, 1972, and Decraemer, et al., 1980b). Suffice it to say, however, that phenomenological models such as have been developed in this chapter -- which yield reasonably flat and broad, continuous spectra that serve to render hysteresis less sensitive to frequency -- have been found to be very useful for defining the constitutive mechanical behavior of striated skeletal muscle. Bearing this in mind, we shall go on in Chapter 5 to look at the mechanics and energetics of muscular contraction in terms of constitutive relationships such as are developed in Chapters 2, 3, and 4.

****

Problem 3-11: a) The four-element viscoelastic model of striated skeletal muscle is strictly linear. How could this model take into account mathematically the *nonlinear* behavior of muscle tissue?

b) Write an equation that might be used based on Figure 3-1 to formulate a *nonlinear, viscoelastic* theory for muscular contraction.

****

References for Chapter 3

See at end of Chapter 4.

Chapter 4

A Nonlinear, Viscoelastic, Stochastic Structural Constitutive Model for Striated Skeletal Muscle

Introduction

As was pointed out in Chapter 2, Nubar's nonlinear theory for muscular contraction accurately predicts such phenomena as passive "strain hardening" and active "compensation" and "decompensation;" but, it does not include any time-dependent or viscous behavior. In terms of the events depicted in Figure 3-4, then, one could surmise that this nonlinear model would only be valid when the time-varying nature of the tissue loading is below 0.015 hertz ($\tau_\varepsilon/T_\omega \leq 0(10^{-3})$), or above 15 hertz ($T_\omega/\tau_\varepsilon \leq 0(1)$) -- i.e., where the tissue response characteristics are essentially "flat" with respect to time. Thus, depending on the relaxation time constant (which is on the order of 0.01 to 0.10 seconds) for muscle, the tissue has a frequency bandwidth of around three decades within which its behavior is significantly time-dependent, and within which one cannot neglect transient viscoelastic effects.

On the other hand, whereas Bahler's viscoelastic theory for muscular contraction accurately predicts such phenomena as passive stress-relaxation, strain retardation (creep) and frequency-dependent phase shifts, and, active "stress-retardation" and "strain-relaxation," it does not take into account any nonlinear behavior. In terms of the events depicted in Figure 2-2, then, it has been found that this viscoelastic model is only valid for muscle lengths of less than 120 percent of the resting length (i.e., $\alpha \leq 0.20$), beyond which point muscle behavior becomes significantly nonlinear, and this nonlinearity cannot be neglected.

Formulation of a Stochastic Constitutive Model

In an attempt to reconcile the limitations of nonlinear theory in the frequency-response bandwidth of muscle tissue, with the limitations of viscoelastic linear theory for large tissue deformation, Decraemer, et al., (1980a and 1980b) developed a nonlinear, viscoelastic model based on the internal structure of soft biological tissue -- viewed as a fiber-reinforced composite material. These investigators develop their model from a *statistical* point of view, wherein a *large number*, N_∞, of fibers -- having individual *initial* (not necessarily "resting") lengths $\ell_i{}^*$ (i = initial) and a common (i.e., the *same*) average cross-sectional area, a -- are assumed to be embedded in a gelatin-like liquid, and to have lengths normally distributed around some mean initial value, ℓ, which has a standard deviation, ρ. The fibers are considered to comprise a total muscle specimen which is deformed ("stretched") from an initial length, L, to some final length, $L_f = L + \Delta L$.

Those muscle fibers for which $\ell_i{}^* > L_f$ (i.e., the "initial" length of the fiber is actually *larger* than the "final" length of the extended total muscle) are assumed to be in a "slack" state. That is to say, they are not load-bearing and the force necessary to further "unfold" them is considered to be negligible. Those muscle fibers for which $\ell_i{}^* < L_f$ (i.e., the fibers which are actually stretched during the extension deformation) are assumed to be the actual load-bearing elements resisting deformation and generating a passive tension.

Now, from the statistical theory for normally-distributed data, if N_∞ samples of such data, having variable values (lengths) $\ell_i{}^*$, are normally distributed around a mean value, ℓ, having a standard deviation, ρ, then the *probability density function* of this distribution is defined by:

$$p(\ell_i^*) = \frac{1}{\rho\sqrt{2\pi}} e^{-\frac{(\ell_i^* - \ell)^2}{2\rho^2}}$$ [4-1]

Equation [4-1] for normally-distributed data gives the *probability* of finding a muscle fiber of initial length ℓ_i^* (ℓ_i^* being *given*, but *variable*) within the population N_∞. Thus,

$$\int_{-\infty}^{+\infty} p(\ell_i^*)d\ell_i^* = 1,$$

i.e., the probability is 100 percent that ℓ_i^* will lie embedded somewhere within the muscle, or, will be within the population N_∞. Going one step further, then, for a *given* value of ℓ_i^* the *number* of muscle fibers in the total population N_∞ (i.e., in the muscle as a whole) which will *have* the instantaneous length ℓ_i^* at any given time, will be equation [4-1] times N_∞, i.e.,

$$n(\ell_i^*) = \frac{N_\infty}{\rho\sqrt{2\pi}} e^{-\frac{(\ell_i^* - \ell)^2}{2\rho^2}}$$ [4-2]

These fibers will be extended by an amount $L_f - \ell_i^*$, assuming (as do Decraemer, et al.) that $\ell_i^* < L_f$ and that all fibers of such initial length are ultimately stretched to a final length L_f. Thus, the *strain* in the group of fibers identified in equation [4-2], can be written as:

$$\varepsilon(\ell_i^*) = \frac{L_f - \ell_i^*}{\ell_i^*}$$ [4-3]

As a first approximation, Decraemer, et al., (1980a) allow each muscle fiber to be purely elastic, having Young's Modulus E_D, so that the force per unit cross-sectional area (i.e., stress) in *each* of the fibers having given length ℓ_i^* can be expressed in the Hookean sense as,

$$\sigma(\ell_i^*) = E_D \varepsilon(\ell_i^*) = E_D \frac{L_f - \ell_i^*}{\ell_i^*}, \qquad [4\text{-}4]$$

and, the corresponding *force per group* of fibers having given length ℓ_i^*, all having the same cross-sectional area, a, is:

$$f(\ell_i^*) = a E_D \left[\frac{L_f - \ell_i^*}{\ell_i^*} \right] \frac{N_\infty}{\rho \sqrt{2\pi}} e^{-\frac{(\ell_i^* - \ell)^2}{2\rho^2}} \qquad [4\text{-}5]$$

Finally, if one assumes a continuous distribution of fibers existing at load-bearing lengths $\ell_i^* < L_f$, then one can integrate equation [4-5] across all such fibers to get the total force, $F(L_f)$, needed to *hold* the muscle specimen at length L_f, i.e.,

$$F(L_f) = \int_L^{L_f} a E_D \left[\frac{L_f - \ell_i^*}{\ell_i^*} \right] \frac{N_\infty}{\rho \sqrt{2\pi}} e^{-\frac{(\ell_i^* - \ell)^2}{2\rho^2}} d\ell_i^* \qquad [4\text{-}6]$$

In their second approximation, Decraemer, et al., (1980b) relax the assumption that each muscle fiber is purely elastic, and allow the existence of internal frictional forces between fibers, or between the fibers and the material in which they are embedded. This introduces into the stochastic model a degree of damping which is accounted for by assuming that the fibers all have identical *linear* (still), but *viscoelastic* properties described by the relaxation function, $G(t)$, which essentially takes over the role of the elastic modulus E_D in the purely Hookean constitutive equation [4-4], in which equation strain, $\varepsilon(\ell_i^*)$ is now also replaced by strain *rate*, $\dot{\varepsilon}(\ell_i^*)$.

As was discussed at some length in Chapter 3, many of the behavioral characteristics of viscoelastic materials may be determined from their responses to step-strain and step-stress inputs -- from which stress relaxation moduli (Problem 3-1) and creep compliances (Problem 3-3), respectively, may be defined; and, from their responses to harmonic strain oscillation inputs -- from which may be defined complex moduli (equation

[3-36]) and complex compliances (equation [3-37]); all of which functions may be expressed in terms of one another because they all relate, ultimately, to the same physical phenomena (c.f., Chapter 3). Indeed, knowing either one of the single-step response functions, $G(t) = L\sigma(t)/\xi_o = \mathscr{R}(t)$, or, $\mathfrak{C}(t) = \xi(t)/L\sigma_o$, allows one to predict the viscoelastic material response to *any* input disturbance within the linear range in which stresses proportional to (shear strain)^3 and strains proportional to (shear stress)^3 can be neglected (Pipkin, 1972). This is because of the linear *Principle of Superposition*, which goes something like this:

Suppose at some specifically given instant of time, t_o, a muscle which had an *initial* length, L, is in equilibrium at an *actual* length, $L_f(t_o)$. Suppose further that at precisely this instant in time, this muscle of length $L_f(t_o)$ is subjected to a *sudden* increase in length (i.e., a "step-strain" input) given by $\Delta L_f(t_o)$. Written in terms of strain, the *fibers* of this muscle, which, at $t = t_o^-$ (i.e., just "prior" to the application of $\Delta L_f(t_o)$), existed at an engineering strain given by $\dfrac{L_f(t_o) - \ell_i{}^*}{\ell_i{}^*}$, experience, at $t = t_o$, a *change* in strain given by:

$$\Delta\left[\frac{L_f(t_o) - \ell_i{}^*}{\ell_i{}^*} \right].$$

Note that fibers with $\ell_i{}^* > L_f(t_o) + \Delta L_f(t_o)$ will be somewhat unfolded, but not yet stretched by this sudden small deformation, and recall that it is being assumed that the small force required to lengthen these non-load-bearing fibers is negligible. Thus, using equation [4-6] modified as described above to account for viscoelasticity, we can write, at the *instant* t_o, the force response:

$$\Delta F(t_o) = G(t_o)\int_{\ell_i{}^* = L}^{\ell_i{}^* = L_f(t_o)} \Delta\left[\frac{L_f(t_o) - \ell_i{}^*}{\ell_i{}^*} \right] \frac{N_\infty}{\rho\sqrt{2\pi}}\, e^{-\frac{(\ell_i{}^* - \ell)^2}{2\rho^2}}\, d\ell_i{}^* \quad \textbf{[4-7]}$$

Note, again, in equation [4-7] that $G(t_o)$ replaces aE_D in equation [4-6], and may be taken out of the integral sign because the integration is on ℓ_i^* rather than on time. Now, in accordance with considerations discussed in Chapter 3, the step-input defined by equation [4-7] will be accompanied by a stress-response that progressively "relaxes" with time (c.f., Figure 3-2A). Thus, for $t > t_o$, the force $\Delta F(t_o)$ -- equation [4-7] -- due to the sudden length increase $\Delta L_f(t_o)$ -- in all muscle fibers with initial length $\ell_i^* \leq L_f$ -- will have *relaxed* to:

$$\Delta F(t, t_o) = G(t - t_o) \int_{\ell_i^* = L}^{\ell_i^* = L_f(t_o)} \Delta \left[\frac{L_f(t_o) - \ell_i^*}{\ell_i^*} \right] \times \frac{N_\infty}{\rho\sqrt{2\pi}} e^{-\frac{(\ell_i^* - \ell)^2}{2\rho^2}} d\ell_i^* \qquad \text{[4-8]}$$

Compared with equation [4-7], equation [4-8] amounts to saying that the tissue response is "time-translation-invariant" (Pipkin, 1972). Let the integral on the right side of equation [4-8] be designated by ΔY_o, so that we may write more simply,

$$\Delta F(t, t_o) = G(t - t_o)\Delta Y_o \qquad \text{[4-9]}$$

Next, consider the stress response to a *two-step history*, i.e., to a step-strain input administered at time t_o, followed by a *second* step-strain input administered at a later time $t_1 > t_o$. Since the response of the material is still considered to be step-wise linear, for small steps, these two inputs, $\Delta L_f(t_o)$, and $\Delta L_f(t_1)$, administered a time interval $\Delta t = t_1 - t_o$ apart, will actually super-impose, such that the *net* stress will be just the *sum* of the individual stress responses corresponding to *each* strain taken separately. Thus, from equation [4-9], we can write:

$$\Delta F(t, t_o, t_1) = G(t - t_o)\Delta Y_o + G(t - t_1)\Delta Y_1 \qquad \text{[4-10]}$$

Coupling effects that depend on *both* ΔY_o and ΔY_1 *jointly* (i.e., on products or powers of these quantities) may occur *physically*, but in the *mathematics* they can only occur in higher-order, nonlinear approximations such as those we will examine later. Thus, carrying this reasoning still one step further, the same arguments that led to the development of equation [4-10] would apply equally well to deformation histories with an *arbitrary* number of discrete step-strain inputs, $\Delta L_f(t_j)$ $j = 0, 1, 2, \ldots$, so that we could generalize this response by writing:

$$F(t) = \sum_j G(t - t_j) \Delta Y_j \qquad [4\text{-}11]$$

Now, the idea is that we can approximate any physically realizable continuous strain history by a corresponding *step* history that involves an arbitrarily large number (depending on the degree of accuracy desired) of arbitrarily small steps. Assuming that the response of the material is such that when two strain histories are close together, so are the stress histories, i.e., the stress corresponding to any given strain history is "nearly" the same as the stress for a close-by (in the "neighborhood") step history, we may pass to the limit in the sum of equation [4-11], to obtain the integral:

$$F(t) = \int G(t - t^*) dY(t^*) = N_\infty \int_{-\infty}^{t} G(t - t^*) \frac{dL_f(t^*)}{dt^*}$$
$$\times \int_{\ell_i^* = L}^{\ell_i^* = L_f(t^*)} \frac{1}{\rho \ell_i^* \sqrt{2\pi}} e^{-\frac{(\ell_i^* - \ell)^2}{2\rho^2}} d\ell_i^* \, dt^* \qquad [4\text{-}12]$$

where: (a) Equation [4-12], which is valid for $t \geq t^*$, is the integrated form of equation [4-8]; (b) $\dfrac{d}{dt^*}\left[\dfrac{L_f(t^*) - \ell_i^*}{\ell_i^*} \right] = \dfrac{1}{\ell_i^*} \dfrac{dL_f(t^*)}{dt^*}$, since ℓ_i^* is assumed not to depend on t^*; (c) the lower limit on t^* is taken to be $-\infty$ in order to be "non-committal" about when the loading began -- although in practice we usually restrict attention to histories with $\Delta L_f = 0$ for all times prior to some starting time; and, (d) the upper limit on t^* takes us up to the "current" time t, where t^*, or, more accurately, $t - t^*$ is a "history of deformation" variable. Note that $G(t - t^*)$ is zero for $t < t^*$ (i.e., there is no "response" prior to the beginning of loading);

$G(t - t^*) = G(0)$ right at the beginning of loading (when $t = t^*$); and, $G(t - t^*)$ is an arbitrary function of the time history parameter, $t - t^*$, for $t > t^*$.

Decraemer, et al. (1980b) now define the function:

$$F^e(t^*) = \frac{N_\infty G(0)}{\rho\sqrt{2\pi}} \int_L^{L_f(t^*)} \frac{L_f(t^*) - \ell_i^*}{\ell_i^*} e^{-\frac{(\ell_i^* - \ell)^2}{2\rho^2}} d\ell_i^*, \qquad [4\text{-}13]$$

which is the viscoelastic equivalent of equation [4-6] in the purely elastic model, and defines the state of the tissue at the start of loading ($t = t^*$).

****

Problem 4-1: Let $F(\ell, t)$ be continuous and have a continuous derivative $\frac{\partial F}{\partial t}$ in a domain of the $\ell - t$ plane which includes the rectangle, $L \leq \ell \leq L_f$, $t_1 \leq t \leq t_2$. Then, for $t_1 < t < t_2$, prove Leibnitz's formula for the derivative of an integral, i.e., that differentiation and integration can be interchanged:

$$\frac{d}{dt} \int_L^{L_f} F(\ell, t) d\ell = \int_L^{L_f} \frac{\partial F}{\partial t}(\ell, t) d\ell \qquad [4\text{-}14]$$

****

Applying Leibnitz's formula [4-14] to the derivative of equation [4-13], one can write:

$$\frac{dF^e(t^*)}{dt^*} = \frac{N_\infty G(0)}{\rho\sqrt{2\pi}} \int_L^{L_f(t^*)} \frac{1}{\ell_i^*} \frac{dL_f(t^*)}{dt^*} e^{-\frac{(\ell_i^* - \ell)^2}{2\rho^2}} d\ell_i^* \qquad [4\text{-}15]$$

and, substituting equation [4-15] into equation [4-12], bearing in mind that $L_f(t^*)$ is not a function of ℓ_i^*, nor are $G(t - t^*)$ and $G(0)$, we get:

$$F(t) = \int_{-\infty}^t \frac{G(t - t^*)}{G(0)} \frac{dF^e[L_f(t^*)]}{dt^*} dt^* \qquad [4\text{-}16]$$

Let $G_r(t - t^*) = \dfrac{G(t - t^*)}{G(0)}$, and divide equation [4-16] by the cross-sectional area, A, of the muscle at rest to arrive at the following constitutive equation expressed in terms of Lagrangian stress, σ, and strain, α:

$$\sigma(t) = \int_{-\infty}^{t} G_r(t - t^*) \frac{d\sigma^e[\alpha(t^*)]}{dt^*}\, dt^* \qquad [4\text{-}17]$$

Several things to observe: First, equation [4-17] here corresponds to Nubar's equation [2-22] in the purely nonlinear model, and Bahler's equation [3-13] in the purely viscoelastic model -- except that the Decraemer model does *not* take into account *active* (i.e., stimulated) muscle behavior (i.e., *excitability*). Second, the function $\sigma^e = \dfrac{F^e}{A}$ describes the *instantaneous, immediate* $(t = t^*)$ stress response of the tissue -- which, for reasons discussed in Chapter 3, is purely elastic (hence the index "e"). This response is then modulated in a relaxation sense by the time function G_r (with $G_r(0) = 1$), which is called the *Reduced Relaxation Function* that describes the relative variation of the stress following a step variation in strain (c.f., Chapter 3).

From the definition of the Relaxation Modulus, $\mathcal{R}$ (Problem 3-1), i.e.,

$$\mathcal{R}(t) = E_{static}F^*(t) = \frac{E_{static}}{E_{dynamic}} E_{dynamic}F^*(t)$$

$$= \frac{1}{1 + v(\tau_\varepsilon)} E_{dynamic}\left\{1 + v(\tau_\varepsilon)e^{-\frac{t}{\tau_\varepsilon}}\right\} \qquad [4\text{-}18]$$

(c.f., equations [3-17], [3-23], [3-50], and Problem 3-8), we can write, more generally,

$$\frac{\mathcal{R}(t - t^*)}{E_{dynamic}} = \frac{1}{1 + v(\tau_\varepsilon)}\left\{1 + v(\tau_\varepsilon)e^{-\frac{t - t^*}{\tau_\varepsilon}}\right\}$$

$$\times H(t - t^*) = G_r(t - t^*), \qquad [4\text{-}19]$$

where $H(t - t^*)$ defines the Heaviside Function, which is zero for $t < t^*$ (before the onset of loading) and unity for $t \geq t^*$. Following the reasoning developed in the Section of Chapter 3 entitled, *The Relaxation Time Spectrum*, we can then extend equation [4-19] to a *network* of Kelvin Models by writing:

$$G_r(t - t^*) = \left[1 + \int_0^\infty v(\tau^*) e^{-\frac{t - t^*}{\tau^*}} d\tau^* \right]$$
$$\times \left[\frac{1}{1 + \int_0^\infty v(\tau^*) d\tau^*} \right] \qquad \text{[4-20]}$$

(c.f., equation [3-52]).

Third, when the viscoelastic response given by equations [4-17] and [4-20] involves *harmonic* strain oscillation inputs, the reduced relaxation function, G_r -- as does the complex modulus of elasticity, $E_{complex}$ (c.f., Chapter 3) -- *also* becomes a complex modulus which depends on ω, which has a "storage" and a "loss" part, and which can be written as:

$$G_{complex}^r(\omega) = G_r{}'(\omega) + iG_r{}''(\omega) \qquad \text{[4-21]}$$

where $G_r{}'$ is the storage part of the complex reduced relaxation function, and $G_r{}''$ is the loss part. Details of the determination of $G_r{}'(\omega)$ and $G_r{}''(\omega)$, based on a Fourier series expansion of σ^e and σ for large t, i.e., in the steady-state condition, and, utilizing equations [4-17] and [4-20], may be found in the work of Decraemer, et al., (1980b), where it is shown that:

$$G_r{}'(\omega) = \frac{\sigma_1(\alpha, \omega)}{\sigma_1^e(\alpha)} \cos \phi_1(\alpha, \omega), \quad \text{and,}$$
$$\qquad \qquad \qquad \qquad \qquad \qquad \text{[4-22]}$$
$$G_r{}''(\omega) = \frac{\sigma_1(\alpha, \omega)}{\sigma_1^e(\alpha)} \sin \phi_1(\alpha, \omega),$$

where: $\sigma_1(\alpha, \omega)$ and $\phi_1(\alpha, \omega)$ are, respectively, the amplitude and phase angle of the fundamental term in the expansion of $\sigma(t) = \sigma[\alpha(t), \omega]$, and

$\sigma_1{}^e (\alpha)$ is the amplitude of the fundamental term in the expansion of σ^e ($\phi_1{}^e = 0$ because σ^e represents a conservative, purely elastic relation).

Finally, to introduce nonlinearities between σ and α, we may let the relaxation function depend on *both* t and α, rather than t alone. As a first approximation, then, we may further write $G(\alpha, t)$ as a product of some function of α only, and some (yet-to-be-determined) function of t only. That is, we may postulate a separation of variables approach (Fung, 1972) that lets the generalized relaxation function introduced earlier be written as:

$$G(\alpha, t) = G_r(t - t^*)\sigma^e(\alpha), \quad G_r(0) = 1 \qquad \text{[4-23]}$$

in which, again, the normalized function of time only, i.e., $G_r(t - t^*)$ is called the *reduced relaxation function*, and the function $\sigma^e(\alpha)$ of α alone is called the *elastic response function*. The elastic response function plays the role assumed by the strain α in the conventional theory of viscoelasticity (Fung, 1972), and the separation-of-variables scheme seems to be a pretty good approximation for α up to about 0.30 (Decraemer, et al., 1980b).

Fung (1972) also shows that (c.f., equation [4-19]):

$$G_r(t - t^*) = \frac{\tau_\varepsilon}{\tau_\sigma} \left\{ 1 + \left[\frac{\tau_\sigma}{\tau_\varepsilon} - 1 \right] e^{-\frac{t - t^*}{\tau_\varepsilon}} \right\} H(t - t^*) \qquad \text{[4-24]}$$

where, again, $H(t - t^*)$ is the "Heaviside Function" designating a unit step increase in stress, i.e., $H(t - t^*) = 0$ for $t < t^*$, $(t - t^* < 0)$, and $H(t - t^*) = 1$ for $t \geq t^*$, $(t - t^* \geq 0)$; $G_r(0) = 1$; and $G_r(\infty) = \frac{\tau_\varepsilon}{\tau_\sigma} =$ the "residual", i.e., the "fraction" of the elastic response that is "left" in the tissue specimen after a "long" $(t \to \infty)$ relaxation. The time constants τ_ε and τ_σ are identical to those defined in Chapter 3, and equation [4-24] is an analog to equation [3-23]. Fung further goes on to present data for the mesentery of a rabbit which suggest that $0.7 \leq G_r(t - t^*) \leq 1$. (Note that in the *human* example considered throughout Chapter 3,

$0.09 \leq G_r(t - t^*) \leq 1$). Moreover, $G_r(t - t^*)$ is a monotonously decreasing function.

As for the elastic response function, i.e., the stress $(k_p + k_s)(\xi_o/A)$ instantaneously generated in the tissue when a step function of stretching ξ_o is imposed on the specimen, Fung points out that, "strict laboratory measurement of $\sigma^e(\alpha)$ according to this definition is difficult, because at an infinite rate of loading, transient stress waves will be bouncing back and forth in the specimen and a recording of the stress response will be confused by these elastic waves." However, since the stress response in a loading process seems to be relatively *insensitive* to the *rate* of loading over a wide range (see Chapter 3), $\sigma^e(\alpha)$ may be *approximated* by the tensile stress response in a loading experiment with a sufficiently *high* (but not infinite) rate of loading. From such experiments, it is found that,

$$\sigma^e(\alpha) \simeq \sigma(t_o),$$

where t_o is *small* (defined such that $t_o \left| \dfrac{\partial G}{\partial t^*} \right| << 1$), but finite, and $\sigma^e(\alpha)$ is defined by dividing equation [4-13] by muscle cross-sectional area, A.

****

Problem 4-2: From equation [4-13] we conclude that $F^e(t^*)$ is a function of L and $L_f(t^*)$ -- or -- in terms of the corresponding viscoelastic model illustrated in Figure 3-1, L, x_d, and x_s. Furthermore, the instantaneous stress generated in the tissue at the start of loading was also shown in Chapter 3 to be equal to $\dfrac{\xi_o(k_p + k_s)}{A}$ (c.f., equation [3-22]), with x_d essentially out of the picture (i.e., fixed and constant) in a step-strain input at $t = t^*$. Thus, to include nonlinear effects in the viscoelastic model of Figure 3-1, one might begin by letting:

$$\begin{aligned} k_s &= k_s(x_s) = k_s[x_s(t)], \text{ and,} \\ k_p &= k_p(L) = k_p[L(t)]. \end{aligned} \qquad \text{[4-25]}$$

Letting k_s and k_p be functions of x_s and L, respectively, and hence, of time, as given by equation [4-25], and, following the same line of reasoning developed in the Introductory section of Chapter 3 (i.e., equations [3-1] to [3-13], *derive* a corresponding *nonlinear* form of equation [3-13] and *show* that your solution *reduces* to equation [3-13] if, indeed, k_s and k_p *are* constant, i.e., if the springs are linear, rather than nonlinear.

****

Problem 4-3: In the nonlinear equation you derived as a solution to Problem 4-2, let $P = 0$ (i.e., consider only the passive behavior of the tissue), and let $\dot{F} = \dot{\xi} = 0$ (i.e., examine only equilibrium states of the muscle). Then, convert the result to corresponding stress, σ, as a function of strain, α. Next, equate *this* result to that for *Nubar's* nonlinear equation [2-22], solved in terms of α for the passive case for $q_l = 0$. From these considerations, *derive* an equation for $\dfrac{k_p}{L}(\alpha)$ to order α^2 and *plot* $\dfrac{k_p}{L}$ vs. α for $0 \le \alpha \le 0.9$ and corresponding values for $r_1, r_2, r_3, E_1, E_2, E_3,$ and $\dfrac{D}{L}$ given in Chapter 2.

****

The Separation of Variables Formulation of Hatze

Since the Decraemer, et al., model is purely passive, i.e., does not take into account tissue excitability, and, since the subsequent quantitative results that these authors obtain are from experiments carried out on the human tympanic membrane, there is nothing further to be gained from examining their work within the context of the nonlinear mechanics of muscle. However, carrying forth the separation-of-variables approach introduced in the previous section, Hatze (1981) *does* develop an active, nonlinear, "myocybernetic" (Cybernetics = the science of control and communication) control model of skeletal muscle that is worth mentioning here as an extension of the basic Decraemer and Fung formulations.

In Hatze's approach, the *passive* behavior of the tissue is treated essentially the same way as was discussed in Chapter 3 for Bahler's model and in this chapter for Decraemer's model. That is, Hatze *also* views the entire muscle as consisting of a network of Kelvin elements linked together in a series arrangement. Each includes three basic structural units:

A parallel elastic spring (PE), a series spring/dashpot loop (SE), and, to account for excitability, a contractile element, CE. Rather than considering the parallel spring to be linear, however, Hatze replaces equation [3-6] by a generalized nonlinear mathematical-series representation of the form:

$$f_2 = \sum_j k_p^{(j)} [\exp(a_j\alpha) - 1]$$ [4-26]

where the constants $k_p^{(j)}$ and a_j are determined by fitting the assumed form of equation [4-26] to experimental data obtained on human muscle *in situ* (see Hatze, 1981), and, calculating as many coefficients and exponential terms as are necessary to ensure a reasonably good fit.

The viscous element in Hatze's model is still assumed to be linear, of the form $c\dot{x}_d$ (see equation [3-1]), but the series elastic spring is again considered to respond exponentially according to an equation of the form:

$$f_1 = k_s e^{a^* \frac{x_s - x_{os}}{x_{ts} - x_{os}}} - 1,$$ [4-27]

which takes the place of equation [3-3], and where x_{ts} is some reference tetanic isometric length for the series element. The various constants, k_s, a^*, x_{os}, and x_{ts} are also obtained from expressions that relate to experimentally observable parameters (ibid.). The reader is directed to Chapter 4 of Hatze (1981) for more details.

The separation-of-variables approach is now applied as follows to the characterization of the contractile element in any typical Kelvin model. First, in a formulation somewhat analogous to Decraemer's statistical model, Hatze lets the force output, P (see Figure 3-1), of the *contractile proteins* of a typical muscle fiber be equal to the *average force output* $F_a(\dot{\zeta})$ of a *typical cross-bridge*, multiplied by the number $N_B\Omega$ of cross-links active in a half-sarcomere, at any instant of time, i.e.,

$$P = N_B\Omega F_a(\dot{\zeta})$$ [4-28]

where N_B denotes the *total* number of cross-bridges present in a half-sarcomere; $\zeta(t)$ is the instantaneous length of a sarcomere at any given time, t; $\dot{\zeta} = \dfrac{d\zeta}{dt}$ is the velocity of the interfilamentary movement only; and Ω is a "weighting function" $(0 < \Omega \leq 1)$ that designates the fraction of *active* cross-bridges. This fraction, in turn, depends mostly on the *active state* of the contractile element CE in the sarcomere (see Chapter 1 and Problems 1-2 and 1-3), the degree of *filamentary overlap* (as reflected in the length-tension characteristics of the tissue, such as is shown in Figures 2-2 and 2-3, and Problem 2-8), and the *velocity* $\dot{\zeta}$ of shortening or lengthening of the contractile element (as reflected in the force-velocity characteristics of the tissue, which shall be examined in greater detail in Chapter 5). Thus, we may write further:

$$\Omega = q^*(\,\bullet\,)k^*(\zeta^*)F_a^*(\dot{\zeta}) \qquad\qquad \text{[4-29]}$$

where $q^*(\,\bullet\,)$ designates a normalized active state function of several variables; $k^*(\zeta^*)$ designates a normalized filamentary overlap function of the normalized sarcomere length, $\zeta^* -- \zeta^* = \dfrac{\zeta}{\bar{\zeta}}$ ($\bar{\zeta} =$ that sarcomere length at which the force output of the fully stimulated and isometrically contracting CE attains a maximum); and, $F_a^*(\dot{\zeta})$ designates a normalized velocity-of-shortening function of $\dot{\zeta}$. Equation [4-29] utilizes the aforementioned separation-of-variables approach, and may be substituted into equation [4-28] to yield:

$$P = q^*(\,\bullet\,)k^*(\zeta^*)f_a^*(\dot{\zeta}), \qquad\qquad \text{[4-30]}$$

which is also in a separation-of-variables format, with $f_a^*(\dot{\zeta}) = N_B F_a^*(\dot{\zeta})F_a(\dot{\zeta})$. Note that the latter is *not* a normalized function.

The Excitation-Dynamics Function

The excitation-dynamics function $q^*(\,\bullet\,)$ is intimately related to the *active state* of the muscle fibers, as discussed in Chapter 1. Thus, from a value of $q_o{}^*$ in resting muscle, $q^*(\cdot) \to 1$ asymptotically as the *maximum* number of potential interactive sites on the Actin filament are exposed by the action of calcium. In-between $q_o{}^*$ and a value of unity, the active state, $q^*(\cdot)$ function is defined to be the relative amount of calcium bound to Troponin. Recall that in the resting state of the muscle, $[Ca^{++}]_o \simeq 5 \times 10^{-9}$ (Chapter 1), with a range of from about 1×10^{-9} to 8×10^{-9} Molar. Recall further that the "threshold state" boundary condition defining the mechanical response level is around $[Ca^{++}]_t = 6 \times 10^{-7}$ when $f_\alpha = 4$ Hz (c.f., problem 1-2), with a range of from 4×10^{-7} to 8×10^{-7} Molar. Thus, the *difference*, $[Ca^{++}] - [Ca^{++}]_o$, between the *actual* free calcium ion concentration, $[Ca^{++}]$, in the sarcoplasm at any given time, and the free calcium ion concentration, $[Ca^{++}]_o$, in the *resting* fiber, for all practical purposes may be assumed to be equal essentially to *just* $[Ca^{++}]$, and may be defined as a function of α-motoneuron stimulation frequency, f_α, by an equation such as [1-2] -- the Sigmoidal Function -- or [1-3] -- the Hill Equation.

In Hatze's formulation, the Ca-concentration-rate-of-change of the active-state-function, $q^*(\cdot)$ is designated by the derivative, $\dfrac{dq^*(\cdot)}{d[Ca^{++}]} = p^*$, where $p^*(0) = 0$. Furthermore, following the reasoning formulated in Problem 1-2, Hatze *also* proposes that "an increment δp^* for a given increment $\delta[Ca^{++}]$ of the free Ca ion concentration [should] be proportional to the difference between the maximum (unity) and the present (q^*) value of $q^*(\cdot)$, controlled by a negative feedback loop." (Ibid., page 33.) And, based on "strong experimental evidence," that such a $\delta p^*/\delta[Ca^{++}]$ relationship should also depend on the length ζ of the CE. Thus, he writes,

$$\frac{dp^*}{d[Ca^{++}]} = r_{11}(\zeta^*)(1 - q^*) - r_{12}(\zeta^*)p^*; \quad q^*(0) = q_o{}^* \qquad [4\text{-}31]$$

where $r_{11}(\zeta^*)$ and $r_{12}(\zeta^*)$ are yet-to-be-determined functions of the normalized length ζ^*, and $q_o{}^*$ denotes the *resting* active state of the fiber, which has a normalized value of around 0.005. One cannot help but notice the similarity between equations [4-31] and [1-1], and between the reasoning that went into the development of equation [4-31], and that which is developed by Nubar in formulating equations [2-1] to [2-13], where, in Nubar's analysis, $q_o = 0.20$ based on *isometric* considerations.

****

Problem 4-4: Substitute the definition of p^* given earlier into equation [4-31], and use the boundary conditions $p^*(0) = 0$ and $q^*(0) = q_o^*$ to solve the resulting second-order differential equation, which yields:

$$q^*(\zeta^*, [Ca^{++}]) = 1 - \frac{(1 - q_o^*)}{m_1 - m_2} \left\{ m_1 \exp m_2 \rho_1(\zeta^*)[Ca^{++}] \right.$$

$$\left. - m_2 \exp m_1 \rho_1(\zeta^*)[Ca^{++}] \right\}$$

[4-32]

where:

$$m_{1,2} = -\rho_2 \pm \sqrt{\rho_2^2 - 1} \qquad \rho_2 > 1$$

$$\rho_1(\zeta^*) = \frac{r_{12}(\zeta^*)}{2\rho_2(\zeta^*)} = \sqrt{r_{11}(\zeta^*)} \neq 0$$

$$\rho_2(\zeta^*) = \frac{r_{12}(\zeta^*)}{2\rho_1(\zeta^*)}$$

****

Because of the role played by depolarization of the T-system in triggering the release of sequestered calcium from the terminal cisternae of the sarcoplasmic reticulum (see Chapter 1), Hatze goes on to propose that $[Ca^{++}]$ in equation [4-32] actually represents the output (delayed response) of an overcritically damped electrical second-order system, the input of which is the depolarizing potential, $V_T\beta^*(t)$, of the T-system, i.e.,

$$\frac{d^2[Ca^{++}]}{dt^2} + \frac{1}{\rho^*(\zeta^*)} \left[s_1 \frac{d[Ca^{++}]}{dt} + s_2[Ca^{++}] \right] = s_3 V_T\beta^*(t)$$

[4-33]

$$[Ca^{++}](0) = \frac{d[Ca^{++}]}{dt}(0) = 0$$

where s_1, s_2, s_3 are constants (see Table 4-I), V_T is about 0.05 (50 milli-volts), and $\rho^*(\zeta^*)$ is a normalized "calcium density function," given by $\rho_1(\zeta^*)/s_4$ (s_4 is also a constant given in Table 4-I):

$$\rho^*(\zeta^*) = \frac{\rho_1(\zeta^*)}{s_4} = \frac{[\overset{v}{\zeta}^Z - 1]}{\left\{\left[\dfrac{\overset{v}{\zeta}}{\zeta^*}\right]^Z - 1\right\}} = \frac{[Ca^{++}(\zeta^*,t)]}{[Ca^{++}(t)]} \qquad [4\text{-}34]$$

for $0.58 \leq \zeta^* \leq 1.8$, and $\rho^*(1) = 1$. In equation [4-34], which Hatze derives from a consideration of the behavior of a *constant total* amount of free calcium ions present in the filamentary-overlap region of a muscle fiber during an *isovolumetric* contraction, $\overset{v}{\zeta}$ and s_4 are experimentally deter-mined constants (see Table 4-I), and the exponent Z (equal to unity for the linear case) gives a degree of freedom that allows for the possibility of the occurrence of nonlinear effects -- such as the collision of the myosin filaments with the Z-lines at short lengths.

****

Problem 4-5: Consider a sarcomere of length $\zeta(t)$ and initial diameter dx, undergoing an isovolumetric contraction, during which shortening from an initial given length ζ_o, its cross-sectional area increases but it maintains its overall cylindrical shape. Let this sarcomere have a total interfilamentary overlap "length" given by $b^*\zeta(t)$, where $0 \leq b^* \leq 1$. From the assumption that the *total amount* of free calcium ions present in the filamentary overlap region remains constant during the contraction, *derive* equation [4-34] above. (Hint: It   helps   to   let $b^* = \left\{\dfrac{\text{constant}}{\zeta^*} - 1\right\}$).

****

Going one step further, the depolarizing potential of the T-system follows directly from the propagation of an *action potential* along the surface membrane, which, in turn, results from the electrochemical trans-mission of the *nerve* impulse, $V_N\alpha^*(t)$ arriving at the motor end plate (c.f., Chapter 1 and Schneck, 1990). Thus, to obtain the response $V_T\beta^*(t)$ in equation [4-33], to the nerve input $V_N\alpha^*(t)$, Hatze (1981) also models the *total* α-motor-neuron-synapse-motor-end-plate-membrane system as a "lumped parameter" second-order system described by:

$$\frac{d^2\beta^*(t)}{dt^2} + s_5 \frac{d\beta^*(t)}{dt} + s_6\beta^*(t) = s_7 V_N\alpha^*(t); \quad \beta^*(0) = \dot{\beta}^*(0) = 0 \quad \textbf{[4-35]}$$

where: s_5, s_6, s_7 are constants (see Table 4-I);
        $V_N = 90$ millivolts; and,

$$\alpha^*(t) \simeq \sin 1000\pi(t - t_i^*), \quad i = 1, 2, \ldots$$
$$\text{for } t_i^* \leq t \leq t_i^* + 0.001, \quad \quad \textbf{[4-36]}$$
$$= 0 \text{ otherwise (refractory)}$$

In equation [4-36], $t^*_{i+1} - t_i^*$ represents the (variable) time intervals at which trains of α-motor-neuron impulses excite the motor end plate; the reciprocal of this quantity thus represents the excitation frequency, f_α (stimulation rate) at which the muscle fibers are being depolarized.

To summarize, then, the *excitation dynamics* of the contractile element of a single muscle fiber goes something like this:

a) An α-motoneuron excites the motor end plate at a stimulation frequency f_α, generating (following an appropriate time delay due to limitations in the rates of the synaptic and membrane chemical reactions involved -- which are herein being neglected) an *end-plate potential* $\alpha^*(t)$ given approximately by a half-sine wave with a half-period of one millisecond, such as is defined by equation [4-36].

b) The end-plate-potential, $\alpha^*(t)$, is propagated along the surface membrane (sarcolemma) of the muscle fiber as a *muscle action potential*, $\beta^*(t)$, which is defined by equation [4-35], and which, following *another* time delay (which is *also* being neglected) -- due to the existence of finite conduction velocities -- eventually depolarizes the T-system.

c) Depolarization of the T-system causes the release of calcium ions, which raise the concentration of free calcium in the sarcoplasm from a negligibly small amount to values which satisfy the governing equations

[4-33] and [4-34]. Again, a small time delay is involved in this *excitation-contraction-coupling* stage, which also involves the protein switch discussed in Chapter 1.

d) The calcium thus released produces an *active state* of the muscle tissue -- i.e., one that allows it to generate a force, as defined by the active state function $q^*(\bullet)$ given in equations [4-32] and [4-31]. This active state is a continuation of the excitation-contraction coupling process, wherein the establishment of a functional actomyosin complex is completed, and the ensuing sliding-filament mechanism is initiated.

e) The constants in equations [4-31] through [4-36] have been determined at 37°C for both fast and slow human muscle fibers (Hatze, 1981) and are tabulated in Table 4-I for $\zeta^* = 1$. Thus, the dynamics of $[Ca^{++}]$ -- as discussed in Chapter 1 and defined by equations such as [1-1] to [1-3] -- together with that of $q^*(\bullet)$ -- as discussed above and defined by equations such as [4-31] to [4-36] -- represent the *excitation dynamics* of the contractile element of a single muscle fiber.

Table 4-I

Hatze's (1981) Values for the Muscle-Specific Constants
Appearing in Equations [4-31] to [4-35]

Constant	Muscle Fiber Type	
$(37°C; \ \zeta^* = 1)$	Fast	Slow
s_1	2.24×10^4	2.24×10^4
s_2	2.50×10^5	0.71×10^5
s_3	8.60×10^{10}	9.20×10^{10}
s_4	1.14×10^5	1.14×10^5
s_5	1.84×10^4	1.84×10^4
s_6	7.36×10^6	7.36×10^6
s_7	10.333	10.333
ρ_2	1.05	1.05
$\overset{\text{v}}{\zeta}$	2.90	2.90

f) The active state of mammalian muscle does not reach its full intensity after just a single stimulus (c.f., the staircase effect, tetanus, and so on); it reaches a *relative peak*, however, some 10 to 12 milliseconds following a single stimulation, and it decays approximately exponentially thereafter. Moreover, in a manner directly analogous to the Logistic Equation [1-1] for Calcium, the relative *increase* in $q^*(\cdot)$ in response to a further stimulus depends also on the then current *value* of $q^*(\cdot)$ -- reaching saturation at some point which is around a stimulation frequency of 100 Hertz for fast, and perhaps one-half to one-third of that amount for slow muscle fibers.

The Kinetics Functions

Having thus defined $q^*(\cdot)$ in equation [4-30], we note from this equation that the active state is further modulated by the length-tension, $k^*(\zeta^*)$, and force-velocity, $f_a^*(\zeta)$, characteristics (or "limitations") of the muscle fiber, before a *net* contractile force P becomes manifest in the tissue. Thus, let us say a few words here about the function $k^*(\zeta^*)$ -- which was addressed in much more detail earlier in this and in Chapters 2 and 3 -- and the function $f_a^*(\zeta)$ -- which will be addressed in much more detail in Chapter 5.

Hatze proposes a mathematical approximation for the function $k^*(\zeta^*)$ which, like Decraemer's, et al. (1980a) equation [4-6], is based on a large number of muscle fibers, N_∞, normally distributed around a mean, and having a statistical distribution with sometimes large values of the variance. *Unlike* Decraemer's model, however, Hatze's approximation is somewhat less intimidating, i.e.,

$$k^*(\zeta^*) = e^{-\left\{\frac{\zeta^*-1}{s_k}\right\}^2}$$

[4-37]

where $k^*(1) = 1$, i.e., the filamentary-overlap function for the whole muscle is *normalized*; and, the parameter s_k -- which is specific for a given muscle -- determines the "peakedness" of the normal distribution curve of the statistically-distributed fibers. Hatze (1981, Chapter 5) discusses several experimental methods for estimating s_k, which is generally in the range $0.28 \leq s_k \leq 0.44$ for most muscles (ibid.).

That the velocity of movement between the actin and the myosin filaments should affect P makes sense for reasons we shall discuss in the next chapter. Suffice it to say here that $f_a*(\dot{\zeta})$ accounts for the "gripping strength" of the cross-bridge attachments (which strength can be higher the *slower* the filaments move relative to one another) -- just as $k*(\zeta*)$ may be thought of as an "interference parameter" for the cross-bridges (c.f., Chapter 3).

From the many empirical relationships that have been proposed to approximate $f_a*(\dot{\zeta})$, Hatze chooses an exponential function that gives a sigmoidal shape to the force-velocity response characteristics of a typical muscle fiber. This function is defined by:

$$f_a*(\dot{\zeta}) = \frac{s_8}{s_9 + e^{-s_{10}F_{10}(\dot{\zeta})}}$$ [4-38]

where s_8, s_9 and s_{10} are, again, experimentally determined constants, and:

$$F_{10}(\dot{\zeta}) = \sinh \left[s_{11} \frac{\dot{\zeta}}{\bar{\zeta}_m} + \frac{s_{11}}{2} \right]$$ [4-39]

In equation [4-39], s_{11} is still *another* constant, and $\bar{\zeta}_m$ denotes the *maximum* shortening velocity of the myostructures at optimum length $\bar{\zeta}$ defined earlier. The constants s_8 and s_9 can be determined in terms of the constants s_{10} and s_{11} from the conditions that:

(a) If the *non-stimulated* fiber is stationary ($\dot{\zeta} = 0$), then its passive force output is also zero $[f_a*(\dot{\zeta})] = 0$; and,

(b) If the *fully-stimulated* fiber contracts against no load $[f_a*(\dot{\zeta}) = 0]$, then its active speed of contraction will be maximum, i.e., $\dot{\zeta} = \bar{\zeta}_m$. Thus, $f_a*(\dot{\zeta})$ will be zero *both* when $\dot{\zeta} = 0$ and when $\dot{\zeta} = \bar{\zeta}_m$ -- in the former case *only* under non-stimulated conditions (i.e., passive, rather than isometric), and in the latter case only under fully-stimulated conditions (but against no load). Hatze goes on to suggest further that the constant s_{11} takes on values between 2 and 5 for human muscle (ibid., page 46), and that s_{10} falls in the range between 0.70 and 2.0 (ibid., page 74).

Substituting equations [4-38] for $f_a^*(\zeta)$, [4-37] for $k^*(\zeta^*)$, and the system [4-31] to [4-36] for $q^*(\bullet)$, into equation [4-30] for P gives a complete set of nonlinear equations which describe the dynamic behavior of the contractile element of a single muscle fiber. Coupled with viscoelastic considerations such as are discussed in the first half of this chapter (i.e., Decraemer's nonlinear stochastic model) one can formulate a rather impressive nonlinear, viscoelastic constitutive model for striated skeletal muscle -- which, alas, cannot be solved in its most general form! This forces investigators such as Decraemer, et al., and Hatze to move from distributed nonlinear models such as have been developed here, to "quasi-linearized," "lumped-parameter" models representing "whole-muscle" properties. In Hatze's own words (1981, pg. 51), "although the distributed system is of value for some applications, it is generally too complex to be employed in the multilink system of the animal body." And, "great difficulties are encountered when an attempt is made to define control parameters for the distributed model."

Thus, as is so typical in so many of these types of formulations, following the elegant development of a sophisticated set of equations to describe a complex physical process, investigators invariably resort to simplification schemes that become necessary in order to *solve* these equations. Unfortunately, such simplification schemes often leave out just enough physics to give the ultimate results limited usefulness, at best. So it is, then, that to date, nonlinear viscoelastic models have shed little more light on our basic understanding of the mechanics of muscular contraction than has already been learned from *separate* nonlinear elastic, or linear viscoelastic theories such as those discussed in Chapters 2 and 3. In particular, they have not elucidated certain "secondary coupling effects" which derive from *interactions* that take place among nonlinear elastic, nonlinear inertial, and nonlinear viscous properties of the tissue, driven by an external stimulus. Such interactions might be expected to be manifest in the nonlinear mechanics of muscle, in the same sense that they are known to generate observable "secondary flows" and other instabilities in the unsteady dynamics of fluids such as blood.

Moreover, related to the dynamics of nonlinear viscoelastic systems are discontinuous instabilities that may lead to *Chaotic* results (Gleick, 1987, Thom, 1975). As Hatze points out (1981, page 43), "While the whole range of negative velocities (shortening) as well as small to moderately large positive velocities (stretches) can be treated using conventional mathematical techniques, this no longer applies to the region of hyperfast extensions, where the discontinuities occur [between the velocity of movement and the force production];" and, on page 48, he re-emphasizes that mathematical theories of muscle dynamics are generally valid only in regions of the velocity-dependence function where no discontinuities occur, i.e., where "no discontinuity in the nature of the system occurs which would give rise to a [thermodynamically irreversible] change in its previous form." This "change" alludes to the essence of the theory of chaos, which is embedded in the notion that the *inherent* nonlinearity of *real* viscoelastic physical systems renders them extremely *sensitive* to the initial conditions of a disturbing influence (Gleick, 1987). Thus, depending on such initial conditions and the nature of the disturbance, a *very small* driving function -- rather than decaying or being damped out (as would be expected of a "well-behaved," stable, continuous dynamic system) -- instead, grows without limit, multiplies, gets amplified, and cascades up through the entire system, causing it to become *unstable, discontinuous, not* predictable or well-behaved -- in short, *chaotic*. The manifestation of dynamic nonlinearity, then, is inherent in the lack of consistent proportionality between the response and the disturbance; and no nonlinear viscoelastic theory to date has been able to take such disproportionality into account.

There is nothing to be gained, then, in pursuing this further at this point, and so, following some closing remarks in the next section, we shall move on in Chapter 5 to examine the mechanics and energetics of muscular contraction.

Closing Remarks

Two aspects of the stress-strain and/or the stress-strain-rate behavior of muscle tissue need to be addressed before one examines the mechanics of contraction. It is important to realize that the characteristics of muscle are very much dependent on temperature and water content. Among other things, the relaxation time constant, the retardation time constant, the elastic moduli, the shear moduli, and other viscoelastic material properties are all very strongly temperature-dependent, as are the viscosity of the fluid in the muscle, the biochemical reactions related to muscle metabolism and contraction, the physical crystalline state of the macromolecules, and the state of patency of the microcirculation permeating the tissue.

For example, since the rate of stress-relaxation is determined by chemical kinetics, and since everything on a molecular scale moves around faster in a hotter environment, one finds that in general, the higher the temperature is, the quicker the material relaxes or complies. Thus, relative to normal body temperature (37°C) the relaxation and recovery time of muscle can be decreased nearly 25 percent by heating, and increased as much as 50 to 150 percent by cooling to very low temperatures. Furthermore, since heat also tends to promote chemical reactions and increased molecular interactions and bonding, one finds that, i) under *equilibrium* conditions the shear and elastic moduli of elastomers increase, i.e., they become stiffer with increasing temperature (a kind of vulcanizing effect), and, ii) the contraction time of muscle decreases with increasing temperature. The latter is due not only to the accelerated biochemical reactions that accompany increases in temperature, but also to the decreased viscous resistance of the tissue fluid at higher temperatures, and to the corresponding capillary dilatation which increases the blood supply to the contractile elements. Thus, again relative to normal body temperature, the *contraction time* of muscle can be decreased almost 15 percent by heating and increased as much as 20 to 85 percent by cooling to very low temperatures.

The fact that cooling can have a much more substantial effect on muscular performance than can heating implies that the normal body temperature of 37°C is in some sense near some optimum maximum for thermodynamic and mechanical efficiency. Moreover, since muscles *generate* heat as they contract, one might reason further that the corresponding *local* increase in temperature actually brings the reacting tissue still closer to its optimum performance level. In any event, temperature effects do play an important role during the contraction process.

To express mathematically the temperature of muscles as a function of the heat generated during contraction, one could write a simple relationship that identifies absolute muscle temperature, T, as a function of its length, L, and the force, F, that it is generating -- assuming all other variables to be held constant. Note that L and F are also functions of time:

$$T = T\left[L(t),\ F(t)\right] \qquad\qquad \text{[4-40]}$$

Then, the rise in temperature, dT, occurring when a muscle of resting length L_{op} contracts by some amount dL, while F changes by some amount dF, is given approximately by the equation:

$$dT = \left(\frac{\partial T}{\partial L}\right)_F dL + \left(\frac{\partial T}{\partial F}\right)_L dF \qquad\qquad \text{[4-41]}$$

The coefficient $\left(\frac{\partial T}{\partial L}\right)_F$, which, in its inverted form, defines the change in muscle length per unit change in temperature when the tension is held constant (an isotonic thermodynamic creep effect) is normally written as:

$$\left(\frac{\partial L}{\partial T}\right)_F = \kappa L_{op}$$

where κ is the linear thermal expansion coefficient of the material.

Similarly, the coefficient $\left(\frac{\partial T}{\partial F}\right)_L$ in its inverted form defines the change in tensile force per unit change of temperature if the length is held constant (an isometric thermodynamic relaxation effect sometimes called the Joule, or Gough-Joule effect),

$$\left(\frac{\partial F}{\partial T}\right)_L = \gamma$$

where γ, the Joule coefficient, is a negative constant up to muscle lengths $L(t)$ three to four times resting length L_{op}. That is, below 300 to 400 percent stretch, muscle tension decreases in direct proportion to increases in absolute Temperature, T, and vice versa.

Substituting the above into equation [4-41], one can write:

$$dT = \frac{dL}{\kappa L_{op}} + \frac{dF}{\gamma},$$

or,

$$\dot{T} = \frac{1}{\kappa}\frac{\dot{L}}{L_{op}} + \frac{1}{\gamma}\dot{F} \qquad [4\text{-}42]$$

where $\frac{dL}{L_{op}} = \alpha =$ muscle strain.

As for the effects of water, studies reveal that a 20 percent decrease in water content of the muscle fiber results in a threefold increase in elastic and viscous stiffness, whereas a 70 percent increase in water content gives no measurable change. It has been suggested that the increase in stiffness might be explained as being due to a reduction in the distance between minute structural elements resulting in an increased number of cross-linkages. The fact that a *higher* water content does *not* affect the dynamic mechanical properties implies that the structural elements are in a state of maximal hydration at the normal osmotic concentration.

One could go on to discuss many other factors upon which the behavior of muscle tissue depends -- factors such as:

(i) the *amplitude,* as well as the frequency of an oscillating disturbance (related to the nonlinear stress-strain characteristics of the tissue);

(ii) the *pressure* as well as the absolute temperature and other thermodynamic variables;

(iii) the *anisotropy* of the material, which causes it to respond differently to stresses applied in different directions, such that there is no longer a simple relation between the elastic constants;

(iv) *elastic after-effects,* which lead to hysteresis under cyclic deformation because, unless sufficient time is allowed for adjustment, tension at a *given length* will always be higher when arrived at by *extension* from a shorter length than by *release* from a longer length (a thixotropic effect illustrated in Figure 3-3 and caused by an increase in cross-bonding and structurization at shorter muscle lengths);

(v) *tethering effects* mentioned briefly earlier -- wherein the external constraints imposed by surrounding tissue affect the muscles' ability to contract as well as its mode of contraction;

(vi) the *age* of the material (see page 77), variations in its *chemical* composition, the influence of *electrolytes,* other *physical* factors -- and so on, and so forth.

However, to discuss all of these factors at great length is not really the intent of this text and the reader is thus referred to the literature for a more comprehensive treatment of these and other issues. Our purpose here is to understand some fundamental principles related to the mechanics and energetics of muscular contraction, which shall be examined in the next chapter, based on the material presented in Chapters 1 through 4.

References for Chapters 2, 3, and 4

1. Alesso, H. P., "Reliability Analysis of the Elementary Catastrophe Theory Model of Muscle Contraction," *Engineering in Medicine* (Institution of Mechanical Engineers), 7(#1):21-30, January, 1978.

2. Alfrey, T., Jr., and Gurnee, E. F., "Dynamics of Viscoelastic Behavior," In: Eirich, F. R., (Editor), *Rheology: Theory and Applica-*

tions, New York, Academic Press, Inc., Vol. 1, Chap. 11, pp. 387-430, 1956.

3. Audu, M. L., and Davy, D. T., "The Influence of Muscle Model Complexity in Musculoskeletal Motion Modeling," *Transactions of the ASME, J. of Biomechanical Engineering*, Vol. 107, Pages 147-157, May, 1985.

4. Bahler, A. S., "The Series Elastic Element of Mammalian Skeletal Muscle," *American Journal of Physiology*, *213*:1560-1564, 1967.

5. Bahler, A. S., "Modeling of Mammalian Skeletal Muscle," *IEEE Transactions on Biomedical Engineering*, *BME-15*:(#4):249-257, October, 1968.

6. Baildon, R. W., and Chapman, A. E., "A New Approach to the Human Muscle Model," *Journal of Biomechanics*, Vol. 16, No. 10, Pages 803-809, 1983.

7. Bawa, P., Mannard, A., and Stein, R. B., "Effects of Elastic Loads on the Contractions of Cat Muscles," *Biological Cybernetics*, Vol. 22, Pages 129-137, 1976.

8. Bawa, P., Mannard, A., and Stein, R. B., "Predictions and Experimental Tests of a Visco-Elastic Muscle Model Using Elastic and Inertial Loads," *Biological Cybernetics*, Vol. 22, Pages 139-145, 1976.

9. Bergen, J. T., (Editor), *Viscoelasticity: Phenomenological Aspects*, New York, Academic Press, Inc., 1960.

10. Boehman, L. I., and Minardi, J. E., "An Irreversible Thermodynamic Analysis of the Energy Conversion Process in an Active Muscle," University of Dayton Research Institute, Technical Report Number TR-71-09, Dayton, Ohio, April, 1971.

11. Bozler, E., "Extensibility of Contractile Elements," In: Remington, J. W., (Editor), *Tissue Elasticity*, Washington, D. C., The American Physiological Society, 1957.

12. Brankov, G., and Petrov, N., "A Thermodynamic Model of Biological Body: Muscle Mechanics," *Trans. A.S.M.E., J. Biomechanical Engineering*, *100*(31):14-19, February, 1978.

13. Buchthal, F., and Rosenfalck, P., "Elastic Properties of Striated Muscle," In: Remington, J. W., (Editor), *Tissue Elasticity*, Washington, D. C., The American Physiological Society, 1957.

14. Buchthal, F., "The Mechanical Properties of Single Striated Muscle Fiber at Rest and During Contraction and Their Structural Interpretation," *Det. Kgl. Danske V. Densk. Selskab. Biol. Meddell*, *17*(#2), pgs. 1-140, 1942, Monograph.

15. Bull, H. B., "Elastic Element of Skeletal Muscle," *Journal of the American Chemical Society, 67*: 2047-2048, 1945.

16. Bull, H. B., "The Elastic Element of Skeletal Muscle," *Quart. Bulletin of the Northwestern University Medical School, 20*:175-179, 1946.

17. Cannon, S. C., and Zahalak, G. I., "The Mechanical Behavior of Active Human Skeletal Muscle in Small Oscillations," *J. Biomechanics, 15*(#2):111-121, February, 1982.

18. Carlson, F. D., "Kinematic Studies on Mechanical Properties of Muscle," In: Remington, J. W., (Editor), *Tissue Elasticity*, Washington, D. C., The American Physiological Society, 1957.

19. Coulter, N. A., Jr., and West, J. C., "Non-Linear Passive Mechanical Properties of Skeletal Muscle," Wright Air Development Division, WADD Technical Report Number 60-636, Wright-Patterson Air Force Base, Ohio, August, 1960.

20. Decraemer, W. F., Maes, M. A., and Vanhuyse, V. J., "An Elastic Stress-Strain Relation for Soft Biological Tissues Based on a Structural Model," *J. Biomechanics*, Vol. 13, pp. 463-468, 1980a.

21. Decraemer, W. F., Maes, M. A., Vanhuyse, V. J., and Vanpeperstraete, P., "A Non-Linear Viscoelastic Constitutive Equation for Soft Biological Tissues, Based Upon a Structural Model," *J. Biomechanics*, Vol. 13, pp. 559-564, 1980b.

22. Eirich, F. R., (Editor), *Rheology: Theory and Applications*, New York, Academic Press, Inc., Volume 1, 1956.

23. Fisher, M. B., and Birren, J. E., "Age and Strength," *J. Appl. Psychol.*, Vol. 31, Pages 490-497, 1947.

24. Fung, Y-C., B., "Stress-Strain-History Relations of Soft Tissues in Simple Elongation," In: Fung, Y-C., B., Perrone, N., and Anliker, M., (Editors), *Biomechanics: Its Foundations and Objectives*, Englewood Cliffs, New Jersey, Prentice-Hall, Inc., 1972, pp. 181-208.

25. Glantz, S. A., "A Three Element Description for Muscle With Viscoelastic Passive Elements," *J. Biomechanics, 10*(#1):5-20, February, 1977.

26. Gleick, J., *Chaos: Making a New Science*, New York, Viking Penguin, Inc., 1987.

27. Gottlieb, G. L., Agarwal, G. C., and Stark, L., "Stretch Receptor Models: I -- Single-Efferent Single-Afferent Innervation," *IEEE Transactions on Man-Machine Systems*, Vol. MMS-10 (No. 1), Pages 17-27, March, 1969.

28. Gutstein, W. H., "A Generalization of Hooke's Law in Muscle Elasticity," *Bull. Math. Biophysics*, *18*:151-170, 1956.

29. Hatze, H., "A Theory of Contraction and a Mathematical Model of Striated Muscle," *J. Theoretical Biology*, Vol. 40, pp. 219-246, 1973.

30. Hatze, H., "A Complete Set of Control Equations for the Human Musculo-Skeletal System," *Journal of Biomechanics*, Vol. 10, Pages 799-805, 1977.

31. Hatze, H., *Myocybernetic Control Models of Skeletal Muscle: Characteristics and Applications*, Pretoria, University of South Africa Press, 1981.

32. Hill, T. L., "Statistical Mechanical Models of Elastic Element in Muscle," In: Remington, J. W., (Editor), *Tissue Elasticity*, Washington, D. C., The American Physiological Society, 1957.

33. Houwink, R., "*Elasticity, Plasticity and Structure of Matter*," New York, Dover Publications, Inc., Second Edition, 1958.

34. Ingels, N. B., "An Electrokinematic Theory of Muscle Contraction," *Ph.D. Thesis*, Stanford University, 1967.

35. King, A. L., and Lawton, R. W., "Elasticity of Body Tissues," In: Glasser, O., (Editor), *Medical Physics, Volume II*, Chicago, Ill., The Year Book Medical Publishers, Inc., Pages 303-316, 1950.

36. Kuhn, W., "Beziehungen Zwischen Molekülgröse, Statistischer Molekulgestalt Und Elastischen Eigenschaften Hochpolymerer Stoffe," *K'olloid-Ztschr.*, Vol. 76, Pg. 258, 1936.

37. Kuhn, W., "Molekülkonstellation Und Kristallitorientierung Als Ursachen Kautschukähnlicher Elastizitä t," *K'olloid-Ztschr.*, Vol. 87, Pg. 3, 1939.

38. Levin, A., and Wyman, J., "The Viscous Elastic Properties of Muscle," *Proceedings of the Royal Society of London*, Ser. B., *101*:218-243, 1927.

39. Mains, R. E., and Soechting, J. F., "A Model for the Neuromuscular Response to Sudden Disturbances," *Journal of Dynamic Systems, Measurement, and Control, 93*(#4):247-251, December, 1971.

40. McElhaney, J. H., "Dynamic Response of Bone and Muscle Tissue," *J. Appl. Physiol.*, 7:1231-1236, 1965.

41. Nubar, Y., "Stress-Strain Relationship in Skeletal Muscle," *Annals of the New York Academy of Sciences*, *93*(Article 21):857-876, October, 1962.

42. Oguztöreli, M. N., and Stein, R. B., "An Analysis of Oscillations in Neuromuscular Systems," *J. Math. Biol.*, Vol. 2, Pages 87-105, 1975.

43. Pasley, P. R., Soechting, J. F., Stewart, P. A., and Duffy, J., "Equations Governing the Force-Deformation Behavior for Partially Stimulated Muscle," *Proceedings of the 23rd Annual Conference on Engineering in Medicine and Biology*, Washington, D. C., Paper Number 6.14, Page 69, November, 1970.

44. Pasley, P. R., Clamann, H. P., Soechting, J. F., Stewart, P. A., Zahalak, G. I., and Duffy, J., "A Quantitative Model for Partially Activated Skeletal Muscle," *Trans. A.S.M.E., J. Applied Mechanics, 41*:849-854, December, 1974.

45. Pipkin, A. C., *Lectures on Viscoelastic Theory*, New York, Springer-Verlag, 1972.

46. Ramsey, R. W., and Street, S. F., "The Isometric Length-Tension Diagram of Isolated Skeletal Muscle Fibers of the Frog," *J. Cellular Comp. Physiol., 15*:11-34, 1940.

47. Ramsey, R. W., "Muscle: Physics," In: Glasser, O., (Editor), *Medical Physics*, Chicago, Year-book Publishers, Volume 1, pp. 784-798, 1944.

48. Ramsey, R. W., "Dynamics of Single Muscle Fibers," *Annals of the New York Academy of Sciences, 47*:675-695, 1947.

49. Remington, J. W., (Editor), *Tissue Elasticity*, Washington, D. C., *The American Physiological Society*, 1957.

50. Schapery, R. A., "Thermomechanical Behavior of Viscoelastic Media With Variable Properties Subjected to Cyclic Loading," *J. Applied Mechanics*, ASME Paper Number 65-APM-15, Pages 1-9, 1965.

51. Schneck, D. J., "A Biomechanical Analysis of Striated Skeletal Muscle," New York University, College of Engineering, Research Division Technical Report, January, 1963.

52. Schneck, D. J., *Engineering Principles of Physiologic Function*, New York, The New York University Press, 1990.

53. Soechting, J. F., Stewart, P. A., Hawley, R. H., Paslay, P. R., and Duffy, J., "Evaluation of Neuromuscular Parameters Describing Human Reflex Motion," *J. Dynamic Systems, Measurement, and Control, 93*(#4):221-226, December, 1971.

54. Stein, R. B., and Oğuztöreli, M. N., "Tremor and Other Oscillations in Neuromuscular Systems," *Biological Cybernetics*, Vol. 22, Pages 147-157, 1976.

55. Stewart, P. A., Duffy, J., Soechting, J., Litchman, H., and Paslay, P. R., "Control of the Human Forearm During Abrupt Acceleration," In: *Symposium on Biodynamic Models and Their Applications*, United States Air Force, Air Force Systems Command, Aerospace Medical Division, Aerospace Medical Research Laboratory, Technical Report Number AMRL-TR-71-29, Paper #26, pp. 671-692, December, 1971.

56. Thom, R., *Structural Stability and Morphogenesis*, Massachusetts, Benjamin, 1975.

57. Truong, X. T., "Viscoelastic Wave Propagation and Rheological Properties of Skeletal Muscle," *American Journal of Physiology*, 226: 256-264, 1974.

58. Truong, X. T., Jarrett, S. R., and Nguyen, M. C., "A Method for Deriving Viscoelastic Modulus for Skeletal Muscle from Transient Pulse Propagation," *IEEE Trans. Biomedical Engineering*, BME-25(#4):382-384, July, 1978.

59. Wallinga-de Jonge, W., Boom, H. B. K., Heijink R. J., and vand der Vliet, G. H., "Calcium Model for Mammalian Skeletal Muscle," *Medical and Biological Engineering and Computing*, 19(#6):734-748, November, 1981.

60. Wilkie, D. R., "Facts and Theories About Muscle," *Progress in Biophysics*, 4:288-323, 1954.

61. Wilkie, D. R., "Measurement of the Series Elastic Component at Various Times During a Single Muscle Twitch," *Journal of Physiology* (London), 134:527-530, 1956.

62. Wilkie, D. R., "The Mechanical Properties of Muscle," *British Medical Bulletin*, 12(#3):177-182, 1956.

63. Wilkie, D. R., "Man as a Source of Mechanical Power," *Ergonomics*, 3:1-8, 1960.

64. Williams, W. J., "Velocity Dispersion in Skeletal Muscle Efferent Nerve Bundle and its Effect Upon Time and Frequency Response," *Medical and Biological Engineering*, 7:283-288, 1969.

65. Woledge, R. C., "The Thermoelastic Effect of Change of Tension in Active Muscle," *J. Physiol.*, Vol. 155, pgs. 187-208, 1961.

66. Yamada, H., *Strength of Biological Materials*, New York, Robert E. Krieger Publishing Company, 1973.

67. Zahalak, G. I., and Heyman, S. J., "A Quantitative Evaluation of the Frequency Response Characteristics of Active Human Skeletal Muscle In Vivo," *Trans. A.S.M.E., J. Biomechanical Engineering*, 101:28-37, February, 1979.

68. Zajac, F. E., III, "The Mathematical Formulation of the Kinematic Properties of Muscle Derived from an Experimental Investigation," *Ph.D. Thesis*, Stanford University, 1969.

Chapter 5

Mechanics and Energetics of Muscular Contraction

Introduction

The constitutive relationships developed in Chapters 2, 3 and 4, provide a theoretical basis for analyzing the ability of muscles to generate forces that eventually produce moments at human joints. This is important for understanding the capability that striated skeletal muscles have to maintain posture and balance, or to cause locomotion of parts or all of the animal body. Both of these functions are accomplished entirely by rotating (or preventing the rotation of) one part of the body relative to another. Indeed, whether one wishes to study gait (walking), athletic performance, various postural configurations, movement in sub-gravity conditions, activities of daily living, dancing, or any other aspect of human endeavor that involves the ability to move, one is ultimately faced with having to examine a type of action wherein muscles generate torques that cause rotation of levers (bones) around fulcrums (joints) or axes of rotation. Thus, equations from which length-tension diagrams such as Figures 2-2 and 2-3, or length-time, tension-time diagrams such as Figures 3-2 and 3-5, are obtained can be used to compute such torques when corresponding information concerning the proper lever-arms is available.

Furthermore, results such as those obtained in the previous three chapters can be used to estimate the energy and power consumption of various types of muscular activity. These quantities are useful not only from the point of view of understanding human performance, but also, and perhaps equally as important from an engineering point of view, for designing prosthetic devices that must replace diseased or amputated muscles or joints. For this and other reasons, it is of interest to develop further some of the theories formulated in Chapters 2-4, in order to derive kinematic, kinetic and energy relationships that will allow us to characterize further the source of power that is ultimately responsible for all of human movement. This we do in the sections that follow.

Kinematics of Muscular Contraction

The science of kinematics concerns itself with the *geometry* of motion, without regard for the *cause* of the motion. Thus, when one speaks of the kinematics of muscular contraction, one is referring to the displacement, velocity and acceleration of a given muscle without concern for the forces or moments that result from or produce said motion. To examine the kinematics of an isotonic twitch, for example, one could start with equation [3-46], which defines muscular displacement as a function of time during the Period of Shortening:

$$\frac{\xi(t)}{\xi(\infty)} = 1 - e^{-(t/\tau_P)} \qquad [5\text{-}1]$$

Expanding this equation in accordance with the definition of ξ, one obtains:

$$\frac{L(t)}{L(\infty)} = 1 - e^{-(t/\tau_P)}\left[1 - \frac{L_{op}}{L(\infty)} \right], \qquad [5\text{-}2]$$

and differentiating equation [5-2] twice with respect to time, one gets corresponding relationships for the velocity and acceleration of the contraction:

$$\dot{L}(t) = \frac{1}{\tau_F} e^{-(t/\tau_P)}[L(\infty) - L_{op}] = \frac{1}{\tau_F}[L(\infty) - L(t)] \qquad [5\text{-}3]$$

$$\ddot{L}(t) = -e^{-(t/\tau_F)}\big[L(\infty) - L_{op}\big]\frac{1}{\tau_F^2} = -\frac{1}{\tau_F^2}\big[L(\infty) - L(t)\big]$$

$$= -\frac{1}{\tau_F}\dot{L}(t)$$

[5-4]

Since $L(t)$ decreases with increasing t for an isotonic contraction, $L(\infty) < L(t)$ and so the velocity of contraction defined by equation [5-3] is negative, which further connotes a concentric contraction. Furthermore, observe that the rate of shortening, $\dot{L}(t)$, has its maximum value, $\frac{1}{\tau_F}[L(\infty) - L(0)]$, at (or at least very shortly after) the start of contraction, when $L(t) = L_{op}$, and that this rate reduces to zero at the end of shortening, when $L(t) = L(\infty)$. Thus, the *rate* of shortening of muscle fibers varies directly with the *amount* of shortening yet to be accomplished -- a parabolic effect characteristic, among other things, of diffusion phenomena.

Although striated skeletal muscles can contract at maximum speeds up to *ten times* their resting length per second, the more common contraction velocities rarely exceed 6 and 2 fiber lengths per second, respectively, for fast and slow human skeletal muscle fibers (Faulkner, et al., 1986). Moreover, under no-load, isolated *in vitro* conditions, this excitable tissue can shorten down to 25% of its resting length. Putting this information into equation [5-3], one concludes that, *at most*:

$$\dot{L}(t)_{max} = -10L_{op}/\text{sec} = \frac{1}{\tau_F}[0.25L_{op} - L_{op}],$$

from which, $\tau_F = 0.075$ seconds $= 75$ milliseconds. This is a reasonable order of magnitude for an isotonic twitch time constant *in vitro*. However, as discussed earlier in this text, such measurements are somewhat artificial because in real life muscles do not exhibit such idealistic behavior. Indeed, even under light loading, connective tissue and surrounding tethering effects prevent any given muscle from shortening down to more than 30 - 40% of its resting length, and under loaded conditions the extent and velocity of contraction drop off dramatically. Intact muscle, for example, shortens maximally to only 60% of its rest length when contracting near maximum capacity. To quantify this somewhat, let us turn our attention to the energetics of muscular contraction.

****

Problem 5-1: For $L(\infty) = 0.25L_{op}$, and $\tau_F = 75$ milliseconds, derive a set of kinematic relationships for displacement, $\dfrac{L(t)}{L_{op}}$, velocity, and acceleration as a function of time, respectively. Plot these functions on rectilinear graph paper and label properly.

****

Energetics of Muscular Contraction

From measurements of heat production in muscle, it has been determined that the total energy involved in the process of contraction includes the effort expended in getting the contractile architecture to function plus the work done by the muscle. Basically, the energy necessitated to cause the contractile architecture to function is *internal work* (strain energy or strain of deformation plus viscous resistance to deformation), which is dissipated as longitudinal and transverse strains associated with overcoming internal muscular and viscous resistance. These may be quantified by referring back to Nubar's constitutive relationships for muscle. Thus, let the total strain energy, ΔU, be written as the sum of two parts: one, ΔU_1 arising from the longitudinal strains, and the other, ΔU_2, resulting from the transverse strains:

$$\Delta U = \Delta U_1 + \Delta U_2 \qquad [5\text{-}5]$$

Strain Energy Due to Longitudinal Deformation

If f is the tensile force required to deform a muscle fiber, and $d\ell$ the corresponding longitudinal deformation taking place during a contraction, then the strain energy associated with the given contraction is defined by:

$$\text{Longitudinal Strain Energy} = \int f \, d\ell \qquad\qquad \textbf{[5-6]}$$

For simplicity, suppose the contractile force in the muscle fiber is constant (isotonic) and equal to some "average" value, $\frac{f}{2}$. That is to say, if the muscle fiber is initially free of stress ($f = 0$), and if we assume, for simplicity, that the force which is ultimately manifest in the tissue increases linearly from zero until it attains its maximum (twitch or tetanic) value, f, then the "average" force acting on the fiber *while* it is undergoing deformation can be approximated by some constant (isotonic) value, $\frac{f}{2}$. This is essentially the same as assuming P to be constant in equations [3-40]-[3-46], and the linearized average, $\frac{f}{2}$, is used just to simplify the mathematics at this point without significantly disturbing the physics of the problem. Then, equation [5-6] becomes $\frac{f}{2} \Delta\ell$ per fiber, and the strain energy, $\Delta U_1{}^{(x)}$, in the ring of fibers located a distance x from the axis of the muscle is given by:

$$\Delta U_1{}^{(x)} = \underbrace{\frac{f}{2} \Delta\ell \frac{1}{dx}}_{\substack{\text{strain energy} \\ \text{per unit length} \\ \text{circumferentially}}} \quad \text{times} \quad \underbrace{2\pi x}_{\substack{\text{circumferential} \\ \text{length}}}$$

$$= \frac{f}{a} \frac{\pi (dx)^2}{4} \pi \frac{\Delta\ell}{dx} x = \frac{\ell \pi^2 L^2 f \Delta\ell}{4a\ell} \beta \, d\beta$$

[5-7]

where: $f = \frac{f}{a} a$, $a = \frac{\pi}{4}(dx)^2$, $x = L\beta$, and $dx = L \, d\beta$. Substituting into equation [5-7] equations [2-9] for ℓ, [2-16] for $\frac{\Delta\ell}{\ell}$, and [2-18] for $\frac{f}{a}$, expanding the result with the further simplifying assumptions that α and β are small enough so that terms of order α^2 or β^4 and higher, or combinations thereof may be neglected, and realizing that $E_2 << E_1$, $x = L\beta$ and $\alpha L = \Delta L$, leads to:

$$\Delta U_1{}^{(x)} = \frac{\pi^2 L^2}{4} E_1 \Delta L \left[2Q\beta^3 + \alpha\beta + \frac{8}{3}\alpha\beta^3 \right] d\beta$$

[5-8]

Integrating equation [5-8] from $\beta = 0$ to $\beta = \dfrac{D}{2L}$ gives the following:

$$\Delta U_1 = \frac{\pi}{8} AE_1\Delta L\left[\alpha\left(1 + \frac{D^2}{3L^2}\right) + \frac{QD^2}{4L^2}\right] \qquad [5\text{-}9]$$

where, $A = \dfrac{\pi D^2}{4}$. Now, from the definition of Q (see equation [2-16]) and N (see equation [2-13]), plus the neglect of terms of order α^2 and higher, and some algebraic rearranging, one may write:

$$Q = \frac{8}{3}\left\{q_o(2 + q_o) - \alpha[2 + q_o(2 + q_o) - 2r_1(1 + q_o)]\right\},$$

which, when substituted into equation [5-9], leads to the result:

$$\Delta U_1 = \frac{\pi}{8} AE_1\Delta L\left\{\alpha\left[1 + \frac{D^2}{3L^2}\right] + \frac{D^2\alpha}{4L^2}\frac{8}{3}\left[\frac{q_o}{\alpha}(2 + q_o) - 2\right.\right.$$
$$\left.\left. - q_o(2 + q_o) + 2r_1(1 + q_o)\right]\right\} \qquad [5\text{-}10]$$

Let: $r_4 = \dfrac{\pi}{12}(2 + q_o)q_o$, and,

$$r_5 = \frac{\pi}{12}\left[\frac{3}{2} + (2 + q_o)q_o - 2r_1(1 + q_o)\right].$$

Then, equation [5-10] becomes:

$$\Delta U_1 = \frac{\pi}{8} AE_1\Delta L\alpha\left[\left(1 + \frac{D^2}{3L^2}\right) + \frac{D^2}{4L^2}\frac{8}{3}\frac{12}{\pi}\left(\frac{r_4}{\alpha} - r_5 - \frac{\pi}{24}\right)\right]$$

Finally, after further simplification, the strain energy due to longitudinal deformation may be written:

$$\Delta U_1 = E_1 A\Delta L\alpha\left[\frac{D^2}{L^2}\left(\frac{r_4}{\alpha} - r_5\right) + \frac{\pi}{8}\right] \qquad [5\text{-}11]$$

Note in equation [5-11] that for an isometric contraction ($\Delta L = 0 = \alpha$), the strain energy, ΔU_1, due to longitudinal deformation also reduces to zero. Thus, ΔU_1, corresponds to the work done *on* muscle tissue to get it to deform by an amount ΔL (like compressing a spring), and represents physically the strain energy associated with *generating* a force, F, at the tendons. That is to say, ΔU_1, also known as the *shortening strain-energy heat*, accounts for the energy required to overcome *internal* viscoelastic resistance in the tissue during an *isotonic twitch*. In that sense, it is contraction energy over and above the heat of activation (see later), or the maintenance heat (see later); and it does not include any net *external* useful work done *by* the muscle as it mechanically moves a resistance F through some displacement ΔL. Such work involves an *additional* expenditure of energy, as described later.

Strain Energy Due to Transverse Deformation

For simplicity, suppose the muscle is considered to be a cylinder of length, L, and diameter, D, which, as a result of some lateral force or pressure distribution, G^*, (force per unit circumferential area) deforms transversely (radially in the Poisson sense) to some new diameter, $D + \Delta D$. Then the lateral strain energy, ΔU_2, may be written approximately as the product of the pressure G^* (assumed to be constant) and the change in volume of muscle, $\pi D \Delta D L$:

$$\Delta U_2 = G^* \pi D \Delta D L \qquad [5\text{-}12]$$

After some algebraic manipulation of equation [5-12], the energy of transverse strain may be related to the variation of the thickness of the muscle by the expression:

$$\Delta U_2 = G A \frac{D}{L} \Delta D, \qquad [5\text{-}13]$$

in which G denotes a pressure factor equal to G^* scaled by the quantity $4\left(\frac{L}{D}\right)^2$, and A is the cross-sectional area of the muscle, $\frac{\pi D^2}{4}$.

****

Problem 5-2: Starting, with equation [2-17] derived in Problem 2-5 for $\frac{D'}{D} = \frac{D + \Delta D}{D}$, and neglecting terms of order q_o^2, $q_o\alpha$, α^2 and higher, use the definitions of N (see equation [2-13]), A_3 (see equation [2-15]), and Q (see equation [2-16]), to show that:

$$\frac{\Delta D}{D} = \alpha + \frac{Q}{4}\left[\frac{3}{4} + \frac{D^2}{3L^2}(r_1 + 2r_2\alpha) \right]$$

Then, further neglecting the terms of order $\left(\frac{D}{L}\right)^2$ and above, and re-placing Q by its value derived to order α from equation [2-22], show that the variation in thickness of the muscle can be written approximately by the equation:

$$\Delta D = \frac{3L^2}{D}\left[\frac{2F}{\pi A E_1} - \frac{\alpha}{2} \right] \qquad \text{[5-14]}$$

****

Substituting equation [5-14] into equation [5-13] yields the following sim-plified relationship for the strain energy due to transverse deformation:

$$\Delta U_2 = 3GAL\left[\frac{2F}{\pi A E_1} - \frac{\Delta L}{2L} \right] \qquad \text{[5-15]}$$

Total Energy of Contraction

Substituting equations [5-11] and [5-15] into [5-5], one can write finally, for the total internal *strain* energy of deformation:

$$\Delta U = \frac{6FGL}{\pi E_1} - A E_1\left[\frac{3}{2}\frac{G}{E_1} - \frac{D^2}{L^2}r_4 + \alpha\left(\frac{D^2}{L^2}r_5 - \frac{\pi}{8} \right) \right]\Delta L \quad \text{[5-16]}$$

Equation [5-16] can be put in the form:

$$\Delta U = H + B\xi \qquad \text{[5-17]}$$

where: $H = \dfrac{6FGL}{\pi E_1}$,

$$B = AE_1 \left[\frac{3}{2} \frac{G}{E_1} - \frac{D^2}{L^2} r_4 + \alpha \left(\frac{D^2}{L^2} r_5 - \frac{\pi}{8} \right) \right], \text{ and,}$$

$$\xi = - \Delta L = - [L_{op} - L(\infty)].$$

If to equation [5-17] is added the *external* useful mechanical work, $F\xi$, that the muscle does as it contracts isotonically, the *total* will represent the amount of energy liberated by the chemical reactions associated with contraction, or, the total *contraction heat*, h:

$$h = H + a_1 \xi \qquad\qquad [5\text{-}18]$$

where: $a_1 = B + F$.

Interestingly, equation [5-18] is in the same *form* as one suggested by A. V. Hill (1938, 1956, 1960) for the energy liberated during muscular contraction -- although there is yet not enough evidence to verify that there is, indeed, a one-to-one correspondence between the terms of Hill's equation and those of equation [5-18]. Nevertheless, both equations suggest that the total heat of contraction consists of two parts: a "heat of activation," H, and a "heat of shortening," $a_1 \xi$. The heat of shortening, as can be seen from the definition of a_1 in equation [5-18], B in equation [5-17], the second term on the right of equation [5-15], and ΔU_1 in equation [5-11], includes a *longitudinal*-strain-energy shortening heat (ΔU_1), a *transverse*-strain-energy Poisson-like heat $\left(\frac{3}{2} GA\xi \right)$, and the work done ($F\xi$) by the muscle during an isotonic twitch. This energy of *shortening* increases with load (i.e., the external resistance against which the tissue is contracting) for a *given* amount of shortening -- a phenomenon known as the *Fenn Effect* after the individual who first described it. The increase is due primarily to the external work term.

In a purely *isometric* twitch contraction ($\xi = 0$) only the heat of activation appears and it is dissipated with no external work being done by the muscle. Moreover, if a muscle is in a state of *tetanic* contraction, having already shortened against an external load, and being *kept* in this shortened condition, then H corresponds to the energy required to *keep* that muscle in its contracted state, continuously supporting the external load in a *given* position.   In this case, the heat of activation for an isometric tetanus becomes the "maintenance heat."   That is to say, the *maintenance heat* is roughly the *sum* of the activation heats corresponding to each successive stimulus that brings a muscle progressively through a series of isotonic twitches to a state of isometric tetanus at some specified length -- i.e., Maintenance Heat $= \Sigma H_i$, $i = 1$ to the total number of stimuli leading to an isometric *tetanus*, where *each* individual H_i corresponds to an isometric *twitch*.   *During* the sequence of successive isotonic contractions that bring the external load to this given position, the energy expended by the muscle includes not only a heat of activation, but also the external *work* done on the moving load and a viscoelastic dissipative shortening heat as well, the latter two comprising the quantity $a_1\xi$.

In his classic studies in muscular contraction, Hill showed that, whereas the rate of release of maintenance heat varies in successive time intervals of a maintained isometric tetanus, H is *nearly* constant *per unit of contraction time*.   This point may be elaborated upon further if one assumes, for the moment, that there *is* a parallel between the value of H defined in equation [5-17] and the corresponding maintenance heat defined by Hill.   Then, denote the time rate of change of the numerical ratio $\dfrac{G}{E_1}$ by $\dot{r}_6$ so that, for duration Δt of the tetanic contraction,

$$\frac{G}{E_1} = \dot{r}_6 \Delta t.$$

The quantity H can thus be written:

$$H = \frac{6FGL}{\pi E_1} = \frac{6}{\pi}\,\dot{r}_6 \Delta t\, FL,$$

and, according to Hill's hypothesis, $\dfrac{H}{\Delta t} = \dfrac{6}{\pi} FL\dot{r}_6 \simeq$ constant for an isometric tetanus, where $F = P$, the isometric (maximum) tension that can be developed by a muscle of length $L = L_{op}$.   In fact, Hill found that the maintenance heat rate at 0°C could be approximated by the constant value:

$$\frac{H}{\Delta t} = \frac{6}{\pi} PL_{op}\dot{r}_6 = 0.325 \frac{PL_{op}}{3} \frac{\text{gram - cm}}{\text{sec}}$$

[5-19]

per gram of muscle

where P is expressed in grams, L_{op} in centimeters and $\dot{r}_6$, in reciprocal seconds. Solving equation [5-19] for $\dot{r}_6$, one gets $\dot{r}_6 = 0.0567$, from which G, and hence G^* may be determined for a given contraction situation, i.e., D, L, E_1 and Δt (see below). Equation [5-19] can also be written as:

$$\frac{H}{\Delta t} = 2.5392 \times 10^{-6} PL_{op} \frac{\text{cal}}{\text{sec}}$$

[5-20]

per gram of muscle

and we note that $\frac{H}{\Delta t}$ decreases with shortening, i.e., with L_{op} or L for a given muscle tension. The maintenance heat rate also varies almost exponentially with temperature. As the temperature increases from 0°C to 37°C (body temperature), the rate of release of maintenance heat increases by about an order of magnitude.

As indicated earlier, the total potential energy lost by a muscle during an isotonic contraction includes not only the heat of activation, but also a heat of shortening which can be divided into a fraction appearing as external work and a fraction lost as deformation heat. The fraction dissipated was previously defined as $B\xi$, so that B corresponds to the fraction of potential energy lost to internal deformation per centimeter of shortening (or per unit length of shortening) at any *given* load. The quantity B has units of force and, in general, depends on the load, F. Again referring to the studies of Hill, he found that B varied from a minimum value of zero under isometric conditions (where $F = P$, $L = L_{op}$, $\xi = 0 = \alpha$ and *no* work is done to deform the tissue), to a maximum value equal to nearly one third of the maximum isometric contractile force, P, under no-load conditions ($F = 0$, $L \simeq 0$, $\alpha \simeq 1$, $\xi \simeq L_{op}$ and *all* of the work goes just into deforming the tissue). Thus,

$$0 < B < \frac{P}{3}.$$

Going one step further, Hill also observed that the variation of B with F is very nearly linear as F decreases to about $\frac{1}{3} P$ and thereafter stays relatively constant as F continues to get smaller. Therefore, one may write further:

$$B = \frac{1}{2}(P - F), \quad \frac{P}{3} \leq F \leq P, \text{ and,}$$

[5-21]

$$B \simeq \frac{P}{3} = \text{Constant}, 0 \leq F < \frac{P}{3}$$

From the definition of B given in equation [5-17], it is apparent that the lateral pressure distribution function, G, which is like a "Bulk Modulus of Elasticity" for the tissue, will also be a function of F, the external load on the muscle, during an isotonic contraction, since,

$$G = G(B, \alpha) = G[B(F), \alpha]$$

for a given muscle. In particular, if:

$q_o = 0.20 \qquad r_1 = q_1 - p_1(1 + q_o) = -0.03$

$p_1 = 0.40 \qquad r_4 = \frac{\pi}{12}(2 + q_o)q_o = 0.12$

$q_1 = 0.45 \qquad r_5 = \frac{\pi}{12}\left[\frac{3}{2} + (2 + q_o)q_o - 2r_1(1 + q_o)\right] = 0.53$

$\left(\dfrac{D}{L}\right) = 0.20$ and $E_1 = 10^8$ dynes/cm^2, then, for

$\alpha = 0$, $B = 0$, $F = P$: $G = 3.2 \times 10^5$ dynes/cm^2, and, for

$\alpha = 1$, $B = \dfrac{P}{3}$, $F = 0$: $G = \dfrac{2}{9}\dfrac{P}{A} - 1.09 \times 10^6$ dynes/cm^2.

If we combine the results above with those obtained previously for an isometric contraction, we conclude that the analysis is self-consistent for a time interval, Δt of order 0.10 seconds or less. That is, Nubar's theory can be reconciled with the experimental findings of Hill, at least in the isometric case, $\alpha = 0$, if:

$$\frac{G}{E_1} = \frac{0.0032 \times 10^8}{10^8} = \dot{r}_6 \Delta t = 0.0567 \, \Delta t,$$

which yields: $\Delta t = 0.06$ seconds. This is not an unreasonable result when viewed in terms of the limitations of both the nonlinear elastic model for muscle and the experimental arrangement used to characterize its isometric behavior. The implication, therefore, is that there *may be* some direct analogy between equation [5-18] and the corresponding one proposed by Hill. Certainly, the matter is worthy of further investigation.

To summarize, the total contraction heat, h, for striated skeletal muscle, can be written as:

$$h = H + (B + F)\xi \tag{5-22}$$

where: $H = H(F, G, L)$ as per equations [5-17] and [5-20],

$B = B(F, G, L, D)$ as per equations [5-17] and [5-21], and the quantity $B + F$ amounts (on the average) to some 350 gram-centimeters (0.0082 calories) per cm² of muscle cross section, per cm of shortening. This sum tends to be somewhat independent of load for small loads.

Various estimates have shown that h accounts for only about 29% of the total energy expended during the contraction, relaxation and recovery phases of an isotonic twitch cycle. This 29% however, translates on the average into some 5×10^{-3} gram calories (2×10^{-2} Joules) of heat energy per gram of muscle, and it contributes to the noticeable rise in temperature that accompanies contraction.

The heat produced during the relaxation phase of muscular activity accounts for an additional 16% of the total heat generated and it is nearly equal to the potential energy stored by the contracting loaded muscle.

In an isometric contraction, this heat is, for all practical purposes, equal to zero in that the muscle gains no potential energy of shortening.

The remaining 55% of the total heat expenditure is associated with events that occur during the period of recovery. Such events take place rather slowly and are concerned with the thermodynamics of the series of chemical reactions that cause Adenosine Triphosphate, Phospho-creatine, Glucose and Adenosinediphosphate to be resynthesized with the release of waste products.

The "Fundamental Equation of Muscle Contraction"

Recall that the heat of shortening for muscular contraction is written as $(B + F)\xi$. Differentiating this expression with respect to time for an isotonic $[F = \text{constant}, \ B(F) = \text{constant}]$ contraction gives:

$$(B + F)\frac{d\xi}{dt} \equiv (B + F)v \qquad\qquad [5\text{-}23]$$

where $v = L$ is the velocity of contraction (assumed constant for a given F). Now, the general form of equation [5-21], together with additional experimental findings suggest that the rate at which shortening energy is released when a muscle contracts under load F can be approximated by an expression of the form: $a_o(P - F)$, where P represents the maximum isometric tension and a_o is a constant of proportionality. This turns out to be a fair approximation, particularly for loads less than $\frac{P}{2}$. Thus, with the identity [5-23], one can write:

$$(B + F)v = a_o(P - F) \qquad\qquad [5\text{-}24]$$

Recalling further that the velocity of contraction is maximum under no-load conditions we can solve for a_o from equation [5-24]. Thus, with $B = \frac{P}{3}$ (see equation [5-21]) and $F = 0$,

$$\frac{P}{3}\,v_{\max} = a_o P,$$

from which:

$$a_o = \frac{v_{max}}{3} \qquad [5\text{-}25]$$

For more realistic loading conditions *in vivo*, and for most muscles, $\frac{a_o}{v_{max}}$ is more generally in the range $0.15 < \frac{a_o}{v_{max}} < 0.25$ (McMahon, 1987), so this value of 0.33 is definitely a light-load, in vitro idealization. Nevertheless, for illustrative purposes, we may substitute equation [5-25] into equation [5-24], expand, and perform some algebraic manipulation to get the result:

$$(B + F)\left(\frac{v}{v_{max}} + \frac{1}{3} \right) = \frac{1}{3}(P + B). \qquad [5\text{-}26]$$

If one assumes that B is relatively constant for light to medium loads and P is a characteristic constant for a muscle of given length (see Figure 2-3), then equation [5-26] is in the form of a hyperbola, $a_1 b_1 = c_1 = $ constant, where:

$$a_1 = B + F = \text{Independent variable,}$$

$$b_1 = \frac{v}{v_{max}} + \frac{1}{3} = \text{Dependent variable, and,}$$

$$c_1 = \frac{1}{3}(P + B) = \text{Constant.}$$

Equation [5-26] is a power equation (force times velocity) which has been termed the "fundamental equation of muscle contraction." To illustrate the hyperbolic nature of this equation let $B = \frac{P}{3}$ for light loading to get, as an example,

$$\left(\frac{F}{P} + \frac{1}{3} \right)\left(\frac{v}{v_{max}} + \frac{1}{3} \right) = \frac{4}{9} \qquad [5\text{-}27]$$

Equation [5-27] is shown graphically in Figure 5-1, where nondimensional velocity, v/v_{max}, is plotted against nondimensional load, F/P.

Although the hyperbola is asymptotic to the lines $\frac{F}{P} = -\frac{1}{3}$ and $\frac{v}{v_{max}} = -\frac{1}{3}$, the only region that is of significance here is that below $\frac{F}{P} = 0.5$ (since only light loading has been assumed) and above $\frac{F}{P} = 0.0$ (since negative loading has no physical meaning within this context -- i.e., muscles cannot "push"). Note further that although certain mechanisms such as the Inotropic Effect can act to move the curve up or down, or to the left or right to new asymptotic values, the basic hyperbolic behavior illustrated remains essentially the same as long as the muscle is *shortening*, i.e., undergoing a *concentric contraction* (above the line $v/v_{max} = 0$ in Figure 5-1), wherein the muscle does *positive work*. In an eccentric contraction (when the muscle does *negative work*) -- i.e., as the curve in Figure 5-1 crosses the zero-ordinate axis and begins to go negative at $F/P = 1.0$ -- the slope of the velocity-force relation, for small lengthening velocities, is suddenly found to become some six times less steep than it was for small shortening velocities (the curve flattens out as it crosses the axis). Furthermore, rather than becoming asymptotic to some negative v/v_{max} axis, this curve, when it reaches the abscissa $F/P = 1.8$ at this flattened, nearly linear slope, now seems to plateau near this value, and remain constant for a while (McMahon, T. A., 1987).

The relative insensitivity of F/P to v/v_{max} when a muscle is forced to lengthen at moderate velocities near $F/P = 1.8$ is called muscle *yielding* (ibid.). At even higher velocities of lengthening, the force may actually drop below the corresponding value of P appropriate for the instantaneous muscle length. That is, the force-velocity curve may actually start *back* towards $F/P \rightarrow 0$ as v continues to increase and the actomyosin architecture becomes essentially nonfunctional.

Equation [5-27] and the corresponding Figure 5-1 imply that muscle power is effectively constant in the sense that the product of force times velocity is invariant. This means that the velocity of muscular contraction is inversely proportional to the load against which it contracts. In fact, this velocity drops dramatically to only 20% of its no-load value as F increases to 50% of the maximum isometric tension, P. Therefore,

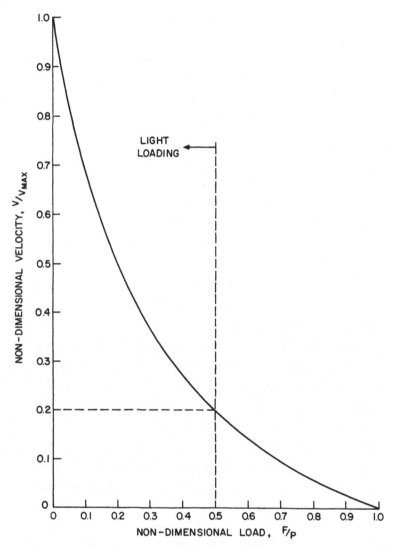

Figure 5-1 The "Fundamental Equation of Muscle Contraction," Describing The Kinetics (Force vs. Velocity) Of An Isotonic, Concentric (Positive Velocity) Contraction.

we again see that expressions such as "fast twitch" or "slow twitch" muscle fibers are only relative from a physiologic point of view, at least in terms of speaking about time-constants for the contractile behavior of such fibers. The "time-to-peak" for fast twitch fibers may, indeed, be much shorter than that for slow twitch fibers -- *relatively* speaking -- but the *absolute* time scales involved depend very much on muscle loading, tethering, mass, fibrous connective tissue content and other variables which are difficult to account for in isolated laboratory preparations. It is not surprising, therefore, to find that τ_F increases with load (see discussion on pages 124-127) and deviates by as much as two orders of magnitude from values obtained in isolated muscle experiments.

Moreover, in such experiments, muscle power has been found *not* to be constant, but to vary *also* with the speed of contraction in a somewhat parabolic manner almost identical to Figure 2-3, where Φ could be replaced as an ordinate by power; α could be replaced as an abscissa by essentially its derivative, which is velocity of contraction; and the curve could be shifted to the right so that it starts at (0, 0). The peak power of $0.096 P v_{max}$ is then found to correspond to a contraction velocity $v = 0.309 v_{max}$, for which the isotonic force generated is $0.309 P$, if $a_o = 0.25$ (McMahon, 1987).

****

Problem 5-3: From equation [5-27], derive an equation for the mechanical power, Fv, produced by a shortening muscle and plot the nondimensional power, $\dfrac{Fv}{P v_{max}}$ vs. $\dfrac{v}{v_{max}}$ for $0 \le \dfrac{v}{v_{max}} \le 1$. From your results, what is the peak power, and for what velocity and corresponding isotonic force does it occur?

****

Physically, the inverse relationship between muscle tension and velocity of contraction has been attributed to two main causes. A major reason seems to be the inability of the tissue to generate successively equal values of tension as the cross-bridges in the contractile elements break and then reform in a shortened condition. Recall that this behavior was discussed in Chapter 2 and is illustrated in Figure 2-3. Essentially, this figure and Figure 5-1 are analogous in that the derivative with respect to time of the abscissa axis, α of Figure 2-3 (which derivative can be clearly seen to decrease with increasing Φ up to $\Phi = 0.5$) is related to the ordinate axis, $\frac{v}{v_{max}}$, of Figure 5-1 and the ordinate axis, Φ, of Figure 2-3 is related to the abscissa axis, $\frac{F}{P}$, of Figure 5-1. The physical reasoning developed to explain the behavior illustrated in Figure 2-3 can thus be applied with equal validity to account at least partially for the corresponding behavior shown in Figure 5-1.

Furthermore, one can see that as the velocity of contraction gets progressively faster and faster, so do the Actin myofilaments slide past the Myosin filaments at steadily increasing speeds. There is thus less and less time available for the cross-bridges to "catch" and get a good "grip" on the fast-moving actin filaments in order to generate a strong pull; and where good contact *is* made at the points of attachment, the contact is broken rapidly, before a maximum pull can be established. Thus, for any *given* instantaneous length of muscle, the instantaneous contractile force that the tissue can generate is a decreasing function of the local relative velocity between its overlapping myofilaments. Expanding upon the tug-of-war illustration suggested on page 40 of Chapter 1, one may view this as being analogous to trying to grab and pull a rope which is moving by you at some given speed. In this case, your body corresponds to the Myosin backbone to which the cross-bridges -- your arms and hands -- are attached; and the rope corresponds to the actin filaments moving by you at some speed v. The faster is v, the less likely you are: (a) to intercept and get a good *grip* on the rope, because it has a tendency to "slip" through your grasp; (b) to hold on to the rope long enough and tight enough to affect a strong *pull*; and (c) to maintain contact with the rope for any significant period of time. In the limit, for a high enough speed, you may not be able to grab the rope at all ($F \rightarrow 0$ for $v \rightarrow v_{max}$).

Going one step further, however, one must also note a second effect which appears to be associated with the fluid viscosity in both the contractile elements and the connective tissue. That is, such viscosity requires internal forces to be overcome and thereby reduces the tendon force that can actually be developed to do external work. It is clear that such an effect is similar to that of viscous friction in a mechanical system, and that it can therefore be modeled as some form of fluid damper, as is done in Figure 3-1. Figure 3-5 then also helps to explain the behavior illustrated in Figure 5-1. That is, a faster velocity of contraction forces the muscle to operate in a time-scale region which falls along the portion of the curves where the viscous damper tends to dominate behavior. The result is that maximum tension never has *time* to develop at fast contraction speeds.

To conclude our discussion of equation [5-24], we should examine, at least qualitatively, some additional aspects of the force-velocity behavior of muscle under *heavy* loading. As long as the external load against which the muscle is contracting is less than the sum of the maximum isometric tension, plus passive elastic restoring forces, that the tissue is capable of generating at any given length and speed, then the ensuing velocity and displacement of the muscle do, indeed, proceed in a "positive" sense from insertion towards origin as the muscle actively contracts. This type of behavior, again, is called a *concentric* contraction and causes the muscle to do positive work in accordance with all of the physical principles which have thus far been discussed.

Now, suppose a muscle of given length is acted upon by some external force which has a magnitude exactly equal and opposite to the passive elastic restoring forces inherent in the tissue plus the maximum active contractile force that it is capable of generating. Then, obviously, an equilibrium situation will result. Assuming the muscle started out at rest, it will *remain* at rest and, by definition, the maximum active contractile force that it will be generating will be that characteristic of an *isometric* contraction. Should the magnitude of the external force increase to offset this equilibrium situation, then one of two things will happen. Either a *new* equilibrium configuration will be established, or the muscle will start to move in a direction opposite to that in which it is attempting to contract.

To establish a new equilibrium configuration, the muscle must be capable of generating a larger isometric tension at its new length, such that when added to the increased elastic restoring forces that accompany a stretching of the tissue, the two will counterbalance the increased external resistance. This, of course, will be possible so long as one is operating to the left of the maximum ordinate on Figure 2-3, which is something less than about 1.3 times the resting length of the muscle. We may refer to this as the "compensating" phase of muscular contraction (c.f., pgs. 72 and 73).

To the right of this ordinate, the tissue is in a "decompensating" stage where the maximum active *contractile* force that it can generate decreases with length. This does not mean that the *total* force in the tissue necessarily decreases (see Problem 2-8), because as Figure 2-2 clearly shows, the *passive* elastic restoring force in muscle tissue continues to rise with stretch. However, if the external resistance rises faster, or to greater values, then despite the fact that the muscle is *contracting* in a direction from insertion towards origin, its insertion is actually moving in a "negative" sense *away* from the origin. This type of behavior is called an *eccentric* contraction and is associated with the muscle doing negative work (i.e., work is being done *on* the tissue) and moving with negative velocity relative to the direction of contraction.

Because the passive behavior of the tissue continues to generate progressively larger restoring forces even as the active contractile behavior drops off to zero, one observes that for eccentric contractions (negative $\frac{v}{v_{max}}$ in Figure 5-1) the ratio $\frac{F}{P}$ actually *exceeds* unity and behaves as already described up to around a value of 1.8. Remember, though, that the total force, F, in this case is almost entirely passive, not active. In fact, we shall see in the next chapter that the *active* contractile behavior of muscle tissue tends to be *actively inhibited* (by Golgi Tendon Organs) when the force manifest in its tendons exceeds by some threshold amount the maximum isometric tension that is characteristic of some given muscle length. Before getting into this, however, let us continue with our consideration of the mechanics of muscular contraction.

Kinetics of Muscular Contraction

The fundamental power equation for muscle contraction (equation [5-24], or, for light loading, equation [5-27]), together with the kinematic relationships [5-2]-[5-4] and constitutive functions such as [2-22], [2-24], [2-27], [3-15], [3-22], [3-26], [3-28]-[3-30], [3-32], [3-41], [3-45], [4-6], [4-12], [4-17], [4-30], and [4-31]-[4-38] of Chapters 2, 3, and 4, can obviously be combined in a variety of ways to yield an arsenal of kinetic equations for muscular contraction. Each set of equations would, of course, define a specific state of the muscle -- i.e., passive, isometric, isotonic, isokinetic, nonlinear, viscoelastic, high-frequency periodic, low-frequency periodic, heavily loaded, light loaded, and so on. One must be careful, however, to combine only those expressions that are based on the *same* assumptions. That is, when an individual has a large array of equations at his or her disposal, there is always the danger that they will be handled in some arbitrary or random fashion, and that the results will therefore not be meaningful. Care must be taken, for example, not to substitute an equation such as [5-27], where v is assumed to be *constant* (isokinetic) for a given isotonic load, F, into the isotonic relation [5-3], where the velocity of contraction clearly *varies* with $L(t)$.

Also, one must keep in mind certain other anatomical and physiologic considerations that contribute in a significant way to the kinematic behavior of the tissue. For example, as has been mentioned, with each stimulation, a motor unit contracts completely or not at all (the so-called "all-or-none" response). *However*, a motor unit does not necessarily develop *maximum tension* each time it contracts; nor are *all* motor units in the tissue necessarily stimulated to contract together each time the muscle functions. That is why one observes such phenomena as graded responses, the staircase effect, summation of contractions, tetanus, and so on (see Chapter 1). The key seems to be related to how much calcium is released with each stimulation. Thus, a second muscle action potential reaching the tissue soon after the first allows *more* calcium to be released while that resulting from the first response is still active (i.e., before it has had a chance to be transported by the calcium pump back into its sequestered state in the cisternae). This, in turn, allows the muscle to generate a more *intense* contraction, and the intensity can keep increasing with each subsequent stimulation up to a tetanic state. Various estimates suggest that about 100 stimuli per second are required for complete tetanus in a fast limb muscle, while 25 to 40 stimuli per second accomplish the same result in slow fibers; and the tension developed in a tetanus is usually about *four times* that of a single twitch. Incidentally, *stretching* muscle tissue *also* facilitates the release of calcium from its sequestered state (by altering the permeability of the sarcoplasmic reticulum and cisternae membranes), which further helps to explain why muscles can generate larger forces when the contraction is initiated from a somewhat elongated state.

It has also been found experimentally that in the passive (unstimulated) state muscle fibers are stressed up progressively from the center out towards the periphery as the external tension on the muscle is gradually increased. By contrast, in the active (stimulated) state the muscle fibers are stressed-up (recruited) progressively from the periphery in towards the center as more and more muscle tension is generated. The *fastest* speeds of contraction measured for striated skeletal muscles have gone all the way up to 24 muscle lengths per second. Average forces developed are usually in the range 1.5 - 3.0 dynes/cm^2; but someone has calculated that if *all* of our muscles, containing an estimated total of 2.7×10^8 individual fibers, exerted their maximum contractile tension in the same direction, at the same time, they could develop an estimated force of at least *25 tons!* Perhaps therein lies the basis of the incredible strength exhibited by those from whom you would least expect it, in emergency situations which demand such strength. Perhaps, also, such a concentrated, coordinated recruitment of all available skeletal muscle tissue explains why those trained in the martial arts can develop such incredible strength when it is needed.

When analyzing any system, the engineer is always concerned ultimately with how efficiently the system does what it is supposed to do.

In the case of muscle, the fact that it converts stored energy into useful work makes it possible to consider it an engine and to determine its efficiency as such. However, although it sounds simple enough in principle -- i.e., efficiency is nothing more than the ratio of the useful work done by an engine to the total energy cost involved in getting it to perform such work -- the determination of the efficiency of muscular contraction is not all that straight-forward. In fact, not only is it difficult to *define* the energy cost of and net work done by contracting muscles, it is almost impossible to *measure* and/or *calculate* these variables to assess the efficiency of the overall process!

Efficiency of Muscular Contraction

The first problem that arises in calculating muscular efficiency has to do with deciding from *where* to start measuring the energy consumption required for contraction. All of our fuel starts with raw materials -- food, water and air. But a good deal of energy is expended in *getting* this fuel from the tank (stomach or lungs) *to* the engine (muscle) in a form suitable for utilization (Schneck, D. J., 1990). Strictly speaking, that energy should be considered as part of the total expended for generating a contraction -- in the sense that only a small fraction of the inherent caloric potential of the food we ingest is actually made available to the fuel cell as a source for doing useful work. Compared to the work muscles actually do, our daily caloric intake of potential energy is enormous, suggesting that the overall efficiency of the system is extraordinarily low (and indeed, it is!).

But, then again, the efficiency of internal combustion engines would *also* be quite low if it was measured relative to the effort required to get crude, unprocessed oil as it comes out of the ground, from the refinery into the automobile tank as usable gasoline. In effect, the human body has its own built-in oil refinery -- taking crude raw materials (food) and converting them into usable fuel (glycogen and simple carbohydrates). To measure its efficiency relative to the total caloric value of the food ingested might thus be somewhat impractical, perhaps even unfair for still another reason.

The problem here is complicated even further by the almost impossible task of discriminating or identifying what percentage of the total energy used for digestion, for pumping blood, for breathing, for chewing and for other metabolic processes, is *directly* concerned with getting oxygen and nutrients *specifically* to striated skeletal muscles for the *sole* purpose of generating a contraction. This type of discrete information is not easily gleaned from the continuous spectrum of processes that are intimately associated with the metabolism of the organism as a whole.

Consider further all of the energy that goes into sending a signal down an α-motoneuron to initiate the contraction process. Is this not also part of the *total* energy required for the muscle to be able to do work? And what about all of the digestive, circulatory, physiological, biochemical and metabolic processes that must precede the muscle action potential so that the somatic nervous system can indeed play *its* part in generating a contraction? Indeed, various estimates suggest that as much as 20% of resting oxygen consumption in mammalian muscle tissue may go entirely for the sole purpose of actively transporting sodium ions via the sodium pump in order to polarize the sarcolemma.

Without belaboring the point, suffice it to say that when we speak of the "efficiency" of muscular contraction, we must qualify this terminology by defining the efficiency *relative* to a certain point in the sequence of events that constitute the overall contractile *process*. We may speak, for example, of a "Gross" efficiency (which is probably on the order of a fraction of one percent) relative to the *total* caloric intake of the body; or we may define a "Net" efficiency (which is much higher) relative to the energy that a muscle expends while at rest (at the basal level muscles are relaxed and basically do no work, but they still require a certain level of metabolic activity and energy just to keep them alive); or, we may define a "Gradient" efficiency which compares the *increment* of additional energy required to the resulting increase in useful work output; or we may define a "Mechanical" efficiency as the ratio of mechanical work done (force times distance) to the total energy available in the muscle fuel cell; or we may define a host of other "efficiencies", such as "Isometric", "Thermodynamic", "Biochemical", "Aerobic", "Anaerobic", "Eccentric", "Work", "Metabolic", "Overall", "Relative", "Concentric", and "Physiologic". In each case, the ultimate quantity of interest is the work *output* of the muscle. The "input" that this quantity is being compared with is what determines the *type* of efficiency that is being considered.

Bearing this in mind, we shall consider here only the *aerobic mechanical efficiency* of muscle, defined as the product of the efficiencies of two component processes, i.e., the appearance of work as the result of the breakdown of high-energy phosphates, and the oxidative regeneration of phosphagens to replenish the first-order fuel cell components. The reader is referred to the literature for detailed descriptions of all of the other types of efficiencies that one can define.

Recall that the total contraction energy, h, for striated skeletal muscle was given by equation [5-22] as:

$$h = H + (B + F)\xi \qquad\qquad [5\text{-}22]$$

Recall further that h includes: (i) the energy associated with the *rate* of buildup of tension within the muscle (accompanied by an internal shortening and deformation of the muscle contractile elements); (ii) the energy associated with *maintaining* tension at the muscle tendons; (iii) the energy *dissipated* as heat through actual shortening; and (iv) the mechanical *work* done by the contracting fibers. Thus, we may define the efficiency of the process whereby work appears as the result of the breakdown of high-energy phosphates by:

$$e_h = \frac{F\xi}{H + (B + F)\xi} \qquad\qquad [5\text{-}28]$$

The ability of a muscle to perform useful work, $F\xi$, varies greatly with the load applied and other factors already discussed. A very light load does not make full use of the mechanical potential of the tissue and so a disproportionate amount of energy is used in simply overcoming the internal frictional resistance of the muscle itself. On the other hand, a very heavy load may cause extremely slow velocities of contraction (see Figure 5-1) which also results in low mechanical efficiency. It has been determined experimentally that the mechanical efficiency of muscle peaks at about one fifth of its no-load (maximum) contraction speed (compare this to the *power* peaking at around 30% of v_{max}). Furthermore, various estimates of the quantities included in equation [5-28] suggest that the efficiency of the production of mechanical work from phosphagen cleavage is of the order of 40% or less, which is about one and one-half times as efficient as internal combustion gasoline engines. But this is a bit misleading because as already mentioned, internal combustion engines do not have to "make" their fuel -- it comes to them in the tank ready to burn.

Thus, to be a bit more realistic, we should also take into account the efficiency, e_p, associated with the synthesis of high energy phosphagens. Recall from Figure 1-8 and previous discussions that ATP and Phosphocreatine can be synthesized either by the direct oxidation (Aerobic) of circulating glucose or stored glycogen (i.e., glycolysis), or by glycogenolysis and the subsequent (Anaerobic) reduction of Fructose Diphosphate to Lactic and Phosphoric Acids. For the present purposes, we shall examine only the *oxidative* process of phosphagen synthesis. In this case, it is known (Schneck, 1990) that the combustion of one mole of glucose yields anywhere from as little as 675,000 calories of energy to as much as 738,000 calories, which is used to manufacture a *net* 34 moles of high-energy Phosphate. Assuming that each mole of phosphagen (ATP) ultimately breaks down to release 7800 ± 500 calories of energy, the 34 moles of ATP synthesized from the oxidation of one mole of glucose would yield a usable $(7800)(34) = 265,200$ calories, at a cost of an average 706,500 calories. The efficiency of this oxidative reaction would thus be:

$$e_p = \frac{265,200}{706,500} \times 100 = 37.54\% \qquad [5\text{-}29]$$

If we now consider glucose to be the "fuel", then the *overall* efficiency of the process whereby work appears as the result of the burning of fuel would be given as the product of equations [5-28] and [5-29]. This is called the *Aerobic mechanical efficiency* of muscle, which is about (0.3754)(0.40), or some 15%. This figure is close to the average efficiency of steam engines, or the lower limit of the efficiency of gasoline engines, so we may conclude that muscle is no more or less efficient than any comparable mechanical device. In fact, the *gross* efficiency of man can vary anywhere between limits less than 10% to just over 40%, depending on the activity and the method of calculation.

The efficiency of muscular contraction is age-dependent. However, in evaluating much of the data available, deVries (1980, pages 366-367) concludes that the *decrease* in muscular efficiency with aging is rather *slight* -- perhaps dropping 2 or 3% from measured values of around 21.9% in the 20-29 age group to 19.6% in the 50-65 age group of adults. This gives a lifetime average of around 21%, which is somewhat higher than the theoretical value of 15% calculated above, but more in line with values of around 22.4% which were obtained experimentally by Komi (1986) in studies performed on muscles generating 60% of peak power during concentric "isotonic" contractions. Muscle efficiency also depends on such other factors as temperature, pH, fatigue, work *rate* (power), conditioning, and state of health, to mention just a few. So, we get back to our original statement -- although it sounds simple enough in principle, the determination of the efficiency of muscular contraction is not all that straightforward -- and it must be interpreted with extreme caution.

****

Problem 5-4: During anaerobic glycolysis, no more than 3 moles of high energy phosphate are synthesized for every mole of glucose ($C_6H_{12}O_6$) converted to Lactic Acid ($C_3H_6O_3$). If the calorific equivalent of Lactic Acid is 230 calories per gram (i.e., 230 calories of energy is released from

Glucose for every gram of lactic acid formed, see Figure 1-8), calculate the *efficiency* of the *synthesis* of phosphagen from glycolysis.
****

Problem 5-5: Of the Lactic Acid produced by the reduction of Glucose, about 80% is synthesized to Glycogen, storing energy equivalent to 33,000 calories per mole of Glucose-Equivalent-Glycogen Unit formed. This energy derives from all of the ATP generated from the oxidation of the remaining 20% of the Lactic Acid formed during Glycolysis (that is, the *combustion coefficient* of lactic acid is 0.20 as shown in Figure 1-8). Assuming that the oxidation of Lactic Acid produces energy equivalent to the oxidation of glucose (i.e., 706,500 calories per 180 grams of Lactic Acid oxidized and the same number of high-energy phosphate moles are synthesized as are per mole of glucose oxidized), calculate the efficiency of the synthesis of Glycogen from Lactic Acid.
****

Problem 5-6: If the Glucose synthesized as described in Problem 5-5 is further oxidized to yield energy for the generation of ATP, and from the results you obtained in Problems 5-4 and 5-5, what is the *overall* efficiency of ATP generation at the expense of *glycolysis*, rather than *direct oxidation*? Compare this with the efficiency of the oxidative reaction indicated in equation [5-29] and comment accordingly (i.e., *explain* your comparison).
****

References for Chapter 5

1. Adler, D., and Mahler, Y., "The Contractile Element Behaviour As Force Generator -- A Well-Defined Representation of the Contractile Element In Hill's Model," *J. Biomechanics, 12*:239-243, 1979.

2. An, K. N., Hui, F. C., Morrey, B. F., Linscheid, R. L., and Chao, E. Y., "Muscles Across the Elbow Joint: A Biomechanical Analysis," *J. Biomechanics, 14*:659-669, 1981.

3. Åstrand, P. O., and Rodahl, K., *Textbook of Work Physiology: Physiological Bases of Exercise*, New York, McGraw-Hill Book Company, 1970.

4. Boehman, L. I., and Minardi, J. E., "An Irreversible Thermodynamic Analysis of The Energy Conversion Process In An Active Muscle," University of Dayton Research Institute, Technical Report Number UDRI-TR-71-09, April, 1971.

5. Crowninshield, R. D., and Brand, R. A., "A Physiologically Based Criterion Of Muscle Force Prediction In Locomotion," *J. Biomechanics, 14*(#11):793-801, 1981.

6. DeVries, H. A., *"Physiology of Exercise for Physical Education and Athletics,"* Dubuque, Iowa, William C. Brown Company, Third Edition, 1980.

7. Elftman, H., "Skeletal and Muscular Systems: Structure and Function," In: Glasser, O., (Editor), *Medical Physics, Volume 1,* Chicago, The Year Book Publishers, Inc., pp. 1420-1430, 1944.

8. Engin, A. E., and Kazarian, L., "Active Muscle Force and Moment Response Of The Human Arm and Shoulder," *Aviation, Space, and Environmental Medicine, 52*(#9):523-530, September, 1981.

9. Faulkner, J. A., Claflin, D. R., and McCully, K. K., "Power Output of Fast and Slow Fibers From Human Skeletal Muscles," In: Jones, N. L., McCartney, N., and McComas, A. J., (Editors), *Human Muscle Power,* Illinois, Human Kinetics Publishers, Inc., 1986, Chapter 6, pgs. 81-94.

10. Hatze, H., and Geyer, J., "Myosim: A Computer Program for Simulating Myocybernetic Models of Skeletal Muscle," Republic of South Africa, National Research Institute for Mathematical Sciences, Technical Report Number NRIMS-TWISK-176, September, 1980.

11. Hatze, H., "Discrete Approximation Of A Continuous Myocybernetic Model of Skeletal Muscle," Republic of South Africa, National Research Institute for Mathematical Sciences, Technical Report Number NRIMS-TWISK-180, November, 1980.

12. Hill, A. V., "The Heat of Shortening and The Dynamic Constants Of Muscle," *Proc. Roy. Soc. London, Section B, Biological Sciences, 126*:136-195, 1938.

13. Hill, A. V., "The Thermodynamics of Muscle," *British Medical Bulletin, 12*:174-176, 1956.

14. Hill, A. V., "Production and Absorption of Work by Muscle," *Science, 131*:897-903, 1960.

15. Jones, N. L., McCartney, N., and McComas, A. J., (Editors), *Human Muscle Power,* Champaign, Illinois, Human Kinetics Publishers, Inc., 1986.

16. Komi, P. V., "The Stretch-Shortening Cycle and Human Power Output," In: Jones, N. L., McCartney, N., and McComas, A. J. (Editors), *Human Muscle Power*, Champaign, Illinois, Human Kinetics Publishers, Inc., 1986, Chapter 3, pp. 27-39.

17. Margaria, R., *Biomechanics and Energetics of Muscular Exercise*, Oxford, The Clarendon Press, 1976.

18. McMahon, T. A., *Muscles, Reflexes, and Locomotion*, Princeton, New Jersey, Princeton University Press, 1984.

19. McMahon, T. A., "Muscle Mechanics," In: Skalak, R., and Chien, S., (Editors), *Handbook of Bioengineering*, New York, McGraw-Hill Book Company, 1987, Chapter 7.

20. Nagelkerke, N. J. D., and Strackee, J., "Fitting the Hill Equation to Data: A Statistical Approach," *IEEE Transactions on Biomedical Engineering*, BME-29(#6):467-469, June, 1982.

21. Nubar, Y., "Stress-Strain Relationship in Skeletal Muscle," *Annals of the New York Academy of Sciences*, 93(Article 21):857-876, October, 1962.

22. Powell, T., "The Validity of Applying Irreversible Thermodynamics To Muscular Contraction," *Phys. Med. Biol.*, 16(#2):233-242, 1971.

23. Ramsey, R. W., "Muscle: Physics," In: Glasser, O., (Editor), *Medical Physics, Volume 1*, Chicago, Year-Book Publishers, Inc., pp. 784-798, 1944.

24. Schneck, D. J., *Engineering Principles of Physiologic Function*, New York, The New York University Press, 1990.

25. Tennant, J. A., "The Dynamic Characteristics of Human Skeletal Muscle Modeled From Surface Stimulation," Stanford University, Information Systems Laboratory, Technical Report Number TR-6303-1, NASA Report Number CR-1691, February, 1971.

26. Tucker, V. A., "The Energetic Cost of Moving About," *American Scientist*, Vol. 63, No. 4, pp. 413-419, July-August, 1975.

27. Wilkie, D. R., "The Relation Between Force and Velocity in Human Muscle," *J. Physiol., London, 110*:249-280, 1950.

28. Wilkie, D. R., "Man As A Source Of Mechanical Power," *Ergonomics, 3*:1-8, 1960.

29. Winter, D. A., *Biomechanics of Human Movement*, New York, John Wiley and Sons, Inc., 1979.

30. Woledge, R. C., and Curtin, N. A., *Energetic Aspects of Muscle Contraction*, Orlando, Florida, Academic Press, Inc., 1985.

31. Zajac, F. E., III, "The Mathematical Formulation of the Kinematic Properties Of Muscle Derived From An Experimental Investigation," Stanford University, Ph.D. Thesis, California, 1969.

Chapter 6

Control of Muscular Contraction

Introduction

Throughout the first five chapters of this book, many factors that act to control muscular contraction have already been mentioned and discussed. To the extent that they address anatomic, physiologic, neural, physical, chemical or thermodynamic variables that constitute the very nature of the tissue, itself, these control factors may be classified as *intrinsic*. Listed in Table 6-I are almost sixty such intrinsic control factors, all of which have at least been touched upon (if not discussed at some length) earlier. While the list is certainly not exhaustive, and although the factors itemized may not be entirely independent of one another, they do constitute an impressive array of constraints on muscular performance. Indeed, the fact that a very complex, intricate, interconnected succession of numerous cascading events must transpire successfully in order for a given muscular contraction to occur makes it possible for this process to be controlled at any one or more of the many sequential steps along the way.

Unfortunately, a significant draw-back of this complicated situation is that the "control" or "constraint" may become a "disease" or "pathologic condition" if it fails to function normally. Thus, corresponding to virtually every discrete step in the contractile process is an associated neuromuscular disorder. Some of these, together with the neuromuscular site at which they impede or totally obstruct the contractile pathways, are summarized in Table 6-II. Observe that six

TABLE 6–I

INTRINSIC CONTROL OF MUSCULAR CONTRACTION

A.   Some Anatomic Factors Limiting The Force That a Muscle Can Produce:

1. Total Number of Fibers and Motor Units
2. Strength of Individual Fibers and Motor Units
3. Size of Muscle (Longer Muscles Generally have more Force–Developing Units)
4. Shape of Muscle (Cross–Sectional and Longitudinal Configuration)
5. Orientation of Muscle Fibers Relative To Muscle Tendon (Fusiform, Unipenniform, Bipenniform or Multipenniform)
6. Geometric Pattern of Arrangement of Muscle Fibers Relative To Each Other (series or parallel)
7. Number of Cross–Bridges Contained in the Filaments
8. Capillary and Vascular Network Permeating the Muscular Tissue
9. External Tethering and Constraints on Tissue
10. Water (fluid) Content of Muscle; Electrolyte Concentrations
11. Amount of Connective Tissue Contained in the Muscle
12. Distribution of Various Types (Fast–Twitch, Slow Twitch, Long, Short) of Muscle Fibers Within Any Given Muscle
13. Anatomic Distribution of α–and–β–Receptors; Terminal Cisternae
14. Ratio of Thin Filaments to Thick Filaments

B.   Some Physiologic Factors Limiting The Force That a Muscle Can Produce:

1. Length–Tension Characteristics of Muscle (Nonlinear Elasticity, Strain–Hardening, Cross–Bridge Crowding, Actin–Myosin Contact Surface)
2. Visco–Elastic Characteristics of Muscle Tissue (Stress–Relaxation, Strain–Retardation, Phase Angle, Magnification Factor, Resonance, Stress–Retardation, Strain Relaxation, Hysteresis, Pre–stress, Relaxation Time Spectrum)
3. Amplitude and Frequency of Contractions
4. Time Scale of Contractions (Latent Period, Hysteresis, Phase Relationships, Refraction)
5. Force–Velocity Characteristics of Muscle (Concentric Contraction, Eccentric Contraction, Kinetics, Work, Power, Efficiency)
6. Type of Muscle (Tonic, Phasic, Kinematics, Time–To–Peak Characteristics, Rate of Shortening)
7. External Resistance (Load Against Which the Muscle is Contracting)
8. Anisotropic Characteristics of Muscle (Direction from which muscle is Loaded)
9. Age of Muscle
10. Material Properties (Density, Viscosity, Poisson Ratios, Stimulation Coefficients, Young's Moduli, Parallel and Series "Spring" Constants, Dashpot Coefficient, Various Time Constants, Relaxation Modulus, Creep Compliance, Elastic and Viscous Moduli)
11. Blood Flow Through Muscle Vasculature

TABLE 6–I (CONTINUED)

C. *Some Neural Intrinsic Control Factors in Muscular Contraction:*

1. Firing Frequency of Alpha–Motoneurons
2. Staircase Effect; Summation of Contractions
3. Graded Contractions
4. "All–or None" Phenomenon For Muscle Fiber Contractility
5. Tetanus or Tetanic Contraction
6. Recruitment of Fibers (Weber's Size Law)
7. Number of Alpha–Motoneurons
8. Refractory Period
9. Nerve Propagation Velocity
10. Excitability or Irritability of Neuro–Muscular Pathways

D. *Some Intrinsic Chemical Control Mechanisms in Muscular Contraction:*

1. Fuel Cell Stores of ATP, ADP, and Phosphocreatine
2. Aerobic (Oxygen) vs. Anaerobic Metabolism of Muscle Tissue
3. Lactic Acid Accumulation (Fatigue)
4. Calcium Concentration in Muscle Tissue Fluid
5. Electrolyte Balance (Magnesium, Phosphorus, Potassium, Sodium, Chlorine)
6. pH (Hydrogen Ion Concentration)
7. Concentration of Acetyl–Choline in the Synaptic Region
8. Chemical Reactions Associated with the Depolarization and Repolarization of the Sarcolemma, the Sarcoplasmic Reticulum, the Cisternae Membranes, and α–Motoneurons, and the Transverse Tubular Network
9. Hormones; Enzymes (Acetylcholinesterase and others)
10. Other Biochemical Constituents such as: Prostacyclin, Prostaglandins, Thromboxane, Serotonin and Various Trace Elements
11. Reactive Hyperemia (Carbon Dioxide and Oxygen Tension in the Blood)

E. *Some Thermodynamic Variables Limiting The Force That a Muscle Can Produce*

1. Temperature Effects on:
   a. Biochemical Reactions (Chemical Kinetics)
   b. Blood Flow (Vasodilatation)
   c. Viscosity of Muscle Tissue Fluid
   d. Viscoelastic Phenomena (Isometric Relaxation and Isotonic Creep with Increasing Temperature)
   e. Heat Transfer Characteristics and Energy Processes
2. Pressure
3. Enthalpy and the First Law of Thermodynamics
4. Humidity
5. Thermal Coefficients (Linear Expansion, Joule, Conduction)
6. Entropy and the Second Law of Thermodynamics
7. Heat of Activation
8. Heat of Shortening
9. Viscosity of Muscle Tissue Fluid
10. Density of Muscle Tissue Fluid

major categories of disease have been classified according to their place of attack in the physiologic system:

(i) The Brain (including such pathologic conditions as Cerebral Palsy, Athetosis, Dystonia, Parkinson's Disease, Encephalitis, Hemiplegia and Multiple Sklerosis);

(ii) The Spinal Cord (including such diseases as Poliomyelitis, Hemiplegia, Multiple Sklerosis, Amyotropic Lateral Sklerosis, Paraplegia, Quadriplegia, Spondylosis and Spondylitis);

(iii) The Motoneuron (including Peripheral Nerve Injuries, Inflammation, Degeneration and/or Compression);

(iv) The Neuro-Muscular Junction (Myasthenia Gravis being the most common affliction);

(v) The Muscle Membrane (taking into account such abnormalities as Myotonia and Muscular Fibrosis); and,

(vi) The Contractile Architecture of the Muscle Itself (including such debilitating and degenerative disorders as Muscular Dystrophy, other diseases that result in muscular atrophy, and Myositis).

Again, Table 6-II is not exhaustive by any means, but it serves to illustrate what might be called *pathologic* control of muscular contraction. Pathologic in the sense that it "controls" the contractile process by impeding it or by destroying the tissues involved. Certainly, this type of control is far from desirable and much work needs to be done in order to eliminate the progressive and degenerative nature of these horrible afflictions. The reader is referred to the literature for a more complete description of these and other types of neuromuscular pathologies.

In the present chapter our attention shall focus on still other means for controlling muscular contraction. To the extent that the processes to be discussed are not inherent characteristics of the tissue, and to the extent that they do not originate within the anatomical, biochemical, physical or physiological limitations or milieu of the musculature itself, these control mechanisms may be classified as *extrinsic*. They have great significance from an engineering point of view because extrinsic control

TABLE 6-II

PATHOLOGIC CONTROL OF MUSCULAR CONTRACTION

Disease	Neuromuscular Site Affected	Type of Affliction
Cerebral Palsy	Brain	Bilateral, symmetric, nonprogressive paralysis resulting from developmental defects in brain or trauma at birth
Athetosis, or, Dystonia	Brain (Caudate Nucleus)	Brain Lesion produces impairment of normal muscle tone leading to slow, repeated, involuntary, purposeless movements
Parkinson's Disease	Brain (Basal Ganglia)	Arteriosclerotic changes in the basal ganglia result in rhythmical muscular tremors, rigidity of movement, peculiar gait patterns, droopy posture and masklike peculiar facial expressions
Encephalitis	Brain	Inflammation of the brain may lead to paralysis, tremor and other neuromuscular disorders
Hemiplegia	Brain or Spinal Cord	Brain or spine lesions destroy upper motor neurons and lead to paralysis of the side of the body opposite to the side of the brain affected
Multiple Sklerosis	Central Nervous System —Cerebrum —Brainstem —Cerebellum —Spine	Patches of demyelinated plaques in the supporting tissue of the brain and spinal cord impede normal transmission of neural action potentials
Poliomyelitis	Spinal Cord	Inflammation of the Gray Matter of the spinal cord destroys the cell bodies of Neurons

TABLE 6–II (CONTINUED)

Disease	Neuromuscular Site Affected	Type of Affliction
Amyotropic Lateral Sclerosis ("Lou Gherig's Disease")	Anterior Horn and Descending Pyramidal Tracts of the Spinal Cord	Degeneration of anterior horn cells and pyramidal tracts leads to progressive muscular atrophy due to destruction of nerves
Paraplegia	Spinal Cord	Spinal Cord Lesions lead to paralysis of lower portion of the body and of both legs
Quadriplegia	Spinal Cord	Spinal Cord Lesions lead to paralysis affecting all four limbs
Spondylosis	Spine	This term is often applied nonspecifically to any degenerative lesion of the spine that results in disc protrusion and impairment of nerve impulse transmission
Spondylitis	Spine	Inflammation of one or more vertebrae interferes with proper transmission of nerve impulses through spine
Peripheral Nerve Injuries Neurapraxia Axonotmesis Neurotmesis	Usually the Nerve Axon	Penetrating wounds or fracture of neighboring bones can damage axons for a transient period of time (Neurapraxia), or can cause peripheral degeneration (Axonotmesis), or can completely sever a nerve (Neurotmesis) leading to paralysis
Causalgia	Peripheral Nerve	Partial Degenerative Lesions of peripheral nerves lead to intense burning pain. In severe cases, the limb affected becomes useless and the patient suffers from persistent pain

TABLE 6-II (CONCLUDED)

Disease	Neuromuscular Site Affected	Type of Affliction
Peripheral Nerve Compression —Carpal–Tunnel Syndrome —Pressure Neuritis of the Ulnar Nerve —Musculo–spiral Radial Nerve Compression	Peripheral Nerve	Arthritic changes, or frequent flexion and extension of joints, where a motoneuron passes through narrow grooves or channels, causes compression of the nerve, followed by tingling, numbness and weakness of the affected muscles
Neuritis —Neuralgia —Hyperesthesia —Parasthesia —Anesthesia	Motoneuron	Inflammation of a nerve leads to pain (neuralgia), altered sensitivity (Hyperesthesia, anesthesia), paralysis and atrophy of the affected muscular region
Myasthenia Gravis	Myoneural Junction	Lack of Acetylcholine or excess of cholinesterase at the myoneural junction prevents the proper transmission of nerve impulses to muscles
Myotonia	Muscle fiber membrane	Congenital Disease leading to tonic muscle spasm and a failure of muscles to relax normally
Muscular Fibrosis	Muscle	Abnormal Formation of Fibrous Tissue leads to myostatic contracture, wherein the relaxed muscle becomes fixed at a shorter length
Muscular Dystrophy	Muscle	Nutritional Disorders lead to progressive atrophy of muscles, beginning at the motor nerve terminals
Myositis	Muscle	Infection, Trauma or Infestation of muscle tissue results in inflammation and impaired function

processes that regulate physiologic function are among the most sophisticated feedback control systems (or servomechanisms) known. There is thus considerable academic interest in studying how they operate. But, perhaps more importantly, a thorough understanding of these servomechanisms is vital to the engineer involved in designing replacement parts for the human machine. Such prosthetic devices should be able to duplicate as closely as possible the real system that they are replacing, and one way to do this effectively is to be completely familiar with how the real system works and is controlled. Thus, we address in the sections that follow some of the major extrinsic mechanisms that control muscular contraction, and this is followed in Chapter 7 by a discussion of some general principles related to the analysis of feedback control systems, and how these are applied to a study of the major pathways concerned with the extrinsic control of muscular contraction.

Control of Muscular Contraction Through Spinal Reflexes

The Myotatic (or Myotactic, or Proprioceptive or Stretch) Reflex

In addition to inherent or "intrinsic" factors that control muscular contraction (Table 6-I), and constraints imposed by disease or malfunction (Table 6-II), there is an important class of control mechanisms that originates *outside* of the natural limitations of the tissue itself. These may be appropriately labelled "extrinsic" to the extent that they involve inputs from the central and autonomic nervous systems and from the endocrine glands. Extrinsic control is concerned with muscle length (spindle receptors), muscle tension (Golgi tendon organs), joint position (Pacinian Corpuscles and Ruffini endings), pain and general body orientation (sensory skin receptors and visual feedback), body temperature ("shivering" reflex), and other factors related to "cross-talk" among the hundreds of muscles that comprise the muscular system. In this section, our attention focuses on the important role played by muscle spindle receptors in initiating the so-called *monosynaptic reflex arc* (MSR), otherwise known as the *myotatic* or *myotactic* or *proprioceptive* or *stretch reflex*. To understand the myotatic reflex, we must first examine the anatomy of muscle spindles.

ANATOMY OF MUSCLE SPINDLES

Lying in parallel with, and interdigitated among the main, or *extrafusal (EF) fibers* located deep within the belly of striated skeletal muscles are numerous structural elements called *muscle spindles*. Depending on its function, a muscle may contain from as few as two muscle spindles per gram of muscle (typical of those generally responsible for gross movements) to as many as 30 spindles per gram (typical of those muscles that are generally involved in more complex, delicate movements). Each muscle spindle services approximately 20 to 25 EF muscle fibers in man; and contains anywhere from as few as three to as many as fifteen smaller packets of *intrafusal (IF) muscle fibers*. The fibers measure 1 to 10 millimeters in length, and the spindles are about 0.10 to 0.25 mm wide at their widest point. They taper at their ends and attach, via a thick encapsulating connective-tissue (fiber) envelope, to the sheaths of the surrounding extrafusal fibers. The pointed ends of the IF fibers attach rigidly to the connective-tissue envelope which, in turn, can be considered to be rigidly attached to the EF fiber sheaths, and this constitutes the *origin* of the tiny IF muscle fibers. Their insertion is discussed below.

There are basically two types of IF fibers: *Nuclear Bag Fibers* (one to three per spindle) which have a maximum diameter of about 25 microns, a length up to one centimeter (usually 7-8 mm), and in which up to a dozen nuclei may be crowded into the central portion of the IF fiber (hence the name, "nuclear bag"); and *Nuclear Chain Fibers* (two to ten per spindle with 4 or 5 being most common) which are so named because their nuclei, although also confined to the midportion of the IF fiber, are fewer in number and are arranged in a single file, forming a chain-like fiber that has about half the thickness (about 12 microns in diameter) and length (about 4 mm) of a nuclear bag fiber. The heavily nucleated, fluid-filled region midway between the tapered ends of the muscle spindle thus forms an outpocketing, or bulge, called the *spindle equator*, while the fibers that ultimately anchor this central portion to the EF sheaths form a contractile region on either side of the equator, which region is called the *poles* of the spindle. This configuration is illustrated schematically in Figure 6-1.

The spindle equator has lost all cross-striations and cannot contract. Instead, its nucleated mid-section houses as well stretch receptors that *respond* to changes in the length, ℓ_e, of the equator. Such changes can be passive, resulting from a generalized change in length, ℓ, of the extrafusal muscle fibers (to which the spindle is attached in parallel), or, they can be active, resulting from a more localized contraction of the spindle poles. The latter is accomplished by innervating the intrafusal fibers with their own set of as many as six motor neurons that originate in the spine, but are under the general control of the brain stem and higher cerebral centers. These spindle motor neurons are much smaller than the major efferent α-fibers (12 - 22 μ diameter) that innervate the main muscle end plate. They are, however, also efferent fibers; they are myelinated motor nerves; they have a diameter ranging from 3 to 7 microns (some investigators extend this range from 1 to 8 microns) and they are called *Fusimotor* or *γ-efferent* fibers.

The γ-motoneurons are classified according to whether or not they innervate the motor end plates of the nuclear-bag fibers, and according to their size. The larger IF motor fibers (5 - 7 microns in diameter) are called γ_1 - or γ-plate fibers because they do innervate discrete motor end plates on *both* the larger nuclear-bag IF fibers (with motor axons called $\gamma_{plate-dynamic}$ or γ_{pd}-fibers) *and* the smaller nuclear chain IF fibers (with motor axons called $\gamma_{plate-static}$ or γ_{ps}-fibers). The smaller IF motor fibers (3 - 5 μ diameter) are called γ_2 - or γ-trail fibers and they innervate *only* the smaller nuclear-chain IF fibers.

If we think of the origin of the intrafusal muscle fibers as being fixed in the sheath of the extrafusal fibers, and if we imagine the insertion of these IF fibers as being on either side of the ends of the spindle equator

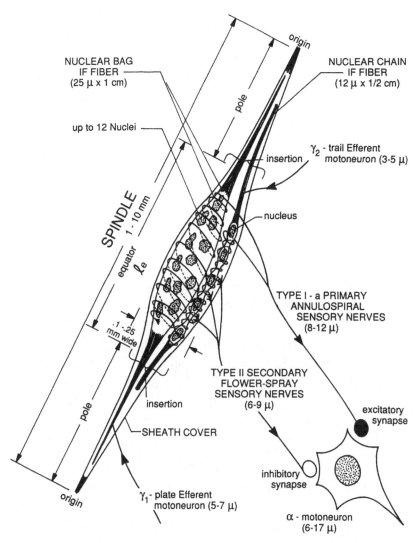

NUCLEAR BAG
IF FIBER
(25 μ x 1 cm)

NUCLEAR CHAIN
IF FIBER
(12 μ x 1/2 cm)

up to 12 Nuclei

origin

pole

insertion

γ_2 - trail Efferent
motoneuron (3-5 μ)

nucleus

SPINDLE
1 - 10 mm

equator
ℓ_e

.1 -.25
mm wide

TYPE I - a PRIMARY
ANNULOSPIRAL
SENSORY NERVES
(8-12 μ)

TYPE II SECONDARY
FLOWER-SPRAY
SENSORY NERVES
(6-9 μ)

insertion

pole

excitatory
synapse

SHEATH COVER

inhibitory
synapse

origin

γ_1 - plate Efferent
motoneuron (5-7 μ)

α - motoneuron
(6-17 μ)

Figure 6-1   Anatomy Of The Striated Skeletal Muscle Spindle (see Figure 6-1), then, clearly, if the IF fibers of the spindle poles contract -- from insertion towards origin -- they will pull on the equatorial region and thus place it in a state of tension. The degree of contraction of the spindle poles depends on the frequency of stimulation of the appropriate gamma fibers. Furthermore, contraction of the nuclear-chain fibers is rapid and almost purely elastic, whereas contraction of the nuclear-bag fibers is slow and quite viscoelastic in character. This has led investigators to postulate that the *dynamic* (phasic) behavior of striated skeletal muscle is influenced or controlled more by the activity of the nuclear bag fibers (innervated by y-plate-dynamic motor neurons), and that the *static* (tonic) control of muscular contraction is more a function of the behavior of the nuclear-chain fibers (innervated both by y-trial and y-plate-static motor neurons).

That is to say, there are basically two types of stretch receptors housed in the multi-nucleated mid-section of the spindle equator. One responds to the *amount* of stretch, and its sensitivity is associated with the activity of the nuclear chain fibers. It relays information pertaining to the length of the muscle. The other type of spindle receptor detects the *rate* of change of muscle length, and *its* sensitivity is associated with the activity of the nuclear bag fibers. In this manner, the central nervous system can *anticipate* the magnitude of the stretch, and, via the y_2 motor neurons, set the sensitivity to such stretch of the nuclear chain fibers. If the velocity of stretch is high, the motion cannot end immediately or instantaneously and therefore the system can *predict* a certain further change in length. In any event, the state of contraction of the spindle poles markedly affects the role of the muscle spindle in controlling muscular contraction, a fact about which we shall have more to say a bit later on.

Continuing, now, with the anatomy of muscle spindles, one observes that entwined around the equatorial region of this structural element are A-type myelinated nerve endings called *annulospiral receptors,* from which Group I (8 - 20 microns in diameter), sensory nerve fibers synapse back to the cell body of the α-motoneuron that innervates the motor end plate of the same muscle. There are no intermediate nerves involved in this *excitatory synaptic* pathway, hence the name *monosynaptic* reflex arc. The name, annulospiral, reflects the fact that these sensory neurons, also called *primary sensory nerves* (myelinated), coil around the nuclear-bag *and* nuclear-chain fibers in the spindle equator, forming an annulus of nerve endings that sense the state of stretch of this mid-portion of the spindle. Since these sensory nerves receive information from *both* the nuclear bag and nuclear chain fibers, their response is a function not only of muscle stretch and/or tension development, but also of the *rate* of muscle stretch and/or tension development. That is, the receptor potential increases in strength in direct proportion to the intensity and rate of change of any given disturbance.

Primary, or type I_a afferent nerve fibers have fast action potential conduction velocities -- on the order of 70-130 meters per second. They share the spindle equator with a second, slower (conduction velocity = 30 to 80 meters per second) group of neurons designated type II (5 - 12 μ in diameter). Type II, or *secondary sensory neurons, or flower-spray nerves*, are so named because of the way the nerve endings "fan out" in spray-like fashion as they course through the spindle equator. These fibers also connect back to the corresponding α-motoneuron in the spine, but they do so polysynaptically (interposing an added time delay) rather than monosynaptically (not shown in Figure 6-1), and they *inhibit*, rather than excite this α-motoneuron.

The significance of having two distinct types of sensory nerves lies in their response-to-strain characteristics, shown schematically in Figure 6-2. Note that the firing frequency (impulses per second) of both nerves increases with the state of stretch (and rate of change of stretch, not shown) of the spindle equator. However, whereas the flower-spray, type II fibers are relatively *insensitive* to stretch, at first, and *inhibit* firing of the α-motoneuron, the annulospiral, type I_a fibers are *extremely sensitive* to stretch, at first, and *excite* the α-motoneuron to fire.

The reason for this inverse behavior shall be discussed further below. For now, we conclude this anatomical description by re-emphasizing that the large fibers from the annulospiral receptors respond to the activity of *both* nuclear-bag and nuclear-chain IF muscle fibers, as well as to passive stretching of the muscle spindle, whereas the flower-spray receptors react primarily to passive stretch and to the activity of the nuclear-chain IF muscle fibers alone. Furthermore, type I_a and II nerve fibers, on entering the spinal cord, synapse not only directly with the anterior motor neurons that supply the same muscle in which the spindles are located, but also send collateral branches through the dorsal spine up to the cerebellum of the brain. The anterior synapses cause instantaneous reflex responses; the signals transmitted dorsally to the cerebellum cause more delayed cerebellar reflexes which are described briefly in the sections that follow. With these anatomical considerations in mind, then, let us examine the stretch, or myotatic reflex arc.

PHYSIOLOGY OF THE MONOSYNAPTIC REFLEX ARC

The main objective of the Myotatic Reflex Arc is to allow a muscle to maintain a *relatively constant length* by contracting in response to being stretched beyond that length. This is an important aspect of postural reflexes and balance and equilibrium considerations. In order to describe how this control is accomplished, let us assume, for the moment, that the α-motoneuron controlling the muscle in question receives *only* inputs from the annulospiral sensory nerve fibers, designated f_{I_a} impulses per second (excitatory $= +$), and from the sensory flower-spray nerves, designated f_{II} impulses per second (inhibitory $= -$). Furthermore, let the firing frequency of the α-motoneuron be simply equal to the sum of these two inputs:

$$f_\alpha = f_{I_a} - f_{II} \qquad\qquad [6\text{-}1]$$

Finally, recall (Chapter 1) that depolarization of the sarcolemma of striated skeletal muscle, followed by contraction of same, takes place only after an impulse of sufficient threshold strength is delivered to the

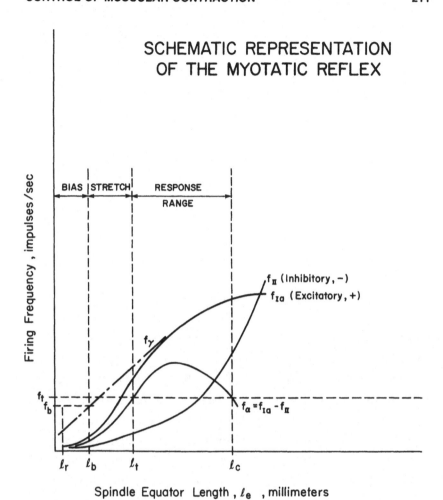

Figure 6-2 Schematic Representation Of The Myotatic Reflex Arc, As A Graph Of Sensory Nerve Firing Frequency vs. Spindle Equator Length

myoneural junction by an α-motoneuron. We shall designate this threshold firing rate as f_t, which is generally of order four cycles per second (4 Hz) for activation of the earliest and smallest motor units of a muscle. Thus, when: $f_\alpha = f_{I_a} - f_{II} = f_t$, the motor unit under the control of f_α will fire and a muscular contraction will be manifest. It has been observed empirically for reasons discussed earlier that the active *force* of contraction is directly proportional to the firing frequency, f_α. Therefore, a plot of f_α vs. muscle strain, α, may be expected to follow closely the active-tension-muscle-strain curve shown earlier in Figure 2-3 and, indeed, it does (compare with Figure 6-2).

Consider, now, a muscle motor unit that exists at some "desired" length which corresponds to a spindle equator length, ℓ_r, for which case $f_{I_a} - f_{II} < < f_t$. If we start to stretch this motor unit passively, the extrafusal fibers (to which the spindle is attached in parallel) will deform, causing a corresponding deformation of the spindle equator. In the early stages of this deformation, the firing frequency (impulses/sec) of the I_a fibers will increase dramatically, while the flower-spray type II fibers will hardly be affected. We may thus write, at first, (see Figure 6-2), $f_\alpha \simeq f_{I_a}$, so the motoneuron will fire at almost the same rate as the sensory neuron. (In reality, the minimum firing rate of the I_a afferent fibers in humans is around 15 impulses per second, but the motor unit still does not fire because inhibitory influences to be discussed later keep the *net* firing frequency of the corresponding α-motoneuron below the threshold for motor unit activation).

When the spindle equator length, ℓ_e, reaches a "threshold" length, ℓ_t, its afferent nerve fibers will exhibit a net firing rate of f_t, and, since this firing rate will be excitatory to the α-motoneuron, the latter will deliver a threshold signal to the corresponding motor unit, causing it to contract. As the motor unit contracts, however, the spindle equator will now be *decreasing* in length, shutting off the whole system. In other words, the stretch of the muscle (ℓ_e increasing) triggers the response (f_{I_a} fibers dominating), which contracts the muscle (an excitatory synapse at frequency f_t is eventually sent to the α-motoneuron), which contracts the spindle

(ℓ_e decreasing), which shuts off the response ($f_{I_a} - f_{II}$ drops below f_t) -- a true feedback control system to monitor muscle length.

Mother nature has installed a *regulator* into this system to prevent contractions from occurring when the muscle has been stretched too far. Recall from the discussion of Figures 2-3 and 5-1 that the ability of a muscle to generate an active tension is limited by the cross-bridge configuration that can be achieved. Thus, when the muscle length exceeds about 1.27 times its resting length, it begins to lose the ability to generate an active contraction of any consequence. The flower-spray sensory nerves therefore serve the function of providing inhibitory pathways that protect motor units from overload by preventing damaging contractions from taking place against strong stretching forces. That is to say, these nerve fibers begin firing at much higher frequencies when the spindle equator length (and hence, the corresponding overall muscle length) begins to exceed safe limits.

Since their effect on the α-motoneuron is inhibitory, the type II fibers seek to *prevent* a contraction from taking place if the muscle attempts to do so from too elongated a state. Indeed, note from Figure 6-2 that by the time the spindle equator length has reached the critical value ℓ_c, f_α has been reduced to f_t. Hence, for $\ell_e > \ell_c$, $f_\alpha = f_{I_a} - f_{II} < f_t$ and the inhibitory effect of the flower-spray sensory nerves is now dominating the response of the motor unit to stretch. Observe further that the net curve of f_α vs. ℓ_e is shaped remarkably similar to the curve of active muscle tension, Φ, vs. muscle strain, α, shown in Figure 2-3. As was explained in the discussion of this figure, muscle tension increases with length, and then drops off again due to anatomical considerations related to the cross-bridge structure of the actomyosin filaments. To compensate for this, and protect the muscle against overload, corresponding α-motoneuron activity first increases with stretch, and then drops off again due to the cumulative effects of excitation (I_a) and inhibition (II). How remarkably self-consistent! The region within which $\ell_t \leq \ell_e \leq \ell_c$ is called the *response range* of the Myotatic Reflex.

Going one step further, mother nature has also installed a means for fine-tuning, or controlling the *sensitivity* of this system. This is accomplished by allowing the spindle equator strain to be adjusted (or "pre-set") independently of the length of the extrafusal fibers, through the action of the gamma-motoneuron fibers. Recall that these fibers act to contract the intrafusal muscle fibers, thereby shortening the length of the spindle poles while stretching the equator. This occurs without materially affecting the overall length of the entire muscle. Referring back to Figure 6-2, suppose the stretched muscle spindle equator *starts out* at a length ℓ_b, rather than ℓ_r, where $\ell_b > \ell_r$, but, where the *rest* of the motor unit is at the same extrafusal length as before. Then, starting from this configuration, less stretch of the extrafusal fibers is required to get the spindle equator to a length ℓ_t than was the case in the previous example. In other words, this muscle is now more *sensitive* to stretch, in the sense that less displacement is required to fire the monosynaptic reflex arc. This is because the spindle equator has been "pre-stretched" by the action of the γ-motoneurons on the IF fibers, and because such action (which has a negligible effect on the length of the entire motor unit) has increased the firing rate of the I_a fibers before *anything* is done to the EF fibers themselves. In effect, the tension created by the pre-stretch excites the equatorial sensory nerve receptors (which are responsive to strain), making them "think" that the extrafusal fibers have been passively stretched, when, in fact, they have not. The result, however, is that less actual passive stretch of the EF fibers is now required to get the alpha-motoneuron to fire, and to generate a contraction of the entire motor unit.

The pre-stretch of the spindle equator is called the *bias* of this transducer. Note (Figure 6-2) that the bigger the bias, the less the passive *stretch* required to produce a contraction of the muscle motor unit ($f_\alpha = f_{I_a} - f_{II} = f_t$). In fact, if *all* of the spindles of a given muscle are biased very close to length ℓ_t, then a mere tap on its tendon, producing a very slight stretch of the muscle, will be followed by an immediate contractile response. This, indeed, would be a very sensitive muscle. There are several examples of such muscles in the human body -- one of which is the quadriceps.

The quadriceps muscle of the thigh inserts just below the knee cap into the shin bone (tibia), and this musculature is responsible for extending the lower leg at the knee. It is also innervated by many very active gamma-motoneurons that are highly excited. This gives the quadriceps a large bias, such that when it is stretched by flexing the knee, a mere tap to its tendon, where it inserts into the tibia, provides just enough additional stretch to fire the monosynaptic reflex arc -- and the leg responds by rapidly extending as the quadriceps contract. This reflex pathway is commonly referred to as the *knee-tendon jerk* (or, simply, the "knee jerk") and is but one example of several such reflexes in humans. Others are found particularly in postural muscles, which are biased to prevent excessive "sway" when gravitational disturbances act to upset balance and equilibrium. Thus, one's ability to "stand up straight" in the face of continuous gravitational influences that constantly act to "knock us down," is attributable to the monosynaptic reflex arc -- which constantly corrects for this disturbance. Interestingly, neurological disorders that affect this reflex pathway manifest themselves by increased postural sway in attempting to stand still -- which makes such sway a valuable quantitative clinical variable for assessing the extent of neurological damage.

One might add, that the gamma-system, being under the general control of higher centers in the brain, also becomes very active during periods of emotional stress and at times when the organism is in a "fight-or-flight" situation. That is, a conditioned perception of danger (fear), a distasteful or hostile situation (anger), an intense desire (such as love), and other emotional responses are transmitted through the forebrain and anterior lobe of the cerebellum to both the Diencephalic Reticular System (Brain Stem) controlling the γ-motoneurons, and the Cerebral Motor Cortex controlling the α-motoneurons. This causes the entire musculature of the body to be supersensitive, being prepared to respond instantaneously to the slightest provocation. Indeed, γ-fiber activity is among those factors that cause one to be "jumpy" when nervous, or to be "hyper-reflexive" (knees shaking) in tense situations, or even to tremble. Some diseases of the musculoskeletal system also produce hyper-reflexivity, while others suppress this response, leading to hypo-reflexivity. Moreover, since all the muscle spindles in a motor unit do not fire simultaneously when an external stretch is imposed upon them, a muscle-spindle-recruitment process occurs, in which both the magnitude and rate (velocity) of muscle stretch influence the activation rate and type of muscle spindle recruited. The reader is referred to the literature for more details.

At this point, it is important to remind ourselves that we have been discussing α-motoneurons as if they receive inputs from only the annulo-spiral or flower-spray sensory nerves attached to their own motor units. It is time, now, to get somewhat more realistic as we recall that type I_a and II nerve fibers synapse not only with their *own* alpha-motoneurons, but they also send *collateral* branches out that cause responses from *other* parts of the body, and vice versa. An examination of the knee-tendon jerk allows us to see why this is necessary, and how mother nature has further provided for every conceivable consequence of a muscular con-traction.

For example, suppose a seated individual crosses his or her legs such that the right leg is flexed over the left leg, the latter being planted firmly on the ground. Now suppose the quadriceps musculature of the right leg, henceforth referred to as the *ipsilateral extensor* (ipsilateral means on the same side), is caused to contract by tapping its insertion tendon. It would be contrary to the intent of the tendon jerk if the *ipsilateral flexors* (the hamstring muscles behind the knee and thigh bone) attempted to contract at the same time, for they would be trying to *flex* the knee while the quadriceps were trying to *extend* it. These muscle groups would thus be working against one another in an undesirable way.

In order to prevent this from happening, the I_a sensory fibers of the ipsilateral extensor send, via an intermediate neuron, an *inhibitory* impulse to the ipsilateral flexor, such that when the former contracts, the latter relaxes. By the same token, the α-motoneuron of the ipsilateral extensor *receives* inhibitory synapses from the ipsilateral flexor when *it* is contracting to flex the knee. This process, whereby when an extensor contracts, its flexor-pair relaxes, and vice versa, is called *reciprocal inhibition,* and its purpose is both clear and necessary.

In a similar fashion, the type II sensory fibers of the ipsilateral extensor, since their purpose is to *inhibit* contraction of their own muscle, send an *excitatory impulse* to the ipsilateral flexor. That is, they attempt to reinforce their efforts to prevent contraction of the extensor by seeking help from the flexor and stimulating *it* to contract instead. The hope here is that the process of reciprocal inhibition will also aid the type II fibers of the extensor. And, of course, the α-motoneuron of the ipsilateral extensor *receives* excitatory synapses (reciprocal excitation) from the type II fibers of the ipsilateral flexor when *its* spindle is attempting to prevent *it* from contracting.

To complicate matters still further, the type I_a, type II and α-fibers of the quadriceps, seeking help when necessary, send excitatory branches to the alpha-motoneurons of the ipsilateral *recruits* and *synergists,* and likewise, the α-motoneurons of the quadriceps *receive* excitatory synapses from its ipsilateral recruits and synergists through the latter's muscle spindles and α-fibers. While the smallest motor units are recruited first at an initial frequency of order 4 Hz, the next-size motor units will generally fire at frequencies ranging from 15 to 60 cycles per second.

Recruitment of motor units (as required, according to the size law) is handled directly by collaterals that branch off the alpha-motoneurons themselves, and this process is further mediated by inhibitory interneurons called *Renshaw Cells.* The purpose of these cells, which can be excited and inhibited by inputs from skin and descending impulses from supraspinal centers, is to inhibit both their own *and* the recruited motor units while they are contracting, generating what has been termed a *silent period* on the electrical record of a muscle engaged in a knee-tendon jerk. By acting as a negative-feedback loop projecting an inhibitory influence on both their originating and nearby motor neurons, Renshaw cells thus regulate the firing behavior of the motoneuronal *pool* for a given muscle. Recruitment of the motor units of an individual muscle tends to go from smaller motor units to larger motor units (Weber's Law), and activation of the fibers seems to progress from the outside of the muscle in, rather than from the inside out.

Now, so far, all that we have described involves only the *ipsilateral* side of the body. To be *still* more realistic, it must be noted that the *contralateral* side of the body, i.e., the corresponding side opposite to the one involved in the reflex response, *also* gets involved in all of this through a variety of cross-pathways, some of which we shall describe later. Suffice it to say at this point that the alpha-motoneuron of any given motor unit, of any given muscle, receives a plethora (as much as ten-thousand bits!) of input information that it sorts, prioritizes and evaluates in a matter of microseconds before the decision to contract (or not to contract) is made. The reader is again referred to the literature for more complete details, for our primary concern at the moment is directed towards establishing techniques that the engineer can use to model and analyze mathematically these very complicated reflex pathways.

Golgi Tendon Organs and the Inverse Myotatic Reflex

As the name implies, the Inverse Myotatic Reflex is just the opposite of the Myotatic Reflex. That is to say, while the main objective of the Myotatic Reflex Arc is to allow a muscle to maintain a relatively constant *length* by *contracting* in response to being stretched beyond that length, the primary goal of the Inverse Myotatic Reflex is to cause a muscle to *relax* when it is being stretched beyond the point where it can generate a contractile *force* capable of overcoming the applied resistance. Recall that when a muscle is in a "decompensating" stage (see Figure 2-3 and associated discussions) the maximum active *contractile* force that it can generate decreases with length. Thus, if it attempts to contract while in this stage, it can potentially become damaged as a result of an overload.

To protect against this happening, mother nature has installed in the tendon of a muscle a special organ in *series* with the motor units (not in parallel, like the spindles). This organ, called the *Golgi Tendon Organ,* is stimulated by *tension* on the muscle tendon (rather than by stretch), and it provides *negative* feedback to the α-motoneurons by sending to them a very strong inhibitory synaptic signal proportional to the actual tension being produced in the muscle. The intent of the Golgi Tendon Apparatus is thus to detect muscle *load,* rather than changes in muscle *length,* and to protect the tissue from being overloaded. That is to say, tendon organs are relatively insensitive to *passive* stretch because they are much *stiffer* (i.e., have a much higher "spring constant," or "Young's Modulus," and so on) than the much-more-compliant contractile elements to which they are attached in series. The latter (including the muscle spindles) thus respond to and absorb most of the passive stretch, and prevent any significant elongation of the tendinous region. However, when a muscle *actively* contracts, the contractile elements *pull* on the tendon organs, and they discharge ("fire") in proportion to the tension that is being developed. The Golgi Tendon organs are thus considered to be *active force detectors,* rather than *passive stretch detectors* (as are the muscle spindles).

Normally, one finds about one Golgi Tendon Organ for every 10 to 15 muscle fibers (this can range from as few as 3 fibers to as many as 25, originating from as many as 15 *different* motor units). There are usually slightly less of these organs in a given muscle than there are spindles (the Tendon-to-Spindle ratio varying between 1:1 and 1:3, where the tendon organs are more numerous in slowly contracting muscles); and they all lie very close to the point at which the muscle fibers insert into the tendon itself. By comparison to the muscle spindle, the 500-micron-long Golgi Tendon Organ is a relatively simple structure which sends impulses *to* the central nervous system but does not receive efferent fibers *from* the central nervous system.

Each Tendon Organ consists of numerous spraylike, thinly-myelinated, B-type, clasplike, granular nerve endings attached to the surface of a bundle of small tendon fibers, the whole being enclosed in a delicate connective-tissue capsule. The afferent fibers from these nerve endings are in the myelinated Group I (12 - 22 microns in total diameter) category and they are the fastest conducting of all the nerve fibers, having speeds of propagation that frequently reach well over 100 meters per second (range 70-130). These are designated type I_b or Group I-B fibers. The I_b fibers synapse back to the α-motoneuron of their own motor unit through an intermediate neuron within the spinal cord. This is thus a *disynaptic* reflex pathway rather than a monosynaptic pathway, as was the case for the Myotatic Reflex. The first synapse is excitatory between the sensory neuron and the interneuron; the interneuron, in turn, has a short axon with a second, inhibitory synaptic ending occurring on the alpha-motoneuron involved. Such inhibition, mediated by afferent fibers from a stressed muscle and acting on motoneurons supplying the same muscle, is known as *autogenic inhibition*.

One theory which has been proposed to explain how the Golgi Tendon Organ works (indeed how many receptors in the body work) is that when the receptor is strained (by a stretch, for instance, or by some tension), the permeability of its membrane to sodium increases. Whether this change in permeability is purely mechanical -- i.e., stretch or deformation causing a widening of minute pores in the organ membrane -- or whether some other electrochemical processes are involved is not entirely clear at this point, but the end result is the same. The nerve-cell endings become depolarized, generating what is known as a *receptor potential*. The receptor potential increases in strength in direct proportion to the intensity and rate of change of the disturbance, and it sends corresponding action potentials through the attached afferent nerve fibers to the spinal cord. Thus, the firing rate of afferent action potentials increases with corresponding increases in receptor potentials. However, if a *constant* stimulus is applied to a physiologic receptor, and this stimulus is maintained, the receptor potential (and consequently the rate of firing of action potentials) will gradually decrease -- a process called *adaptation* (Schneck, D. J., 1990).

Some receptors adapt very rapidly and are consequently sensitive almost entirely to *changes* in stimulus (i.e., they are rate-sensitive or so-called phasic-type frequency transducers as discussed earlier). Other receptors adapt hardly at all, and all gradations in between are seen (i.e., these are amplitude-sensitive, or so-called tonic-type transducers). Golgi tendon organs have the characteristics of both types of transducers. That is to say, they monitor *total* muscular force, which, as we have seen, is a function of (i) the instantaneous length of the muscle (tonic); (ii) the velocity of shortening (phasic); and (iii) the degree of fatigue (cyclic); and, (iv) they are also sensitive to the rate of change of force (phasic).

Golgi Tendon Organs, then, *inhibit* the motoneurons going to the same muscle -- just the opposite of the myotatic reflex -- hence the name, *inverse* myotatic reflex. But that is not all these Organs do. As was the case for the type II fibers of the muscle spindle, the type I_b fibers of the tendon organ also attempt to reinforce their inhibitory influence on their own (agonist) α-motoneuron by *exciting* the α-motoneuron of the antagonist pair on the ipsilateral (same) side. Again, the intent here is to get some help through the process of reciprocal inhibition and other cross-pathways to be discussed later, in an effort to prevent an active contraction of the agonist against a sensed overload. And, of course, the ipsilateral agonist correspondingly *receives* excitatory synapses from the I_b fibers of the ipsilateral antagonist.

Moreover, type I_b fibers send (and the agonist alpha-motoneuron receives) collateral branches through which the ipsilateral synergist muscle groups are also inhibited from contracting. And finally, for reasons to be discussed later, the type I_b fibers (as do the type II fibers of the ipsilateral agonist), while inhibiting their own muscle, also send an excitatory synapse to the corresponding agonist on the *contralateral* (opposite) side of the body, via neural pathways that constitute what is called *Phillipson's Reflex*. We alluded to these cross-pathways briefly toward the end of the section dealing with the Physiology of the Monosynaptic Reflex Arc, and again a couple of times in this section. They shall become clearer when we describe the Nociceptive Reflex Pathway in the next major section of this chapter.

To summarize the respective roles of the Myotatic and Inverse Myotatic Reflexes in controlling muscular contraction, we shall describe

an interesting sequence of events that involve *both* the muscle spindle and
the Golgi Tendon Organ. These events occur in a phenomenon which
has come to be known as the *Clasp Knife Reflex*.

THE CLASP KNIFE REFLEX

Consider what happens if one begins to stretch a muscle that is at rest,
and continues to do so, forcibly, regardless of the response of the tissue.
That is, suppose one generates deliberately an eccentric contraction, and
forcibly overcomes any resistance offered (actively or passively) by the
muscle. At first, a great deal of resistance would be encountered, and this
resistance would increase throughout the initial phase of stretch. This is
because, with the muscle spindle equator below length ℓ_c, and the muscle
strain less than around 0.3 (see Figure 2-3), the stretch would be taking
place within the response range of the Myotatic Reflex (see Figure 6-2),
and we would be operating in the *compensating* range of the active response characteristics of the muscle. Thus, the muscle would be actively
contracting in response to being stretched, and the person doing the
stretching would encounter resistance far above what might be expected
from purely passive viscoelastic forces.

Now if one persists and forcibly continues pulling on the tissue, two
things happen: first, the spindle equator length exceeds ℓ_c, putting the
muscle in the response range where the type II fibers begin to dominate;
and second, the Inverse Myotatic Reflex begins to come into play as
muscle tension goes beyond some one-to-two-hundred grams-force. At
this point, all active resistance to additional deformation seems to disap-
pear and the stretched muscle seems to elongate freely, offering only
passive elastic resistance. What is happening, of course, is that the
alpha-motoneurons activating this muscle are being totally inhibited from
generating any contractile response (in accordance with the mechanisms
studied thus far) and so we are effectively just pulling on a passive "rubber
band". Because this reflex phenomenon was first observed during attempts to flex forcibly the rigid limb of a decerebrate animal, and because

the resistance of the limb resembled that of a spring-loaded folding knife blade as one attempts to close it, the reflex came to be known as the Clasp Knife Reflex.

The Myotatic and Inverse Myotatic Reflexes (including reciprocal inhibition, autogenic inhibition, Phillipson's Reflex, Renshaw Cell mediation and the Clasp Knife Reflex) are extrinsic control pathways that are associated with the performance of the muscle *itself*. That is, they are directly concerned with the length of the muscle, its velocity of contraction, the force it is generating, and the number of times it has contracted in the process of carrying out a specific task consciously involving the positioning or locomotion of the joint spanned by the muscle itself. There are several other extrinsic controls (which we shall examine in somewhat less detail) that involve the musculoskeletal system, but their intent is to compensate for something *else* that is going on in the physiologic organism, rather than to position or cause locomotion per se of the involved structure.

For example, muscles are called upon to help control body temperature (by shivering). They also help the organism respond to a "flight-or-fight" situation; to painful stimulants applied to its skin; and to the efforts of the cardiovascular system to get blood back to the heart (by extravascular compression). All of these, and more, are activities that one might classify as being "peripheral" to the *main* functions of the musculoskeletal system. They are "spin-offs", if you will, that exploit the positive features of a very sophisticated force-generator. The first of these that shall be examined is called the Flexion, or Nociceptive Reflex.

The Flexion or Nociceptive Reflex Arc

At some time or other, most of us have experienced the unpleasant sensation of stepping on a tack, or putting one foot into an unexpectedly hot bath tub. The response is virtually instantaneous -- the affected foot reflexively pulls away from the source of the discomfort. This response to piercing, pinching, burning, strong electrical voltages or other sources of noxious stimulation is called the *Flexion* or *Nociceptive* (noceo is Latin for "injure" or "hurt") Reflex Arc. The flexion reflex originates in specialized pain receptors located chiefly in the skin. These receptors have C-type unmyelinated nerve endings, to which are attached either deep myelinated afferent nerve fibers less than 12 microns in total diameter (mostly of the Group A-II-β classification), or cutaneous myelinated A-III-δ or unmyelinated C-IV-δ afferent nerve fibers of diameter 1 to 5 microns. As shown in Table 6-III the classification of nerve fibers into types such as A, B, C, I, II, III, IV, α, β, γ, δ, and ε, has to do with the diameter of their respective axon (or axon plus surrounding sheath, e.g., α, β, γ, δ, ε); to whether or not the nerves are myelinated (e.g., A, B, C); to the speed with which they transmit action potentials (e.g., I, II, III, IV); to the intensity of stimulus required to generate a receptor potential, and so on (see Schneck, D. J., 1990).

The Flexion reflex involves multi-synaptic pathways that are excitatory to the flexor muscles of the affected limb. Thus, when you step on a tack, your knee joint will flex due to the reflexive contraction of the hamstring muscles, and, hopefully, your foot will be withdrawn from the source of the discomfort. The same thing will happen if you step into a scalding hot bath tub. And, as before, while your knee is flexing, the ipsilateral extensors (the quadriceps musculature) are being encouraged to relax through the process of reciprocal inhibition.

But the reflex pathway does not stop there. If you are standing, and you flex, say, your right knee, something else must happen if you are to maintain your balance. The weight of your body must shift to your left leg *and*, your left leg had better not be bending at the same time, or you will fall. Thus, to complete the picture, the afferent nerves that are responsible for the Flexion Reflex send collateral fibers to the *contralateral* side of the body, *inhibiting* this side from flexing while the *ipsilateral* side is doing so. This inhibition is accomplished by a double-barreled approach. First, the motoneurons that innervate muscles which cause flexion of the limb on the other side of the body are directly inhibited. Second, the motoneurons innervating muscles which cause *extension* of

TABLE 6—III

AXON TYPES

Fiber Type And Diameter (Microns)	A (Myelinated) 1 — 22				B (Thinly Myelinated) ≤ 3.0	C or IV (Unmyelinated) 0.3 — 1.3			
	I (Muscles) 12 — 22	II (Somatic) 6 — 12	III (Motor) 1 — 6			s.C (Sympathetic) 0.3 — 1.3		d.r.C (Dorsal Roots) 0.4 — 1.2	
	(α)	(β)	3 — 7 (γ)	1 — 5 (δ)		1 — 1.3 (δ)	0.3 — 1.0 (ε)	1 — 1.2 (δ)	0.4 — 1.0 (ε)
Conduction v (m/sec)	70 — 130	30 — 80	10 — 50	5—30	3 — 15	0.7 — 2.3	0.7 — 2.3	0.6 — 2	0.6 — 2.0
Action Potential Spike ($msec$)	0.4 — 0.5				1.2	2.0			
R^*_m	50,000 to 50 Megaohms per cm.				30,000	180,000 to 9,000 Megaohms per cm.			
C^*_m	8.9 Picofarads per cm.				≈ 200	80 to 400 Picofarads per cm.			
Absolute Refractory τ ($m\,sec$)	0.4 — 1.0				1.2	2.0			
Activation to Threshold (mv)	20 — 30				40	50			
τ^*_m	445 to 0.445 msec per cm^2				6	14.4 to 3.6 seconds per cm^2			

the contralateral limb are simultaneously *excited* (which, incidentally, further reinforces the contralateral inhibition through ipsilateral reciprocal innervation on the contralateral side). The left knee is therefore firmly "locked" in place, to take the weight of the body as the right knee flexes.

The contralateral component of the ipsilateral flexion reflex is called the *Crossed Extension Reflex*, and it illustrates an arrangement which is called *Double Reciprocal Innervation*. That is, while the agonists on one side of the body are being excited, the corresponding ones on the other side are being inhibited, and, simultaneously, while the antagonists on one side are being inhibited, those on the other side are being excited. We have alluded several times already to the role of contralateral inputs to ipsilateral performance, and vice versa. Suffice it to say, in summary, that the ipsilateral agonist alpha-motoneuron also receives:

(i) Inhibitory synapses from the contralateral agonist I_a fibers, Λ-II-β, A-III-δ, and C-IV-δ-fibers; and from the contralateral antagonist II fibers;

(ii) Excitatory synapses from the contralateral agonist I_b and II fibers; and from the contralateral antagonist I_a fibers.

Note that inhibition of the ipsilateral agonist (the hamstring muscles in our example) by the type Λ-II-β, A-III-δ, and C-IV-δ-fibers of the contralateral agonist makes it easier for the right leg to extend (i.e., helps the quadriceps musculature). This is precisely what the knee-jerk is trying to accomplish via the myotatic reflex. Thus, the contralateral input to the ipsilateral flexor aids the extensors on the ipsilateral side in carrying out the stretch reflex. This phenomenon is called *Myotatic Reflex Facilitation*, wherein the side of the body *opposite* to the one experiencing the reflex actually makes it easier for the whole process to transpire.

The Myotatic Reflex, the Inverse Myotatic Reflex and the Nociceptive Reflex are all examples of so-called *Spinal Reflex patterns*. These are basically self-contained in the sense that even with the spinal cord cut from its connection to the brain, they continue to operate. In other words, the brain and higher centers are not directly involved in the essential reflex pathways, although the cerebellum may help to mediate in some of them. There is a whole separate category of reflex responses which *are* mediated more directly through the encephalon itself and involve the musculoskeletal system. Some of these are described below.

Control of Muscular Contraction Through Higher Centers

Thermoregulation

Because the breakdown of ATP to ADP is a highly *exergonic* reaction, muscles serve as a very convenient source of heat. This fact is exploited by the hypothalamus, which functions as the temperature control center of the human body. First of all, hypothalamic thermoreceptors can monitor blood temperature directly as it courses through the Pre-Optic Anterior thermoregulatory center (which apparently responds to heat stress) and the Posterior thermoregulatory center (which apparently responds to cold stress). Secondly, cold sensors in the spinal cord are intimately connected with the posterior hypothalamus. Third, peripheral cutaneous temperature sensors in the skin (Krause's end-bulbs respond to cold, Ruffini Corpuscles respond to warmth) also have intimate connections with both the anterior and posterior hypothalamus.

Fourth, mucosal peripheral sensors on the tongue and in the nose, the latter providing sensory information via the Trigeminal, or V'th Cranial Nerve, are important in relation to diving and nasal circulatory reflexes. And finally, central visceral thermodetectors, the most important of which lie in muscles, the gastrointestinal tract, the kidney, the urinary tract, and the ventricular wall of the heart, all provide important temperature information to the central nervous system via afferent pathways that ultimately converge on the hypothalamus. The latter acts as a comparator and decides whether body temperature is too low or too high. If it is too low, the hypothalamus discharges, via efferent pathways, excitatory synapses to alpha-motoneurons, initiating the *Shivering Reflex*. Hopefully, the heat thus released will bring the body temperature back to acceptable levels. Shivering is but one of several mechanisms by which thermoregulation (or homothermosis) is accomplished in physiologic systems. The others are not immediately relevant to the subject matter of this text (see Schneck, D. J., 1990, and other literature references on the subject).

Proprioception

Human joints contain transducers (proprioceptors) that sense the orientation of a limb in space, even when there is no visual feedback to the person whose limb it is! This can be easily demonstrated by so-called "appreciation of passive movement" and/or "sense of position" maneuvers. In the former, a person is blindfolded and one of his or her fingers or toes is grasped by the side (to minimize cues from pressure). The respective toe or finger is then moved up or down and the person with normal sensibility can discriminate the precise direction of quite small angular displacements. Sense of position maneuvers include: without looking, bringing the extended forefinger of either hand to touch the tip of one's nose, or placing a limb in an unusual position and, with eyes closed, duplicating this posture with the other limb, or passively moving one arm and bringing it to rest with finger extended, then touching the extended forefinger with the forefinger of the other hand (the finger-to-finger test), or any of a number of other such demonstrations. All of these illustrate the action of *Pacinian Corpuscles* (pressure transducers), Meissner's Corpuscles ("touch" receptors), *Ruffini Receptors*, and Golgi Endings.

The Pacinian corpuscle consists of an encapsulated soft core containing sensitive nerve endings, to which is attached the axon of a sensory neuron. The core is surrounded by confocal elliptic layers of connective tissue (called lamellae), with the distance between successive lamellae increasing as one moves radially outward from the center. The major diameter of the outermost lamina is about 1.2 millimeters, with the minor axis measuring about 0.8 mm. The spaces in between the lamellae are filled with a viscous liquid having properties similar to those of water.

The sensory neuron that is stimulated by the soft core is a single myelinated (Type Λ) nerve fiber (5-8 microns in diameter, Type II- β) that loses its myelin sheath once it enters the capsule, within which its diameter decreases to 2 - 3 microns.

Pacinian Corpuscles function as direction-sensitive, rate-sensitive pressure transducers. When pressure applied in a particular direction compresses the outermost lamella, displacing it by as little as 0.20 to 0.50 μ, this stimulus is transmitted to the core, causing compression of the innermost lamella. This compression decreases the transmembrane potential of the nerve terminals (i.e., depolarizes the neural endings), giving rise to an appropriate receptor potential which is directly proportional to the strength of the stimulus, its rate-of-change *and* to its direction. The action potential that is generated as a result of the receptor potential is transmitted via afferent pathways to the Thalamus, the Anterior Lobe of the Cerebellum, and the Cerebral Motor Cortex of the brain. The pattern of signals thus transmitted from joint receptors and relayed to the sensorimotor cortex reports the exact position of the respective joint and associated limbs. This information, unlike that from stretch receptors in the muscles, actually does reach consciousness.

Joint receptors are of four basic types: Ruffini Endings, which, as previously mentioned, have the dual role of responding both to temperature (warmth) and to pressure; Pacinian corpuscle endings, described above; Golgi endings; and, free (sometimes called Meissner's) nerve endings. These different joint receptors respond optimally over different portions of the total range of joint movement. Although not nearly as much is known about the organization of reflex patterns associated with higher centers in the brain, as is known about spinal reflexes, the commands which cerebral centers send to lower levels as a result of proprioceptive inputs are also guided by feedback principles to be discussed later.

While the basic *principles* of operation of proprioceptors are essentially understood, and some attempts to analyze these transducers mathematically have met with modest success, the intimate *mechanisms* involved in these processes are not yet completely known and much more work remains to be done. The same can be said of the kinesthetic processes that control balance and equilibrium, which are described below.

Kinesthesis

Located in each mammalian ear is a specialized set of sense organs that are responsive to linear acceleration of the organism, to angular acceleration and to vibration. Known collectively as the *Labyrinth* or *Vestibular Organ*, these special senses are intimately connected to postural reflexes that orient the body in space, and provide feedback information concerning its kinematic relationship to its environment. The Labyrinth consists of two major parts: the *semicircular canals* (of which there are three oriented mutually orthogonal to one another), and two *Otolith Organs* (the *Saccule* and the *Utricle*), as shown schematically in Figure 6-3.

THE SEMICIRCULAR CANALS

Hollowed out of the temporal bone of the skull is a series of canals called the *bony labyrinth*. Part of this bony labyrinth consists of three semicircular, mutually orthogonal, interconnected arches called the semicircular canals. When the head is bent backwards 30°, the lateral horizontal canal is in a plane parallel to the ground. In this position (the nose is to the left in Figure 6-3), the superior (towards the head) canal lies in a vertical plane that has an axis of symmetry which is tilted forward (anterior) 45°, to the vertical, and the posterior (towards the rear) canal is in a vertical plane that tilts backward 45° with respect to the vertical. Thus, where the radii of curvature of these canals meet locates the center of an orthogonal coordinate system having each radius as a respective axis. The semicircular canals contain *endolymph*, a fluid found in most all of the sensory organs in the inner ear. They also contain a weblike gelatinous material that acts as a partition between the endolymph and the hair-like sensory receptors of the organ. This layer of gelatinous material is called the

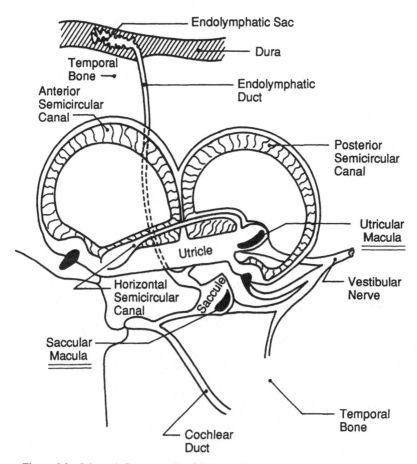

Figure 6-3   Schematic Representation Of The Architecture Of The Semi-Circular Canals

cupula. Thus, any motion of the endolymph is transmitted through shear to the cupula, and thence, elastically through the cupula to the sensory receptors.

The semicircular canals have a common origin at the utricle, one of the two otolith organs (see Figure 6-3). Near this junction, there is an outpocketing, called the *ampulla,* in each canal. Inside the ampulla lies the *crista acustica,* an elevated area within which is contained the cupula itself. The crista acustica is where the sensory receptors of the organ are also located. These are very fine hair cells which communicate with nerve fibers that ultimately combine to form the *vestibular branch* of the *eighth cranial nerve.* This nerve enters the brain and terminates in the vestibular nuclei, situated at the boundary of the pons and medulla. From there, connections are made to the spinal column, cerebellum, reticular formation, nuclei of the third, fourth, and sixth cranial nerves and, through the thalamus, to the sensory projection area for equilibrium in the temporal lobe of the brain. Branches of the eighth cranial nerve also pass directly to the cerebellum.

The bony labyrinth is fixed rigidly to the temporal bone of the skull and thus moves with it if the head is rotated. However, the endolymph in the semicircular ducts initially lags behind this motion due to the inertia of the fluid. The endolymph thus exerts a shearing force on the elastic cupula, causing the sensory hair processes embedded in it to be deformed in a direction opposite to that of the rotation. This deformation is transduced into nerve action potentials which are delivered directly to the brain to provide information concerning the angular motion of the head.

If, however, the motion is maintained at a constant rate, the endolymph eventually "catches up" with the movement of the skull, the hair processes straighten up, the nerve action potentials cease, and the vestibular receptors in the brain are led to believe that the head has actually *stopped* turning. One concludes, therefore, that these receptors actually sense angular *acceleration* and/or *deceleration,* rather than angular velocity, and, in the absence of any other reference information (such as visual inputs), can be misled into thinking that the organism is not rotating when, in fact, it is. This is a particularly dangerous situation that arises when pilots fly into clouds, such that their horizon and other visual reference points are no longer available to orient them in space. These pilots may experience disorientation and vertigo if they rely on their vestibular senses (rather than their instruments) to tell them how their aircraft is oriented in space. And since the vestibular senses can be wrong, the end result can be tragic to the pilot.

Conversely, the inertial properties of the endolymph can cause one to think that he or she *is* rotating when, in fact, this is not the case. This occurs when a rotating body is stopped suddenly, and is the cause of dizziness. The fluid in the canals continues to move for some time after the head has stopped. Incidentally, certain chemicals such as drugs or liquor, which alter the viscosity of the endolymph, can cause the semicircular canals to be more "sensitive" to movement and lead to consequent dizziness at much lower thresholds. Some central nervous system disorders can also cause this.

THE OTOLITH ORGANS

The otolith organs contain vessels called *maculae* (macula, singular) which are also filled with endolymph. The macula contained in the utricle (i.e., the *utricular macula*) lies on the floor of the utricle in a plane parallel to that of the horizontal semicircular canal. This vessel is a common storage area for the endolymph that is used by the canals. The *saccular macula* lies on the medial wall of the saccule in a plane orthogonal to the utricular macula.

Each macula is composed of two distinct parts: a rigid upper portion and an elastic lower portion. The upper portion consists of calcium carbonate crystals (called *otoconia*) also embedded in a thin, weblike gelatinous membrane called the *otoconial membrane.* Extending below the otoconial membrane, this same weblike gelatinous material (which is identical to the substance that makes up the cupula of the semicircular canals) goes on to form the more elastic cupular membrane of the otolith organs, which is devoid of the calcium carbonate crystals. Finally, the cupular membrane is attached to the wall of the respective otolith organ.

Projecting outward from the utricular (or saccular) wall through the cupular membrane are discrete bundles of sensory hairs which, again, serve as the transducers of these vestibular organs. These sensory hair bundles originate from a 25-micron-thick supporting tissue layer in the wall of the otolith organ, pass through a 5 to 8 micron-thick subcupular zone and terminate in the 10 - 15 μ-thick cupular membrane. The latter bounds the 15 - 20 - μ - thick otoconial membrane on one side; endolymph bounds it on the other side. The average surface area of each macula in humans is approximately 2 square millimeters.

The utricular and saccular walls are both fixed rigidly to the temporal bone of the skull through a 100-micron-thick layer of connective tissue. Thus, any linear movement of the skull results in a corresponding movement of the wall of the otolith organs. Due to the viscoelastic properties of the cupular membrane, however, this motion will not be transmitted directly to the otoconial membrane. Rather, the latter, due to its rigid body inertia, will lag the motion of the skull, producing a shearing action on the cupular membrane. Again, as before, this shearing action deforms (bends) the sensitive hair bundles, causing them to generate action potentials which are also sent via the 8th cranial nerve to higher centers. There, the trains of nerve action potentials are integrated to provide linear velocity and acceleration information. Each hair bundle is directionally sensitive, so that different shearing directions produce different trains of action potentials in different hair bundles.

Just as the semicircular canals provide *angular* kinesthetic information to higher centers, the otolith organs provide to these centers *linear* kinesthetic information, as well as slow vibration responses. Some of the things that are done with this information are described below, where we discuss two of the major so-called "Labyrinthine reflex pathways" associated with the vestibular sense organs -- i.e., *Nystagmus* and the so-called "*Righting Reflex*".

LABYRINTHINE REFLEXES

During rapid angular acceleration around the vertical axis of the body, a series of reactions resulting from sensory information received through the semicircular canals affects the muscles of the eyes, neck, limbs and trunk. As the head turns in one direction, the eyes turn in the *opposite* direction (perfectly synchronized with the head) in order to maintain the gaze at a fixed point in space, and to maintain visual contact with the environment, i.e., to "track" a target. However, if rotation of the head continues in the same direction, beyond the point where the eyes can still sight on their original target, then they quickly swing in the *same* direction as the head rotation to fix upon a new point. Then they hold this new point in view as before, until *it* goes out of range, whereupon they sight on still another new point ... and so on. This alternate movement of the eyes, i.e., a *slow fixation deviation phase* followed by a *quick refixation phase,* is termed *nystagmus.* It is definitely a reflexive action caused by *acceleration* of the semicircular canal apparatus, because if rotation is continued for some time at a constant rate, the nystagmus reaction disappears -- only to reappear again if there is any angular acceleration or deceleration. Nystagmus may occur spontaneously if there exist pathologic lesions that affect the sense organs or the neural pathways connecting the labyrinth with the motor nuclei innervating the eye muscles.

Signals transmitted by the vestibulospinal tracts are important for maintaining the tone of antigravity muscles, and for maintaining equilibrium and balance as the body falls to one side, forward or backward. Most of us, for example, have experienced the tendency to "grab" for support after tripping or inadvertently starting to fall; or sensed the tensing up of the lower back and leg muscles if the body begins to sway or lean too far in any given direction. We have seen people, as they fall off to sleep in a sitting position, suddenly jerk their head up and become erect if their body begins to slump too far from an equilibrium position. All of these illustrate *righting reflexes,* which represent control of α-motoneurons that comes from interconnections between the vestibular nuclei of the brain, the reticular formation, and the cerebellum, via impulses sent through the reticulospinal and vestibulospinal tracts. The classic righting reflex, of course, can be demonstrated in the intact cat by dropping it, blindfolded, with its legs pointed upward. The cat turns with almost incredible speed and lights deftly on all fours.

Subconscious Control -- Dreaming

At this point, it should be obvious to the reader that each and every α-motoneuron of the human body is inundated with a multitude of influences, up to 10,000 of them at any given time, some excitatory and some inhibitory, as summarized in Table 6-IV. The motoneuron simply adds up all of the messages that impinge upon it, and the net sum is what determines whether or not the neuron will, itself, fire at a frequency of sufficient threshold strength to call for a muscular contraction.

An interesting "aside" in this respect has to do with musculoskeletal function during sleep. When one is dreaming about something that involves locomotion of the body, the motor cortex actually sends excitatory messages to the corresponding musculature that can accomplish this movement. However, subconscious centers in the brain, realizing that the individual is sleeping, send equally intense inhibitory synapses to the same muscles, effectively "short-circuiting" the attempts of the excitatory messages to generate contractions. This is why people frequently report that during a dream, they seem unable to run quickly or otherwise perform the tasks that they are dreaming about. If someone is chasing them in a dream, for example, the other individual seems to have no trouble at all in hot pursuit, but the individual being chased can't seem to get his or her legs to move. This sluggishness is the manifestation of the inhibitory pathways that are blocking actual motor function.

Inhibitory signals are associated with subconscious thought processes that are related to the appearance of θ - waves (4-8 cycles/sec) in a cortical electro-encephalogram. They do not always work, however, and

TABLE 6–IV

EXTRINSIC NEURAL CONTROL OF STRIATED SKELETAL MUSCLE CONTRACTION

Input From	Reflex Involved	Excitatory	Inhibitory
Autogenetic Fibers			
I–A	Myotatic Reflex	X	
I–B	Inverse Myotatic Reflex		X
II	Autogenic Inhibition		X
Renshaw Cells ⎰ ⎱ — — — — — Autogenic Inhibition			X
Skin Receptors			
Ipsilateral A–II–β, A–III–δ, C–IV–δ ⎱ — — — ⎰ Nociceptive Reflex	To Flexor ⎱		To Extensor ⎰
Contralateral A–II–β, A–III–δ, C–IV–δ ⎱ — — — Crossed Extension Reflex	To Extensor ⎰	Double Reciprocal Innervation	
Contralateral A–II–β, A–III–δ, C–IV–δ ⎱ — — — ⎰ Myotatic Reflex / Facilitation			To Flexor
Ipsilateral Agonist			
α–Motoneuron ⎰ Recruitment / Synergism	X / X	
Renshaw Cells ⎰ — — — — — — — ⎰ Recruitment / Synergism		X / X
I–A	Synergism	X	
I–B	Synergism		X
II	Synergism	X	
Ipsilateral Antagonist			
I–A	Reciprocal Inhibition		X
I–B	Reciprocal Excitation	X	
II	Reciprocal Excitation	X	
α–Motoneuron	Reciprocal Inhibition		X
Contralateral Agonist			
I–A	Crossed Inhibition		X
I–B ⎱ ⎰ — — — — — Phillipsons Reflex			
II ⎰		X / X	
Contralateral Antagonist			
I–A	Crossed Excitation	X	
I–B ⎱ ⎰ — — — — — Phillipsons Reflex			
II ⎰			X
Higher Centers			
Thermoregulation–Shivering Reflex		X	
Proprioception–Conscious Control		X	X
Kinesthesis – – Righting Reflex / – – Postural Reflexes / Labyrinthine Reflexes / – – Nystagmus ⎰ — — — — —		X	X
"Will" and Conscious Control		X	X
Subconscious Control – – "Dreaming"		X— — equal to — — — — X	

that is why some people do walk in their sleep, or perform other motor functions corresponding to whatever it is they happen to be dreaming about. In the latter case, the excitatory pathways are allowed to proceed, unimpeded by subconscious inhibition.

Be that as it may, the ultimate control over all of the processes that affect the alpha-motor-neuron is at the conscious level. Whether one considers this to be a fortunate or an unfortunate situation, the fact is that an individual can "over-ride" every one of the servomechanisms that we have thus far described. Thus, he, or she, through conscious control of the Cerebral Motor Cortex, the Pyramidal System and the Extra-Pyramidal System, has the final say as to whether or not a contraction will take place. This is bad in some ways -- people pull muscles in their back; strain, sprain, tear or otherwise injure their musculoskeletal system by over-or-improper-use -- but it is also desirable in many ways. We *should* have the ability to consciously control how and when we will move, and for what purposes. This is part of what makes life interesting and productive. But is this control absolute and unbounded? Or is it in some sense predictable (able to be deduced *a priori*), such that conscious control of musculoskeletal function may *not* be as voluntary as we might be led to believe?

"Will" -- The Ultimate Control -- Or Is It??

In the realm of continuum mechanics, the deductive analytical approach to problem solving generally begins with the stipulation that certain fundamental governing laws of nature must be satisfied, viz.:

(i) Conservation of Mass (commonly referred to as the Continuity Equation);

(ii) The Laws of Newtonian Mechanics expressing, in an inertial coordinate system, relationships which must exist between external forces and moments and corresponding rates of change of linear and angular momentum, respectively;

(iii) Conservation of Energy (the first law of thermodynamics); and,

(iv) The Second Law of Thermodynamics.

If the problem is one of rigid body dynamics, these basic laws, together with appropriate initial and boundary conditions, normally suffice to describe a given situation -- provided the number of independent equations, j, generated exactly equals the number of unknown quantities, n, introduced by these equations. In that case, the n unknowns may be determined uniquely by solving simultaneously the j independent equations that contain them.

Consider what happens, however, if $n > j$. In the absence of any additional information, this situation is indeterminate in the sense that it hypothetically allows there to be an infinite number of solutions to the problem. That is, by assigning arbitrary values to $(n - j)$ of the unknown quantities, one is left with $n - (n - j) = j$ unknowns and j equations, from which the remaining j unknowns may be determined. But, since the unknowns one chooses to define, as well as the values assigned to these, can be purely arbitrary, there are obviously many possibilities, each leading to a different solution for the "family of parameters" $(n - j)$. In many cases, such a parameter-dependent family of solutions may be perfectly acceptable, but in others, it may not. Thus, in order to alleviate this situation, investigators make some attempt to reduce the number of unknown quantities in a systematic fashion. This may involve utilizing one or more of the following strategies (see Schneck, D. J., 1990):

   (i) Making certain simplifying assumptions based on sound and logical physical reasoning, or a dimensional analysis of the problem, or the imposition of mathematical continuity requirements;

   (ii) Introducing additional boundary conditions or constraints (e.g., choosing values for a governing parameter) in order to get a more specific solution for a special case;

   (iii) Performing careful laboratory experiments to define some unknown quantities from actual data rather than by guessing;

   (iv) Finding some functional scaling relationship among certain of the variables (such as by similarity schemes, nondimensionalization, or functional dependence methods) so that they may be combined into parameters that are less in number than the original n unknowns; and,

(v) Utilizing approximation and scaling techniques to examine asymptotic or perturbation solutions. (Note that this is a special case of (i) or (ii) above).

Quite often, indeterminate formulations for rigid-body problems may be made determinate by relaxing the rigid-body assumption and considering the behavior of specific materials. For this purpose, subsidiary laws or "constitutive" relationships (for example, like those developed in Chapters 2, 3 and 4 of this text) are introduced to make the governing physical laws specific for a particular type of material. Common examples of these are the perfect gas law, Newton's law of viscosity for a fluid, Hooke's law for an elastic solid, and a wide variety of additional stress-strain or stress-strain-rate equations that are functions of individual material properties. These constitutive equations allow one to examine the deformation characteristics of specific media subjected to given loadings, which, after the further imposition of compatibility conditions and mathematical continuity requirements based on physical reasoning, may be sufficient to set up a "well-posed" problem. Well-posed in the sense of the number of unknown quantities being equal to the number of governing equations and the possibility for obtaining a physically meaningful and realizable solution.

Application of any of the above methods categorizes the problem-solving technique as being an *inductive* one, i.e., concluding what happens in a *general* case from an arsenal of results obtained for *specific* cases. In physiological research, inductive reasoning has traditionally been the rule, rather than the exception, since mathematical formulations of human body function inevitably lead to more unknown quantities than there are equations to describe them (Schneck, D. J., 1990).

For example, the problem with *deductive* analysis of musculoskeletal mechanics has always been that the resulting equations are indeterminate. This is because there are S unknown moments at the joints, where S exceeds precisely the number of equations, j, available from basic continuum mechanics. The degree of indeterminateness is thus $S = n - j$, where n equals the total number of unknown quantities. This degree is reduced by the number of constraints, r, as described later, so that the problem is left with $S - r$ degrees of freedom. That is to say, it is possible to ascribe values to $S - r$ of the primary unknowns, and still satisfy the laws of mechanics and the constraints. This situation is generally attributed to the fact that the unknown moments are capable of being generated at "will" by the normal individual through control of his/her muscles, and that "will" renders a problem indeterminate because it is an undefinable variable. Or *is* it?

In 1961, Nubar and Contini postulated the following: "A mentally normal individual will, in all likelihood, move (or adjust his posture) in such a way as to reduce his total muscular effort to a minimum, consistent with the constraints." In other words, it appears likely, and feasible that, whether conscious or subconscious, the patterns of motion of an individual seem concerned with the reduction of exertion to a minimum at all times, consistent with the task assigned and other restrictions. When the individual takes the shortest path between two points, when he or she settles into a preferred position while sitting or drifting off to sleep, when s(he) adjusts his or her stance according to some particular rhythmic pattern while swinging a hammer -- in all of these cases one might surmise that the individual is instinctively obeying some governing law which gives him or her a need to economize physical activity -- or, suffer the consequences of overexertion, which may include discomfort, fatigue, pain, and so on.

Of course, this is not necessarily true in an absolute sense, but in a relative sense consistent with certain constraints. For example, there may be a broken bone or other disability which constrains movement; there may be a desire to maintain some prescribed velocity or step length while walking; there may be patterns of motion derived from culture, habit and experience that dictate how an individual will behave in a given situation, and many more. The point is, however, that these constraints can frequently be well defined both physically and mathematically (see later), and that within and subject to these constraints, the minimum-energy principle will guide a person's desire or "will" to perform a given function in a prescribed manner.

If Nubar is right -- and there is every reason to believe that he *is* -- then the ultimate control of muscle function at the conscious level is not an *undefinable* "will," per se, but a "will" that is the manifestation of an underlying principle of least energy, which *is* definable. That is to say, viewed within the context of such an "optimization" scheme, the analysis of musculoskeletal function can exploit methods of, for example, variational calculus in order to develop more *equations* to describe such function, rather than to resort to the techniques mentioned earlier that basically attempt to reduce the number of *unknowns*. Let us look at a simple example to see how this might work:

Nubar and Contini (1961) attempted to predict the postural configuration most likely to be assumed by an individual asked to stand on one leg, with the other leg held just slightly off the ground at a prescribed distance (the "constraint") from the stationary leg. In this case, it was assumed that the human figure is made up of only five articulated body segments: One rigid head-torso-link (segment 3), two rigid arm-links attached at the shoulder joints (segment 4 is left arm, segment 5 is right arm), and two rigid leg-links attached at the hip joints (segment 1 is left leg, segment 2 is right leg). The segments have, respectively, total lengths, ℓ_i ($i = 1, 2, 3, 4, 5$), individual weights W_i, acting through their respective center of gravity, d_i (located with respect to one end of the body segment), and make angles α_i with respect to the vertical, as shown in Figure 6-4.

****

Problem 6-1: Draw a free-body diagram first of the entire human body shown in Figure 6-4, and then of each of the segments separately. From the free-body diagrams derive the following set of equilibrium equations for the postural configuration shown in the figure:

$$M_1 - C_1 \sin \alpha_1 = 0 \qquad\qquad \text{[6-2]}$$

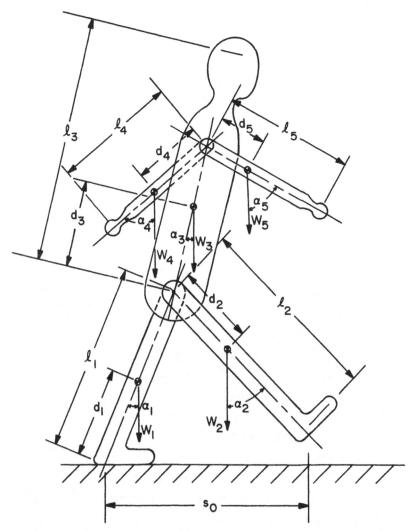

Figure 6-4 Sagittal Plane (Two-Dimensional) Representation Of A Five-Linkage Model Of The Human Body

$$M_2 - C_2 \sin \alpha_2 = 0 \qquad\qquad \text{[6-3]}$$

$$M_4 + C_4 \sin \alpha_4 = 0 \qquad\qquad \text{[6-4]}$$

$$M_5 - C_5 \sin \alpha_5 = 0, \quad \text{and} \qquad \text{[6-5]}$$

$$M_1 + M_2 + M_4 + M_5 + C_3 \sin \alpha_3 = 0 \qquad\qquad \text{[6-6]}$$

where:

$M_1 =$ The moment generated by the musculature at the left hip joint;

$M_2 =$ The moment generated by the musculature at the right hip joint;

$M_4 =$ The moment generated by the musculature at the left shoulder joint;

$M_5 =$ The moment generated by the musculature at the right shoulder joint;

$C_1 = d_1 W_1 + \ell_1 [W_2 + W_3 + W_4 + W_5]$;

$C_2 = d_2 W_2$

$C_3 = d_3 W_3 + \ell_3 [W_4 + W_5]$

$C_4 = d_4 W_4$

$C_5 = d_5 W_5$, and the angles α_1, α_2, α_3, α_4, and α_5 are defined on Figure 6-4.

****

Observe that the five equations derived in Problem 6-1 contain nine unknown quantities: M_1, M_2, M_4, M_5, α_1, α_2, α_3, α_4, α_5, making the problem one of fourth-order indeterminateness (it is assumed that the constants C_1, C_2, C_3, C_4 and C_5 can be calculated for a given individual from values tabulated in Anthropometric charts). Thus, as predicted, the indeterminateness of the problem, four, is equal exactly to the number of joints involved in the movement: right shoulder, left shoulder, right hip, left hip -- because, presumably, the joint torques, M_1, M_2, M_4, and M_5, can be generated "at will". We can reduce this indeterminateness by constraining the motion to require the right leg to be held a fixed distance, s_o, in front of the left leg. This allows us to generate one additional constraint equation as follows. From Figure 6-4:

$$s_o = \ell_1 \sin \alpha_1 + \ell_2 \sin \alpha_2,$$

or, using equations [6-2] and [6-3],

$$s_o = \ell_1 \frac{M_1}{C_1} + \ell_2 \frac{M_2}{C_2} \qquad \text{[6-7]}$$

which still leaves a third-order indeterminate problem.

Now, as mentioned earlier, one way to reduce this indeterminateness might be to measure in the laboratory the kinematic quantities α_1, α_2, α_3, α_4 and α_5 for s_o given, and, from these, inductively calculate M_1, M_2, M_4 and M_5 from the set of equations [6-2] through [6-7], where two of these would now reduce to identities. The joint torques so calculated would thus yield a family of results, depending on the measured (or assigned) values for the angles α_i. Just such a technique is discussed at length elsewhere (Schneck, 1990) -- using as an example a simple forearm flexion. One may also find many literature references that exploit this method, since, until very recently, it was among the very few that would make a problem of this type mathematically tractable (see, for example, Davis, R. B., III, 1986).

To solve this problem in a purely *deductive* way employing the method of least energy, Nubar and Contini (1961) define an energy function, U^*, as follows:

$$U^* = (\beta_1 M_1{}^2 + \beta_2 M_2{}^2 + \beta_3 M_4{}^2 + \beta_4 M_5{}^2)\Delta t \qquad \text{[6-8]}$$

where the β's are so-called "sensitivity coefficients" and Δt is the time duration of muscular exertion. The sensitivity coefficients are assumed to be constant for all joints for all normal individuals under normal conditions, and they allow one to account for the physical condition of a joint, or for how an individual favors them in the prescribed motion. The joint torques are squared to insure that the energy function will always be positive regardless of whether the moments are positive or negative. And finally, since equation [6-8] will ultimately be differentiated, one can increase its generality by tacking on an arbitrary constant to account for muscle "tone" with the joint at rest. We leave it out here for convenience.

Proceeding according to the variational method of Lagrange multipliers, we now form the function:

$$w = U^* + \lambda s_o,$$

there being only one constraint to deal with in this problem.

If there were *several* constraints, $s_i(x, y, z, t)$, $i = 1, 2, 3, \dots, r$, one would instead form the function:

$$w = U^* + \sum_{i=1}^{r} \lambda_i s_i \qquad\qquad [6\text{-}9]$$

where the λ_i are constants (Lagrange multipliers), as yet undetermined in value. Now, the calculus of variations is concerned with maximizing or minimizing functions of points in function spaces (so-called "functionals"), and its physical application relates to the existence of particles capable of an equilibrium state wherein some energy function has its smallest value. Typically, this energy function will depend on several variables, where the variables themselves are related by one or more equations which represent constraints on the problem. Thus, in principle, variational calculus can be used to generate extra equations which constrain the system to minimize a given energy function. The extreme values of w can be obtained by setting $dw = 0$, as in the following.

****

Problem 6-2: Substitute equation [6-8] for U^* and equation [6-7] for s_o into the un-numbered equation for w given above. For simplicity, let $\beta_1 = \beta_2 = \beta_3 = \beta_4 = 1.00$, and take Δt to be constant. Then, set $dw = 0$

and, treating M_1, M_2, M_4 and M_5 as independent variables, with λ constant, collect coefficients of dM_1, dM_2, dM_4 and dM_5 to get:

$$2M_1\Delta t + \lambda \frac{\ell_1}{C_1} = 0 \qquad \text{[6-10]}$$

$$2M_2\Delta t + \lambda \frac{\ell_2}{C_2} = 0 \qquad \text{[6-11]}$$

$$2M_4\Delta t = 0 \qquad \text{[6-12]}$$

$$2M_5\Delta t = 0 \qquad \text{[6-13]}$$

Note that we now have added four additional equations and one more unknown (λ) to our list, giving us a well-posed problem in closed form, containing ten equations for ten unknown quantities.

****

Problem 6-3: Using the principle of least energy as developed above, together with the following data, compute and sketch the posture most likely to be assumed by an individual required to stand in such a way that the right leg is 20 inches in front of the left leg and raised just slightly off the ground. The frame-work of an individual 5 feet - 9 inches in height and weighing 160 pounds may be taken to be:

$$W_1 = W_2 = 30 \text{ pounds}$$
$$W_3 = 80 \text{ pounds}$$
$$W_4 = W_5 = 10 \text{ pounds}$$
$$\ell_1 = \ell_2 = 37 \text{ inches}$$
$$\ell_3 = 18 \text{ inches}$$
$$\ell_4 = \ell_5 = 30 \text{ inches}$$
$$d_1 = d_2 = 18.5 \text{ inches}$$
$$d_3 = 9.9 \text{ inches}$$
$$d_4 = d_5 = 15 \text{ inches}$$
$$s_o = 20 \text{ inches}$$

What are the values of the moments generated at the joints for the configuration determined above and what is the sum of the squares of these moments (i.e., a measure of the total effort involved)?

****

Nubar and Contini's results, taking into consideration the simplicity of both their human body model and the sample posture they examined, were quite reasonable in defining an equilibrium position of minimum effort. In fact, so reasonable that others have pursued the approach with great success, using somewhat different methods.

For example, Beckett and Chang (1968) and Beckett and Pan (1971) utilized a Hamiltonian formulation to analyze gait by minimum energy considerations. In this method, the energy function is defined in terms of the kinetic (T^*) and potential (V^*) energies of the musculoskeletal system. Both T^* and V^* are expressed in terms of angular coordinates q which specify the configuration of the system during each instant of time (much like the α's do in the previous example). Minimization of the energy function relative to constraint functions $h_{(i)}$ (also written in terms of coordinates q) is accomplished again by the use of Lagrange multipliers. In this case, a new potential energy function, $\overline{V} = V^* - \lambda h_{(i)}$ is introduced to include the condition of constraint, and the joint moments, M_S, are calculated from the Lagrangian relationships:

$$M_S = \frac{d}{dt}\left[\frac{\partial T^*}{\partial \dot{q}_S} \right] - \frac{\partial T^*}{\partial q_S} + \frac{\partial \overline{V}}{\partial q_S} \qquad \text{[6-14]}$$

In the equation above, the subscript S identifies the joint under consideration ($S = 1, 2, 3, \ldots$), the coordinate q_S is the corresponding angular position of the skeletal part associated with that joint, and the dot over the q indicates differentiation with respect to time.

Among the interesting conclusions that Beckett, Chang and Pan came to regarding the minimum energy principle as it applies to human gait is that, for a given individual, there is a natural gait at which he or she can travel a given distance with a minimum of effort. Given the parameters of the body, one can determine this gait by pure deductive analysis and it turns out to be somewhere near 80 steps per minute for the average person. Above this cadence, the energy consumed to travel the same distance increases, as it does also for cadences below 80 steps per minute. The authors find their results to be in good agreement with the reported findings of several experimental studies available in the literature.

The finding of an optimum gait frequency based on a deductive analysis of musculoskeletal function is particularly interesting in view of our discussion in Chapter 3 of the viscoelastic behavior of muscle tissue. Recall in that chapter that -- based on the rheologic and energy-dissipating characteristics of muscle -- we concluded that there may be some optimum frequencies at which physical exertion should be accomplished in order to maximize performance and minimize energy expenditure. The self-consistency of these results is thus quite encouraging, and strongly suggestive of the fact that some optimization scheme does, indeed, govern physiologic function -- making the mathematical treatment of "will" quite manageable.

Still a third approach which makes use of minimum energy principles is the optimization scheme proposed by Chao and An (1978) to study the mechanics of the human hand. Instead of defining an energy function, these authors present a generalized theory of muscle force distribution as optimized with respect to individual muscle strength limitations during the performance of a given task. The principle, however, is the same, i.e., to minimize effort. Furthermore, their conclusions are consistent with the underlying theme of all such analyses, i.e., that viewed in terms of minimum effort, the seemingly indeterminate problems associated with musculoskeletal dynamics do offer unique solutions that take into account the mysterious variable called "will." In this respect, again, applied mathematicians have made unique contributions to the study of human locomotion.

The human organism is indeed, a remarkable machine. But, then again, it should be! It is the perfected product of millions of years of evolution. The machine that is the 20th century model Homo Sapiens has survived attack from the environment, from hungry predators, and from pathological processes by which it could conceivably have been annihilated. At least today, *this* model is the fittest. It has learned to optimize its performance and to economize on energy expenditures. It has brought into delicate balance homeostatic and immune mechanisms that can ward off environmental threats and disturbances. It even has a built-in ability to modify itself in response to environmental changes that might otherwise make it obsolete. In short, the human machine has learned to do what it needs to do to survive.

Within this context, it is not unreasonable to suspect that economy of effort, as a means for efficient survival, carries over into our activities of daily living, i.e., into the "choices" we make as to how certain tasks are to be performed. Given this supposition, human performance can then be analyzed in a deductive sense, with the variable "will" being handled through a variety of optimization or variational methods. This not only seems reasonable, but, in fact, probable, especially when viewed in terms of "control" mechanisms such as pain, fatigue and discomfort. While somewhat abstract in its present level of development, the concept is certainly deserving of additional input and discussion. Thus it is left to be pondered further.

Chemical and Hormonal Control of Muscular Contraction

What we have examined to this point are only those factors that act as *inputs* to the cell body of the α-motoneuron. To the extent that they excite or inhibit the neuron, they attempt to control whether or not it will fire. But, recall that the firing of an α-motoneuron does not, in and of itself, guarantee that a contraction will follow. Indeed, the α-motoneuron must fire at a frequency sufficient to deliver a stimulus of *threshold* strength to the motor end plate. The stimulus must not arrive when the motor unit is in a *refractory* (repolarizing) state. All *transmission* and *synaptic* pathways must be intact. Membrane *permeability* characteristics of the sarcolemma must favor the proper *transport* of mass, both for depolarization and for substrate uptake and product removal in the case of biochemical reactants. *Blood flow* rates through the tissue must be in phase with corresponding metabolic requirements.

Fuel (Glycogen, Glucose, ATP, Oxygen, and so on) must be available in a retrievable form. The *enzymes* required for catalyzed reactions must be *present* in sufficient quantity and in a *functional*, active state. *Calcium* must be present and released from entrapment in the cisternae. The Actomyosin *cross-bridge* filament configuration must engage so as to produce the required "ratcheting" action. And so on, and so on.

In other words, one may view the activation of an α-motoneuron as being a *necessary*, but not *sufficient* condition for muscular contraction. And to the extent that such activation must be followed by the successful accomplishment of a long, complex, intricately interconnected sequence of numerous cascading events, further control can be manifest through at least all of the mechanisms mentioned above and shown (numbered 1-20) schematically in Figure 6-5. This control tends to be more chemically and hormonally-mediated, rather than neurologically mediated as is the case for all of the reflex systems discussed earlier. Thus, in the sections which follow, the mechanism of action of some of the more important chemical and hormonal regulators of muscular contraction will be described.

Control Through the Endocrine System

Because striated skeletal muscles receive only sympathetic nerve innervation, and not much, at that, most hormonal control of muscular contraction originates through the endocrine system and its ten or so constituent glands. The endocrine system is closely linked, both developmentally and functionally, to the nervous system -- so much so that in effect it serves functionally as an extension of it. This intimate connection between the nervous and endocrine systems allows psychic influences to modify hormonal activities.

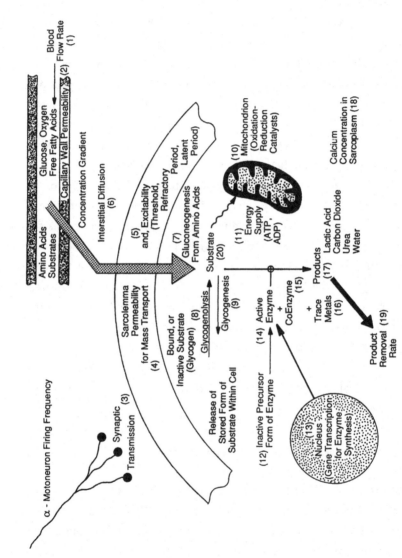

Figure 6-5 Schematic Representation Of Some Of The Mechanisms Through Which Hormones Can Control Muscular Contraction

However, whereas nerves function through synaptic connections *directly* on tissues, hormones are secreted by particular endocrine organs into the systemic circulation, which, in turn, *carries* these substances to their sites of action, or "target organs" elsewhere in the body. Here, they regulate membrane permeability, mass transport, reaction rates of specific enzyme-catalyzed processes, and whatever else it is they are supposed to do to integrate the activities of the various parts of the body into those of a coordinated unit (Schneck, D. J., 1990).

Not all ten of the endocrine organs, which include: The Hypothalamic region of the brain, the Hypophysis (Pituitary Gland) located just beneath the brain, the Thyroid Gland lying on either side of the trachea, the Parathyroid Glands located behind and just below the Thyroid, the Adrenal (or Suprarenal) Glands sitting on top of the kidneys, the Islets of Langerhans of the Pancreas, the Ovary, the Testis, the Pineal Gland lying at about the middle of the brain, and the Placenta -- have secretions that directly affect striated skeletal muscles. Those that do, however, the hormones involved, and their effect on the physiology of muscular contraction are summarized in Table 6-V.

In particular, note how many of them influence the fuel cell -- by controlling the *delivery* (blood flow rate), *uptake* (membrane permeability and mass transport processes), and *utilization* (Glycogenesis, Glycolysis, Gluconeogenesis, Aerobic and Anaerobic Metabolism) of glucose. If one were tempted to generalize, one could say that reflexive (neural) control of muscular contraction acts through inputs to the cell body of the α-motoneuron -- to determine whether or not an *active state* is to be established -- whereas hormonal control of muscular contraction acts through the utilization of fuel for the generation of energy in the system -- to determine whether or not a *contractile state* of the tissue is to be accomplished. This is somewhat simplistic, however, especially considering the fact that hormones *also* have direct and indirect effects on the reflex arcs, themselves. These will not be dealt with in this particular work.

In addition to their influence on the fuel cell, itself, hormones can regulate synaptic transmission at the neuro-muscular junction, the

TABLE 6–V
Hormonal Control of Muscular Contraction

Hormone	Effect On Striated Skeletal Muscle
1. Thyroxin (T_4) and Triiodothyronine (T_3) (Thyroid Gland)	a) Increased Glucose Uptake and Utilization b) Increased Oxygen Uptake and Consumption c) Increased Nitrogen Retention d) Increased Glycogenolysis e) Increased Gluconeogenesis f) Decreased ATP Synthesis g) Decreased Oxidative Phosphorylation h) More Heat (Calorigenic Effect) i) Increased Metabolic Rate j) Less Work (Muscle Weakness, Lethargy)
2. Insulin (Pancreas)	a) Increased Glucose Uptake and Utilization b) Accelerated transport of Amino Acids into Muscle Cells c) Increased rate of Glycogenesis d) Increased Rate of Lactic Acid Production Through Anaerobic Glycolysis e) Increased Rate of Carbon Dioxide Production Through Aerobic Oxidation f) Increased Membrane Transport Characteristics g) Increased Activation of the Enzymes Required for Glucose Metabolism h) Helps Muscle Fibers Utilize Ketones Properly for Fuel i) Enhances the Incorporation of Amino Acids into Muscle Protein
3. Growth Hormone (GH) (Pituitary Gland)	a) Decreased Glucose Uptake and Utilization (hyperglycemia) b) Increased Mobilization and Uptake of Fatty Acids c) Increased Uptake and Utilization of Amino Acids d) Decreased Oxygen Uptake and Consumption e) Increased Glycogenesis f) Enhanced Protein Synthesis g) Enlargement of Muscle Mass with No Corresponding Increase in Contractile Behavior

TABLE 6–V (CONTINUED)	
Hormone	*Effect On Striated Skeletal Muscle*
4. Glucocorticoids, principally, Cortisol (Adrenal Cortex)	a) Decreased Glucose Uptake and Oxidation b) Increased Catabolism of Muscle Protein into Amino Acids c) Decreased Incorporation of Amino Acids into Muscle Proteins (Anabolism) d) Decreased Cellular Uptake of Amino Acids e) Increased Fatty Acid Mobilization f) Increased Liver Gluconeogenesis g) Reduced Cell and Capillary Permeability (Anti–Inflammatory and Anti–Allergic effects)
5. Mineralocorticoids, principally, Aldosterone (Adrenal Cortex)	a) Increased Sodium Concentration b) Decreased Potassium Concentration c) Increased Blood Volume (Anti–Diuretic Effect) d) Decreased Blood Flow (Vasoconstriction Effect; Vascular Smooth Muscle Contraction; Increased Peripheral Resistance) e) Increased Blood Pressure (Vasopressor Effect) f) Electrolyte and Water Balance g) Increased Muscle Excitability
6. Anti–Diuretic Hormone (ADH) (Hypothalamus, Pituitary Gland)	a) Increased Blood Volume b) Increased Blood Pressure c) Decreased Blood Flow Rate (Vasocon–striction, Contraction of Vascular Smooth Muscle) d) Increased Peripheral Resistance
7. Epinephrine (Mainly) (Adrenal Medulla)	a) Activates The Phosphorylase Enzyme Required for Glycogenolysis (Excitatory to Muscle) b) Increased Contractile Response During Tetanic Stimulation or in Fatigue c) Increased Force and Amplitude of Contraction (Inotropic Effect in Cardiac Muscle which Raises Systolic Blood Pressure Only) d) Increased Resistance to Fatigue; Increased Frequency of Contraction (Chronotropic Effect in the Heart Raises Heart Rate) e) Immediate, But Short–Lived Increase in Oxygen Uptake and Utilization

TABLE 6–V (CONCLUDED)	
Hormone	*Effect On Striated Skeletal Muscle*
7. Epinephrine (Continued)	f) Anaerobic Metabolism; Lactic Acid Build–up; Decreased pH; Inhibition of Smooth Muscle Contraction g) Vasodilatation; Drop in Diastolic Blood Pressure; Decreased Peripheral Resistance h) Increased Systolic Pressure (c) Plus Decreased Diastolic Pressure (g) Equals An Increase in Pulse Pressure. Combined With a Decreased Peripheral Resistance (g) and an Increased Heart Rate (d), There results an Increased Cardiac Output and an Increased Blood Flow Through The Muscles
8. Norepinephrine (Mainly) and Sympathetic Innervation (Adrenal Medulla)	a) Increased Muscular Blood Flow in Response to Exercise and Alarm b) Glycogenolysis Enhancement During Increased Response to Exercise and Alarm c) Increased Force of Contraction (Systolic Blood Pressure Increase) d) Decreased Blood Flow In Response To The Need To Raise Blood Pressure e) Primary Vasoconstrictor in Striated Skeletal Muscle (Increased Peripheral Resistance) f) Increased Diastolic Blood Pressure (due to Vasoconstriction) g) Anoxia (Glycogenolysis Inhibition) When Vasoconstriction Occurs h) Increased Membrane Permeability to Sodium i) Reduced Refractory and Latent Periods j) Increased Contractile Response to Stimulation
9. Thyrocalcitonin (Thyroid Gland)	a) Inhibition of Bone Resorption, Calcium Release and Utilization in Response to Hypercalcemia b) Impaired Muscle Contractile Apparatus and Function
10. Parathormone (Parathyroid Glands)	a) Stimulates Bone Resorption b) Inhibits the Deposition of Calcium in bone c) Enhances Kidney Reabsorption of Calcium d) Makes Muscles Hyperirritable in Response to Hypocalcemia

excitability of the sarcolemma, sarcoplasmic reticulum, and transverse tubular network (through their effect on electrolyte and water balance), other cellular metabolic processes (through their ability to activate or deactivate enzyme systems), and the very anatomy of the contractile architecture (through their effect on protein synthesis).

It is particularly noteworthy to mention that Epinephrine (but *not* norepinephrine to any great extent) prolongs the contractile response of skeletal muscle during tetanic stimulation and increases the response of the muscle after partial fatigue. It is believed that this effect transpires through the activation by epinephrine of the phosphorylase enzyme that is responsible for catalyzing the breakdown of glycogen (glycogenolysis) into Glucose-1-Phosphate, which is subsequently oxidized to generate energy for muscular contraction (see Figure 1-8).

In resting skeletal muscle, the phosphorylase enzyme normally exists mainly in the inactive, or "b" form. It is partly converted to the active, or "a" form when the muscle is stimulated to contract, and then is deactivated as the muscle fatigues. Epinephrine has the ability to reactivate this enzyme by augmenting the activity of the cyclizing enzyme which increases the concentration of cyclic Adenosine Mono-Phosphate. The latter, in turn, activates the kinase responsible for converting inactive phosphorylase "b" into active phosphorylase "a" required for glycogenolysis -- thereby increasing the contractile response of muscle during tetanic stimulation or in fatigue. This sequence of events occurs both in striated skeletal muscle and in cardiac muscle, as well, and it has the effect of increasing the force, amplitude and frequency of muscular contraction (chronotropic and inotropic effects).

The increased manufacture of hexose phosphates by glycogenolysis as described above causes the concentration of glucose to rise dramatically as the liver, too, via a liver phosphatase, manufactures more glucose. The net result is that epinephrine, in physiologic counterpoise to the action of Insulin, acts as a hyperglycemic agent. Contributing, as well, to this hyperglycemia is the fact that the epinephrines (more epinephrine than norepinephrine) also reduce the rate of glucose utilization by the peripheral tissues. This is accomplished mainly by the promotion of lipolysis in adipose tissue (due to activation of a tissue lipase), with the consequent release of free fatty acids into the blood stream. Fatty acids interfere with the uptake and oxidation of glucose by body tissues, thereby promoting hyperglycemia.

An immediate, but short-lived increase in oxygen consumption follows the administration of epinephrine. Thus, muscular contraction soon becomes anaerobic and the muscle glycolytic cycle begins to produce much lactic acid. This results in a lactacidemia, which drops the pH of the blood and inhibits the motility of smooth muscle tissue. *Both* epinephrines actually inhibit several kinds of smooth muscle, to a degree correlated with the degree of glycogenolysis induced.

Relaxation of vascular smooth muscle tissue leads, in general, to vasodilatation, thereby increasing the flow of blood through the organ involved, decreasing the corresponding peripheral resistance, and dropping the blood pressure in the blood vessels. This occurs especially in the coronary circulation feeding the musculature of the heart and is attributed mainly to the action of *epinephrine*. *Norepinephrine*, on the other hand, has the ability to constrict arterioles and precapillary sphincters, especially in the skin, mucosa, splanchnic bed, kidneys, cerebral areas, and skeletal muscles and limbs, thereby producing a generalized *vasoconstriction*, anoxia and *no* glycogenolysis. This, however, does not occur in the heart, as norepinephrine is *also* a vasodilator in the coronary circulation.

Both epinephrines raise blood pressure, pulse rate and cardiac output due to their stimulatory effects on the contractile response of skeletal and cardiac muscle. However, epinephrine raises only the *systolic* blood pressure because of its vasodilator effect in skeletal muscle (decreased peripheral resistance during diastole). Norepinephrine, on the other hand, raises both the systolic and diastolic pressures, and hence exhibits a greater total pressor activity than does epinephrine because it also *increases* peripheral resistance by its vasocontrictor action. The increased diastolic pressure due to norepinephrine commonly results in reflex slow-ing of the heart, whereas after epinephrine, tachycardia (speeding of the heart) is typical.

Both epinephrines tend, in general, to be stimulatory in the vascular system but inhibitory in the viscera. When they are excitatory, the activity of the two compounds is of the same order of magnitude, with epinephrine usually somewhat the more potent. In inhibitory effects, epinephrine is frequently, but not always, much more active than norepinephrine. Some of the other interesting effects of these two hormones are to:

   i. Excite (constrict) the Iris Dilator muscles of the eyes,
   ii. Excite the Nictitating (winking) membrane muscles,
   iii. Excite the sphincters of the gastrointestinal tract and bladder, the splenic capsule and the pilomotor muscles,
   iv. Inhibit motility in the gut,
   v. Relax the bronchial musculature,
   vi. Inhibit the uterus of a non-pregnant animal, but excite the uterine musculature of a pregnant animal,
   vii. Increase secretion by the anterior pituitary gland of Adreno-corticotrophic hormone (ACTH), Thyrotrophin and Gonadotrophins,
   viii. Decrease the secretory activity of the salivary glands,
   ix. Increase sweating, and,
   x. Promote Male Ejaculation.

Because the action of the epinephrines can be excitatory in some cases and inhibitory in others, their mechanism of action is believed to be distinct from the nerves, the nerve endings and the contractile fibers themselves. Rather, it is likely that specialized receptors in the muscle cells respond to and affect the desired contractile state of any given motor unit. This is typical of most tissues that respond to Autonomic and/or Adrenal secretions (Schneck, D. J., 1990). Tissue receptors that respond to, or can be activated by norepinephrine (and/or, epinephrine) are called Adrenergic Receptors, or α-receptors if they elicit an *excitatory* response when stimulated. If they elicit an *inhibitory* response under the influence of epinephrine and/or norepinephrine, they are called β-Adrenergic-Receptors. The hormones tend to elicit their response by activating enzyme systems that catalyze biochemical reactions whose products are either excitatory or inhibitory to specific physiologic processes.

In the same sense that anatomical "intrinsic" neuromuscular control mechanisms may lead to a host of pathologic conditions (see Table 6-II) when they fail to work properly, so, too, can pathologic "control" of muscular contraction be manifest through diseases that attack the various "extrinsic" endocrine glands -- afflictions such as Diabetes Insipidus, Hyperthyroidism, Diabetes Mellitus, and so on. Table 6-VI lists but a few of the many disabling conditions that can attack the endocrine system, and, through the consequences of such attack, the contractile behavior of striated skeletal muscle.

Control Through the Sympathetic Nervous System

The Sympathetic Nervous System is that branch of the Autonomic Nervous System that originates from preganglionic neurons located in the Thoracic and Upper Lumbar spinal segments of the Central Nervous System. It is thus sometimes called the Thoracolumbar Division of the Autonomic Nervous System. Its axons leave the spinal cord via the corresponding ventral roots located from the level of T_1 (the first thoracic vertebra), down to the level of L_2 and L_3 (the second and third lumbar vertebrae, respectively). The other division of the Autonomic Nervous System is the Parasympathetic Nervous System, but striated skeletal muscles receive no direct Parasympathetic Innervation and the latter has little, if any, direct, first-order effects on muscular contraction.

The Sympathetic Nervous System functions primarily through the transmitter substance, Norepinephrine (or, noradrenaline), which is released from the post-ganglionic terminals of its nerve fibers. Nerve endings which liberate norepinephrine when properly stimulated are said to belong to *Adrenergic* nerve fibers. Chemical substances that are not Norepinephrine, per se, but which can mimic the same physiological responses that are normally attributable to the action of this hormone are called *Sympathomimetic* substances (for example, Hydroxyamphetamine, Phenylephrine, Ephedrine, Isoproterenol, Caffeine, and Methoxamine).

TABLE 6–VI

SOME ENDOCRINE DISORDERS THAT AFFECT MUSCULAR CONTRACTION

Disease	Endocrine Organ Affected	General Effects
Hypothalamic Dysfunction	Hypothalamus	Hypothalamic disorder leads to Diabetes Insipidus, Adiposity, Genital Dystrophy, Disordered Carbohydrate Metabolism, Defective temperature regulation, autonomic attacks and disorders of sleep
Simmonds Disease	Pituitary Gland	Atrophy of this Gland causes loss of function of the Thyroid, Adrenal Gland and Gonads, upsetting metabolism, and causing premature aging and emaciation
Diabetes Insipidus	Pituitary Gland	Inadequate secretion of Vasopressin leads to Polyuria (dehydration) and Polydipsia (great thirst), hypotension, decreased blood volume and associated symptoms
Marie's Disease (Acromegaly)	Pituitary Gland	Excessive Growth Hormone release in middle—aged persons leads to elongation and enlargement of bones of the extremeties and the head (Gigantism)

TABLE 6–VI (CONTINUED)

Disease	Endocrine Organ Affected	General Effects
Gulls Disease (Myxedema)	Thyroid Gland	Hypofunction of the Thyroid Gland in older children and adults leads to muscular weakness, prolonged tendon reflexes, intolerance to cold, lethargy, and many associated symptoms
Graves Disease (Plummers Disease) (Toxic Goiter)	Thyroid Gland	Hyperfunction of the Thyroid Gland leads to elevated metabolic rate, intolerance to heat, weakness, fine muscle tremors, tachycardia, negative nitrogen balance and other associated symptoms
Addisons Disease	Adrenal Gland	Deficiency in the secretion of adrenocortical hormones leads to weakness, fatigability, hypotension, hypoglycemia, and many associated symptoms
Pheochromocytoma (Paraganglioma)	Adrenal Gland	Chromaffin Cell tumors of the sympatho—Adrenal system leads to hypertension tremor, palpitations, abdominal cramps, headaches, sweating and apprehension
Cushings Syndrome	Adrenal Gland	Hypersecretion of Glucocorticoids leads to protein loss, fatigue and weakness, capillary fragility, diabetes mellitus, wasting of muscles, and hyperglycemia

TABLE 6–VI (CONCLUDED)

Disease	Endocrine Organ Affected	General Effects
Diabetes Mellitus	Pancreas	Failure of Beta Cells of the Pancreas to secrete an adequate amount of Insulin leads to a disorder of carbohydrate metabolism, lipid and protein usage
Hyperpancreatism	Pancreas	Abnormal pancreatic secretion leads to hypoglycemia, acute fatigue, weakness, marked irritability, restlessness, malaise, delirium and possible death
Hypoparathyroidism (Tetany)	Parathyroid Gland	Insufficient secretions from this gland lead to increased excitability of the musculature to mechanical stimulation and fibrillary twitchings, followed by jerky muscular contractions, and some tetany
von Recklinghausens Disease (Osteitis Fibrosa Cystica)	Parathyroid Gland	Hyperfunction of this gland leads to "Moans" (pain), "Stones" (Kidney) and "Bones" (Lesions and Demineralization) plus muscle weakness and nerve damage

The major cardiovascular and metabolic effects of Norepinephrine were already mentioned above -- i.e., this hormone is known to:

a) Dilate arterioles in skeletal muscle by relaxing vascular smooth muscle tissue (as lactic acid builds up); and thus, increase the flow of blood through the musculature in response to exercise and alarm -- bringing nutrients and oxygen, and removing waste products and carbon dioxide;

b) Constrict striated skeletal muscle vasculature by acting as "α-moto-neurons" to stimulate smooth muscle contraction when baro-and-chemo-receptor mechanisms call for an increase in peripheral resistance to raise the blood pressure (Guyton, 1981);

c) Stimulate the breakdown of Glycogen in skeletal muscle (Glycogeno-lysis) to activate the fuel cell in response to exercise and alarm;

d) Produce Anoxia and inhibit Glycogenolysis in muscle tissue when a vasoconstriction, rather than a vasodilatation has occurred;

e) Enhance the mobilization of fatty acids (lipolysis) for fuel, from fat depots by activating a fat tissue lipase enzyme; and,

f) Increase membrane permeability to Sodium Ions, thus permitting a more rapid depolarization of the sarcolemma to the threshold firing level for the muscle. This amounts to reducing both the refractory period and the latent period of the contractile response to stimulation.

Again, observe that the action of norepinephrine can be excitatory in some cases and inhibitory in others, suggesting the existence of specialized receptors (membrane protein molecules) that respond in different ways to the presence of this hormone.

The skeletal muscle of the body represents up to 35 to 40% of the total body mass and yet, in the inactive state, the blood flow through all of the skeletal muscles is only about 15 to 20% of the total cardiac output. This is because, with the body at rest, this tissue has a very low metabolic rate. When muscle becomes active, its metabolic rate can increase as much as 50-fold, and blood flow in individual muscles can increase as much as 20-fold, due at least in part to the action of norepinephrine. Other chemical constituents that act to increase blood flow through this tissue are discussed below.

Control Through Other Chemical Substances

The list of chemical substances other than those already discussed, which have a direct or indirect influence on the contractile behavior of striated skeletal muscle, would fill volumes! Indeed, there are chemical substances that act as enzyme inhibitors, and those that act as enzyme activators. There are chemical substances that affect biological cell membrane permeability (increasing or decreasing such permeability). There are chemical substances that act as α-adrenergic stimulators, or α-adrenergic inhibitors, or β-adrenergic stimulators, or β-adrenergic inhibitors. Some chemicals suppress the enzymic destruction of biochemical substrates, while others affect nuclear gene transcription for enzyme synthesis. There are chemicals that enhance, inhibit, retard, accelerate, mediate and otherwise affect just about each and every aspect of all of the processes required to generate a muscular contraction. Obviously, we cannot get side-tracked at this point to list or discuss all of them; but some deserve at least to be mentioned to the extent that they either occur naturally in the physiologic system and play a somewhat major role in controlling muscular contraction -- or, they affect aspects of the contractile process the control of which we have not yet dealt with to any great extent. Those that we shall concentrate upon here are chemical substances that are primarily involved in regulating blood flow through muscular tissue, or in controlling electrolyte distribution and activity, or in affecting synaptic transmission.

SOME CHEMICAL FACTORS REGULATING BLOOD FLOW THROUGH MUSCLES

Vascular smooth muscle tissue requires (as does skeletal muscle) oxygen in order to remain contracted and to generate a vascular "tone". A *lack of oxygen* causes relaxation of smooth muscle, allowing the blood pressure to dilate passively muscular blood vessels, thereby increasing the flow of blood through these tissues. In fact, a 75% drop in oxygen concentration (due, for example, to an increased rate of tissue utilization) can increase blood flow through a muscle capillary bed by a factor of three. So can an *increase in Carbon Dioxide concentration*. This is a process called *reactive hyperemia*.

By blocking the breakdown of ATP into ADP (see Chapter 1), the anaerobic accumulation of *Lactic Acid* either in skeletal or smooth muscle tissue can stop the contraction in a process called *fatigue*. Thus, Lactic Acid build-up during periods of excessive skeletal muscle exertion, as well as an increase in the concentration of *Adenosine*, *Adenosine Phosphate compounds* and *Adenine Nucleotides*, all act to relax vascular smooth muscle tissue, resulting, again, in an increased flow of blood through muscle capillary beds.

The same occurs locally when there is an accumulation of *Potassium*, *Magnesium* and/or *Hydrogen* ions (decreased pH), but for different reasons. The latter positively-charged ions may *inhibit Calcium* from leaving the cisternae by simply repelling electrostatically this also-positively-charged ion. Since smooth muscle tissue also requires Calcium-release in order to activate its contractile architecture, the electrostatic entrapment of Ca^{++} in the cisternae reduces vascular tone and leads to vasodilation. Indeed, Calcium-Chelators and Calcium Channel Blockers are used clinically to increase blood flow through diseased or occluded arteries because of their ability to "relax" the walls of such blood vessels. Examples of clinical calcium inhibitors are Verapamil, Nifedipine, Diltiazem, Lidoflazine, and Chlorpromazine.

Conversely, chemical substances that *promote* the release of sequestered intracellular calcium and increase the influx of this ion into the sarcoplasm can induce contracture -- with or without a corresponding depolarization of the sarcolemma. An example of such a substance is *Histamine*. The latter is released by damaged tissue cells to constrict arterioles and dilate veins. It also dilates capillaries, constricts bronchial smooth muscle and increases gastric secretions. The mode of action of Histamine is through control of membrane permeability characteristics (e.g., Calcium "Channels"), increasing such permeability to Calcium.

Acting also on membrane permeability are groups of substances called *Kinins*. These are small polypeptides that are split off from an α-globulin in plasma or tissue fluids by proteolytic enzymes, and they are powerful vasodilators. They are capable of influencing smooth muscle contraction; inducing hypotension; increasing the blood flow and permeability of small blood capillaries, and inciting pain. One kinin in particular, *Bradykinin*, is believed to be present in exocrine glands, but its physiologic significance is still under investigation.

A group of substances also manufactured in cell membranes and released (as is Histamine) when the tissue is injured are the *Prostaglandins*. There are a very great number of these substances which have been identified and they are classified into various "Series" or "Groups". In general, prostaglandins of the E-series are vasodilators (i.e., they increase blood flow through tissues), whereas those of the F-series are vasoconstrictors, and those of the G-and-II-series affect muscle membrane activity.

Thromboxane A_2, also released from cell membranes, induces platelet aggregation and vasoconstriction, whereas *Prostacyclin* (also manufactured in cell membranes) is a powerful inhibitor of platelet aggregation and causes vasodilatation in various vascular beds. Thus, just as "for every action, there is an equal and opposite reaction," it seems that for every *vasoactive* Prostaglandin, there appears to be an equal and opposite *vasoinhibitory* Prostaglandin! And, just as there are clinical anti-histamines which counteract the activity of Histamine, there are clinical Prostaglandin Inhibitors which counteract the activity of (mainly) the vasoactive Prostaglandins. Examples of some of these are Aspirin, Sulphinpyrazone (inhibits Thromboxane A_2, in particular), Fenoprofen, Indomethacin, Phenylbutazone and Tolmetin, but there are many others.

The enterochromaffin cells of the gastrointestinal tract and other abdominal structures give rise to a powerful smooth muscle stimulant and vasoconstrictor called *Serotonin* (5-Hydroxytryptamine, or 5-HT). This derivative of the amino acid Tryptophan is transported in the blood by Platelets and is commonly found in the brain and in other tissues. Since, depending on the state of the circulation, it may also sometimes produce vasodilatation, its exact role in vascular control is somewhat poorly understood at present, especially as it relates to blood flow through striated skeletal muscles.

SOME CHEMICAL FACTORS ASSOCIATED WITH ELECTROLYTE DISTRIBUTION AND ACTIVITY IN STRIATED SKELETAL MUSCLES

We have already mentioned the role of Potassium, Magnesium and Hydrogen ions in affecting vascular smooth muscle tissue to produce vasodilatation. *Magnesium* ions can also *inhibit* vascular tone through their effect on cyclic-AMP, as well as their repulsion of Calcium. Cyclic-AMP is involved in activating many of the enzymes required for the biochemical reactions associated with a contractile response. It also appears to be essential for the normal sequestering of Calcium and for mediating the effects of must hormones. By blocking the activity of Cyclic-AMP, excessive Mg^{++} can relax muscle tissue. Conversely, a deficiency of Magnesium can lead to hyperactivity of Muscles, which is an effect similar to that produced by *Caffeine*. That is to say, Caffeine tends to cause a significant release of Calcium from entrapment in cisterns, by a Calcium-induced mechanism. The same is true of the substances *Procaine* and *Thymol*.

Both Magnesium ions and Calcium ions activate the ability of the protein actomyosin to act as a catalyst (ATP-ase) for the breakdown of ATP. Such ATP-ase activity is also exhibited by the protein Myosin alone (but not Actin), although the hydrolyzing ability of Myosin acting as an ATP-ase is activated only by Calcium (not Magnesium). Indeed, Magnesium ions actually *inhibit* the ability of Myosin to act as a catalyst. The action of ATP-ase in splitting ATP also requires the presence of Sodium ions, Ammonium ions and Potassium ions. This allows still further chemical control of muscular contraction in that substances (such as *Ouabain* and other *Cardiac Glycosides*), which inhibit or otherwise impede Sodium and Potassium Transport, also impede muscular contraction by affecting the NH_4^+-Na^+-and-K^+-dependent ATP-ase activities of cells.

Some trace elements, such as Manganese, Cadmium and Lanthanum attach themselves to the sarcolemma on the extracellular fluid side, and, because they, too, are positively charged, they replace Calcium, Sodium and Potassium on membrane binding sites. Thus, Mn^{++}, Cd^{++} and La^{+++} are inhibitory towards muscular contraction, and are also vasoinhibitory. Although they, themselves, do not penetrate muscle cells, they prevent Ca^{++}, Na^+ and K^+ from getting in. Lithium (Li^+), on the other hand, is vasoactive because it promotes the movement of Calcium from the extracellular fluid space into the intracellular fluid space.

Finally, some chemical substances, such as 2,4-Dinitrophenol, Digitalis, Deslanoside, Digitoxin, Gitalin, and Lanatoside C, act as metabolic inhibitors that break down the active Sodium Pump, thus preventing membrane repolarization and inhibiting muscular contraction. Various cardiac glycosides also do this. It should be clear by now, that proper contraction of striated skeletal muscles depends quite heavily on the proper distribution and activity of electrolytes (Na^+, K^+, Ca^{++}, Mg^{++}, Cl^-, NH_4^+), Trace Elements (Mn^{++}, Cd^{++}, La^{+++}, Li^+), Hormones, pH, and so on. Any chemical substances that upset or otherwise interfere with this distribution and activity may have a profound effect on the contractile process. The last of these which we shall discuss at this point are those substances that interfere with synaptic transmission.

SOME CHEMICAL FACTORS THAT AFFECT
SYNAPTIC TRANSMISSION

Recall that stimulation of an α-motoneuron causes the release of the transmitter substance, Acetylcholine, from the nerve endings of the neuron. In fact, this same transmitter substance is released from the terminals of the nerves of the Parasympathetic Nervous System, and it is this substance that initially depolarizes the motor end plate and/or elicits the characteristic responses of parasympathetic nerve stimulation. Chemical substances that are not, in themselves, Acetylcholine, but which can elicit the same response, are called Cholinergic substances, or Parasympathomimetics. They promote the accumulation of acetylcholine at skeletal muscle sites by inhibiting the destruction by the enzyme Acetyl Cholinesterase of the transmitter substance released from the α-motoneuron terminals. That is to say, once stimulated, the motor neuron releases Acetylcholine from its nerve endings (c.f., Chapter 1), and, once the latter has initiated depolarization of the motor end plate, it is promptly destroyed by the enzyme Acetyl Cholinesterase. Cholinergic substances deactivate this enzyme. They can also slow down the synaptic transmission characteristics by altering the concentration gradients that drive Acetylcholine across the synapse. These substances thus tend to increase the irritability of the sarcolemma, but decrease the synaptic transmission time (which tends to increase the latent period following stimulation). Parasympathomimetics, such as Neostigmine, Ambenonium, Pyridostigmine, Edrophonium, Carbachol, and Pilocarpine have been used with some success in improving the muscular performance of persons who have Myasthenia Gravis.

A chemical substance which *competes* with Acetylcholine for receptor sites on the muscle membrane is *Curare*. Curare-like substances form an inactive complex with the sarcolemma, thus blocking neuromuscular transmission and facilitating skeletal muscle relaxation. Some muscle relaxants (neuromuscular blockers), such as Gallamine, Metocurine, Pancuronium, and Tubocurarine work this way. Others, such as Decamethonium, Hexafluorenium Bromide and Succinylcholine prolong the time it takes for the motor end-plate to depolarize once stimulated. Still others, such as Meprobamate, Valium, Librium, Trancopal, Quiess, and Tybamate, are tranquilizers that act as central nervous system depressants to relax skeletal muscle from higher centers.

And so the list goes on and on -- generating a veritable "Physicians Desk Reference," as it were, of biochemical and pharmaceutical substances that directly or indirectly affect the contraction of muscles.

Concluding Remarks

Reading back through both this chapter and Chapter 1, and realizing that:

(i) As complicated as all of the reflex pathways may sound, they are probably even *more* complex because not all of the interneurons and associated collaterals have been entirely defined as yet;

(ii) The material presented is not even exhaustive in terms of all of what is known regarding chemical, neurological and hormonal effects on striated skeletal muscle contraction;

(iii) There are undoubtedly many more biochemical substances involved in musculoskeletal control than have even been identified, isolated, purified and structurally characterized as yet; and,

(iv) We have said very little about how striated skeletal muscle contraction fits in (in a systems "sense") to the other physiologic processes (e.g., digestion, circulation, and excretion), which invariably regulate the ultimate contractile properties of this tissue,

it is a wonder that muscles contract at all!! Imagine all of the complicated circuitry that must perform flawlessly for a muscle to contract properly. Now imagine all that can go wrong (both directly and indirectly), and marvel at the challenges that face researchers in trying to cure and/or manage neuromuscular diseases.

Before getting too overwhelmed, however, one should be made aware that what seems to be emerging from studies conducted in this area is that muscular control is managed by a hierarchy of sophisticated feedback control systems built one upon the other. Moreover, all of them seem to lend themselves to being described by control systems theory, which suggests an important role for the engineer in this field. Some attempts in this direction are discussed in the next chapter.

References for Chapter 6

1. Allen, J. B., "Cochlear Models - 1978," *Scand. Audiol. (Suppl.)*, Vol. 9, Pages 1-16, 1979.

2. An, K. N., Kwak, B. M., Chao, E. Y., and Morrey, B. F., "Determination of Muscle and Joint Forces: A New Technique to Solve the Indeterminate Problem," *J. Biomech. Engrg., Trans. ASME,* Vol. 106, pp. 364-367, 1984.

3. Barineau, D., and Schneck, D. J., "Improvements in the Control of Robotic Motion Simulations Using the ATB Model," Virginia Polytechnic Institute and State University Technical Report Number VPI-E-88-38; Blacksburg, Virginia, 1988.

4. Beckett, R., and Chang, K., "An Evaluation of the Kinematics of Gait by Minimum Energy," *J. Biomechanics,* Vol. 1, Pages 147-159, 1968.

5. Beckett, R. E., and Pan, K. C., "Analysis of Gait Using a Minimum Energy Approach," Aerospace Medical Research Laboratory, Technical Report Number AMRL-TR-71-29, Paper Number 33, Pages 823-841, December 1971.

6. Boyd, I. A., Eyzaguirre, C., Matthews, P. B. C., and Rushworth, G., *The Role of the Gamma System in Movement and Posture,* New York, The Association for the Aid of Crippled Children, Revised Edition, 1968.

7. Chao, E. Y., and An, K. N., "Graphical Interpretation of the Solution to the Redundant Problem in Biomechanics," *J. Biomech. Engrg.,* Vol. 100, No. 4, Pages 159-167, ASME Paper Number 77-Bio-1, August, 1978.

8. Crowe, A., and Matthews, P. B. C., "Further Studies of Static and Dynamic Fusimotor Fibres," *J. Physiol.,* Vol. 174, Pages 132-151, 1964.

9. Crowe, A., and Matthews, P. B. C., "The Effects of Stimulation of Static and Dynamic Fusimotor Fibres on the Response to Stretching of the Primary Endings of Muscle Spindles," *J. Physiol.,* Vol. 174, Pages 109-131, 1964.

10. Crowninshield, R. D., "Use of Optimization Techniques to Predict Muscle Forces," *J. Biomech. Engrg.,* Vol. 100, Pages 88-92, 1978.

11. Crowninshield, R. D., and Brand, R. A., "A Physiologically Based Criterion of Muscle Force Prediction in Locomotion," *J. Biomech.,* Vol. 14, pp. 793-801, 1981.

12. Davis, R. B., III, "Musculoskeletal Biomechanics: Fundamental Measurements and Analysis," In: Bronzino, J. D., (Editor), *Biomedical Engineering and Instrumentation -- Basic Concepts and Applications,* Boston, PWS Publishers, 1986, Chapter 6, pp. 180-221.

13. Deutsch, S., and Micheli-Tzanakou, E., *Neuroelectric Systems*, New York, New York University Press, 1987.

14. DeVries, H. A., *Physiology of Exercise*, Chapter 5, "The Nervous System and Coordination of Muscular Activity," Dubuque, Iowa, William C. Brown Company Publishers, Third Edition, Pages 77-106, 1980.

15. Gardner, E. D., *Fundamentals of Neurology*, Chapter 10, "The Control of Muscular Activity," Philadelphia, W. B. Saunders Company, 1968.

16. Ghosh, T. K., "Dynamics and Optimization of a Human Motion Problem," Ph.D. Thesis, Florida University, Gainesville, Florida, 1973.

17. Gottlieb, G. L., and Agarwal, G. C., "Role of Stretch Reflex in Voluntary Movements," In: *Proceedings of the Eleventh Annual Conference on Manual Control*, NASA, Ames Research Center, Technical Report, NTIS Accession Number, N75-33689, Pages 192-203, May, 1975.

18. Granit, R., *Receptors and Sensory Perception*, New Haven, Connecticut, The Yale University Press, 1955.

19. Granit, R., "Systems for the Control of Movement," *Congr. Int. Sci. Neurol. Brussels*, Vol. 1, Pages 63-99, 1957.

20. Gurfinkel, V. S. and Pal'Tsev, E. I., "Reflex Reaction of Antagonist Muscles During an Evoked Tendon Reflex," *Neirofiziologiia* (Russian), Vol. 5, Number 1, Pages 70-76, January/February, 1973.

21. Guyton, A. C., *Textbook of Medical Physiology*, Philadelphia, W. B. Saunders Company, Sixth Edition, 1981.

22. Hardt, D. E., "A Minimum Energy Solution for Muscle Force Control During Walking," Ph.D. Thesis, MIT Department of Mechanical Engineering, 1978.

23. Hardt, D. E., "Determining Muscle Forces in the Leg During Normal Human Walking -- An Application and Evaluation of Optimization Methods," *J. Biomech. Engrg.*, Vol. 100, Pages 72-78, 1978.

24. Hardy, J. D. (Editor), *Temperature: Its Measurement and Control in Science and Industry*, New York, Reinhold Publishing Corp., Vol. 3, 1963.

25. Houk, J., and Henneman, E., "Responses of Golgi Tendon Organs to Active Contractions of the Soleus Muscle of the Cat," *J. Neurophysiol.*, Vol. 30, No. 3, Pages 466-481, May, 1967.

26. Houk, J. C., Rymer, W. Z., and Crago, P. E., "Dependence of Dynamic Response of Spindle Receptors on Muscle Length and Velocity," *J. Neurophysiol.*, Vol. 46, No. 1, Pages 143-166, July, 1981.

27. Houk, J., and Simon, W., "Responses of Golgi Tendon Organs to Forces Applied to Muscle Tendon," *J. Neurophysiol.*, Vol. 30, No. 6, Pages 1466-1481, November, 1967.

28. Hoyle, G., *Muscles and Their Neural Control*, Somerset, New Jersey, John Wiley and Sons, Inc., 1983.

29. Ito, F. Komatsu, Y., "Transduction and Encoding Mechanisms in Muscle Spindle," *Nagoya. J. Med. Sci.*, Vol. 42, Nos. 3-4, Pages 37-48, March/April, 1980.

30. Jacob, S. W., Francone, C. A., and Lossow, W. J., *Structure and Function in Man*, Philadelphia, W. B. Saunders Company, Fifth Edition, 1982.

31. Jones, G. M., and Watt, D. G. D., "Observations on the Control of Stepping and Hopping Movements in Man," *J. Physiol. (London)*, Volume 219, Pages 709-729, 1971.

32. Jones, R. W., "Biological Control Mechanisms, Section 3. Muscular Control Systems: Spinal Reflexes," In: Schwan, H. P., (Editor), *Biological Engineering*, New York, McGraw-Hill Book Company, Chapter 2, Pages 87-204, 1969.

33. Kleeman, C. R., and Cutler, R. E., "The Neurohypophysis," *Annual Review of Physiology*, Vol. 25, Pages 385-432, 1963.

34. Krieger, D. T., "Endocrine Functions of the Hypothalamus," *N. Y. State J. of Medicine*, Vol. 59, No. 4, Pages 643-648, Feb. 15, 1959.

35. Lennerstrand, G., "Position and Velocity Sensitivity of Muscle Spindles in the Cat, I. Primary and Secondary Endings Deprived of Fusimotor Activation," *Acta Physiol. Scand.*, Vol. 73, Number 3, Pages 281-299, July, 1968.

36. Lundberg, A., "Control of Spinal Mechanisms from the Brain," In: Brady, R. O., (Editor), *The Basic Neurosciences, Volume 1, The Nervous System*, New York, Raven Press, Pages 253-265, 1975.

37. Magdaleno, R. E., and Ruer, D. T., "A Closed-Loop Neuromuscular System Explanation of Force Disturbance Regulation and Tremor Data," In: *Proceedings of the Fourth Annual Conference on Manual Control,*, NASA, Washington Center, Technical Report, NTIS Accession Number, N70-14876 04-05, Pages 527-541, May, 1969.

38. Matthews, P. B. C., "Muscle Spindles and Their Motor Control," *Physiological Reviews*, Vol. 44, Number 4, Pages 219-288, April, 1964.

39. Matthews, P. B., and Stein, R. B., "The Regularity of Primary and Secondary Muscle Spindle Afferent Discharges," *J. Physiol. (London)*, Vol. 202, Number 1, Pages 59-82, May, 1969.

40. Merton, P. A., "How We Control the Contraction of Our Muscles," *Scientific American*, Vol. 226, Number 5, Pages 30-37, May 1972.

41. Milsum, J. H., "Optimization Aspects in Biological Control Theory," In: Sumner N. Levine (Editor), *Advances in Biomedical Engineering and Medical Physics*, Volume 1, New York, Wiley-Interscience Publishers, Pages 243-278, 1968.

42. National Aeronautics and Space Administration, *Biomedical Research in Space*, NASA CR-3487, Falls Church, Virginia, BioTechnology, Inc., 1981.

43. Nishi, K., and Sato, M., "Depolarizing and Hyperpolarizing Receptor Potentials in the Non-myelinated Nerve Terminal in Pacinian Corpuscles," *J. Physiol. (London)*, Volume 199, Number 2, Pages 383-396, December 1968.

44. Nubar, Y., and Contini, R., "A Minimal Principle in Biomechanics," *Bull. Math. Biophysics*, Vol. 23, pages 377-391, 1961.

45. Patriarco, A. G., Mann, R. W., Simon, S. R., and Minsour, J. M., "An Evaluation of the Approaches of Optimization Models in the Prediction of Muscle Forces During Human Gait," *J. Biomechanics*, Vol. 14, No. 8, pp. 513-525, 1981.

46. Pedotti, A., Krishnan, V. V., and Stark, L., "Optimization of Muscle Force Sequencing in Human Locomotion," *Math. Biosci.*, Vol. 28, Pages 57-76, 1977-1978.

47. Penrod, J., Day, D., and Singh, F., "An Optimization Approach to Tendon Force Analysis," *J. Biomechanics*, Vol. 7, Pages 123-129, 1974.

48. Rambourg, A., Clermont, Y., and Hermo, L., "Three-Dimensional Structure of the Golgi Apparatus," *Methods Cell Biol.*, Vol. 23, pp. 155-166, 1981.

49. Ruch, T. C., and Patton, H. D., *Physiology and Biophysics*, Philadelphia, W. B. Saunders Company, Nineteenth Edition, 1966.

50. Schmidt, R. A., "Proprioception and the Timing of Motor Responses," *Psychol. Bulletin*, Vol. 76, No. 6, pp. 383-393, Dec., 1971.

51. Schneck, D. J., "Deductive Physiologic Analysis in the Presence of 'Will' as an Undefined Variable," *Mathematical Modelling*, Vol. 2, Pages 191-199, 1981.

52. Schneck, D. J., "Principles of Bioenergetics and Metabolism in Physiologic Systems," Virginia Polytechnic Institute and State University, College of Engineering, Department of Engineering Science and Mechanics, Biomedical Engineering Program, Technical Report Number VPI-E-83-42, Pages 1-45, November 1, 1983.

53. Schneck, D. J., "Principles of Mass Transport Across Biological Membranes," Virginia Polytechnic Institute and State University, College of Engineering, Department of Engineering Science and Mechanics, Biomedical Engineering Program, Technical Report Number VPI-E-83-07, Pages i-vi and 1-66, March 15, 1983.

54. Schneck, D. J. *Engineering Principles of Physiologic Function*, New York, The New York University Press, 1990.

55. Schroeder, J. M., Kemme, P. T., and Scholz, L., "The Fine Structure of Denervated and Reinnervated Muscle Spindles: Morphometric Study of Intra-Fusal Muscle Fibers," *Acta Neuropathol (Berl.)*, Vol. 46, Numbers 1-2, Pages 95-106, April 12, 1979.

56. Vallbo, A. B., "Human Muscle Spindle Discharge During Isometric Voluntary Contractions - Amplitude Relations Between Spindle Frequency and Torque," *Acta Physiologica Scandinavica*, Vol. 90, No. 2, Pgs. 319-336, February, 1974.

57. Williams, W. J., "A Systems-Oriented Evaluation of the Role of Joint Receptors and Other Afferents in Position and Motion Sense," *Crit. Rev. Biomed. Eng.*, Vol. 7, No. 1, Pages 23-77, 1981.

58. Yao, B. P., "Investigations Concerning the Principle of Minimal Total Muscular Force," *J. Biomech.*, Vol. 9, pp. 413-416, 1976.

59. Zelen'a, J., and Soukup, T., "The Development of Golgi Tendon Organs," *J. Neurocytol.*, Vol. 6, No. 2, Pages 171-194, April 1977.

Chapter 7

Mathematical Modelling of Neuromuscular Control Systems

Introduction

Striated skeletal muscles fall into the general category of devices called "transducers". These are elements of a system that transmit energy, but in so doing, convert that energy (i.e., "transduce" it) from one form into another. The energy that enters the transducer is called its *input*. In the case of striated skeletal muscles, the input is electrochemical energy associated with the muscle fuel cell, which is activated by an action potential initiated by an alpha-motor-neuron. The energy that leaves the transducer is called its *output*. In the case of striated skeletal muscles, the output is either the external work associated with an isotonic contraction (i.e., the integral of force times distance), or the internal work associated with an isometric contraction (the latter ultimately manifesting itself as external heat energy), or some combination of both. Thus, basically, muscles transduce electrochemical energy into thermomechanical energy.

The ratio of the output of a transducer to the corresponding input is related to a quantity called the *Transfer Function*, K_t, of that transducer. Most commonly, K_t is defined to be the ratio of the *Laplace Transform* of the output to the Laplace Transform of the input (see problem 7-2). If this is the case, then the real part (absolute value) of this *complex* transfer function is called the *Gain* of the transducer; and the imaginary part (Argument) is called the *Phase* of the transducer. Thus, for example, viewed as a simple open system, the total force, F_u (output) generated in

one motor unit (controlled system = transducer), innervated by an
α-motor neuron (controlling system) firing at a frequency f_α, (input) could
be written first as a generalized independent *function* of f_α, i.e.,

$$F_u = F_u(f_\alpha);$$

and then, in differential form, the Laplace-transformed *change* in F_u could
be written as a function of the Laplace-transformed *change* in f_α using the
concept of a motor-unit transfer function, i.e.,

$$dF_u = \frac{\partial f_u}{\partial f_\alpha} df_\alpha = K_t df_\alpha, \qquad [7\text{-}1]$$

from which,

$$K_t = \frac{dF_u}{df_\alpha}.$$

As discussed in Chapter 6, however, in reality f_α is not entirely independent of F_u or muscular displacement ξ. Indeed, through a variety
of reflexive mechanisms, normal and abnormal extrinsic control factors
(including "will"), and normal and abnormal intrinsic control factors, the
input to a muscle depends very much on its output. Thus, from a control
engineering point of view, the tissue must be examined as a *closed* system,
such as is illustrated in Figure 7-1 (see later).

The Canonical Form of a Feedback Control System

A specific distinction of feedback control systems is that they all may be
made to fit a particular pattern, such as that shown in Figure 7-1. For a
rather in-depth discussion of this Figure, especially as it relates to the
physiologic concept of *Homeostasis*, the reader is referred to the work of
Schneck, D. J. (1990), and others. Suffice it to say here that, in a global
sense, u_r represents a reference signal to which the system attempts to
conform. In terms of musculoskeletal mechanics, this signal may be

thought of as some "desired level of activity" -- such as a prescribed postural configuration, a required movement, an instinctive reaction, and so on. In many instances, this goal, or desired level of activity will be constrained by the then-current envelope of performance capability, and, by the *cost* of achieving it. The latter is a very interesting concept which was addressed in the previous chapter.

The desired level of activity, u_r for muscle function is, again in a global sense, established within the Central Nervous System -- either at the level of the Spinal Cord, or in "Higher" Brain Centers, such as those of the Cerebral Cortex that dictate conscious effort. These reference quantities are ultimately manifest upon the muscle as the "controlled element" of the muscular system. The output, u (force, and/or, displacement, and/or, some combination of both of these and/or their time-derivatives), is monitored ("fed-back" to a comparator and controller of the system) in order to assess system performance relative to the reference standard (and, perhaps, to *set* the standard, see Schneck, D. J., 1990). Depending on whether u is less than, bigger than, or equal to u_r, and how fast and how consistently u is changing relative to u_r, the comparator and controller of the system issues forth a "controlling", or command signal, u_c to rectify this situation.

In a generic sense, with the muscle being the "controlled" system, u_c would represent the activity f_α of an alpha-motoneuron, the latter representing the "controller" of the system, which is responding to a "desired" level of activity, u_r. If $u = u_r$, everything is fine and nothing happens. But rarely, if ever, is this the case, for we live in an environment that is constantly challenging ("disturbing", u_d) the equilibrium of our physiologic systems; and if the environment is not doing it, we do it ourselves by the very life styles that we lead. Therefore, as Figure 7-1 depicts, controllers in feedback control systems are continually making corrections u_c in order to bring the output u of controlled elements to within an acceptable range of u_r, when the equilibrium of the system is being constantly upset by some disturbance, u_d -- such as gravity or the external resistance against which any given muscle is contracting.

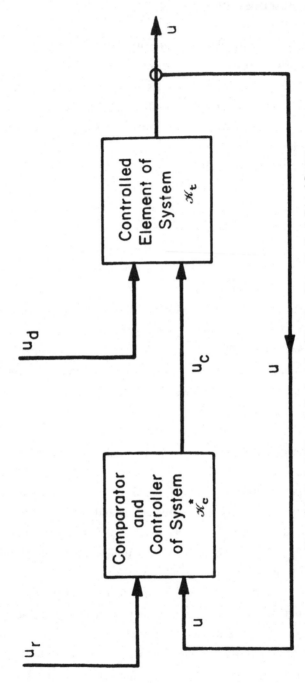

Figure 7-1 Typical Schematic Configuration Of A Closed-Loop Feedback Control System

We should mention that there is some *envelope* of u_d within which u_c will be effective in bringing u to within some acceptable range of u_r. Outside of this envelope, the system will "break down" (get sick or suffer some physiologic disability), or, some nonlinearity will intervene (K not constant) which may allow the system response to "jump" to a new output range (in a sense, "condition" itself to u_d). Thus, with these brief considerations in mind, let us examine some processes that control musculoskeletal performance, to the extent that they have been quantified in accordance with the theory presented here, and with the ultimate goals of not only shedding some more light on disease processes, but also of highlighting factors that are important in designing synthetic implants. Using as a basis for analysis the canonical representation shown in Figure 7-1 for a generic feedback control system, we shall examine first the α-motoneuron as the *controlling* element of the system (in accordance with our discussions in Chapter 6), and then the motor unit as the *controlled* element of the system (in accordance with our discussions in Chapters 1 through 5). We begin, after the following problems, with the stretch reflex.

****

Problem 7-1: Since we want the intensity of the controlling signal to be proportional to the deviation of u from u_r, we may write:

$$u_c = K_c(u - u_r) \qquad\qquad [7\text{-}2]$$

which is called Proportional Control. For simplicity, let $K_c = -1$, such that $u_c = u_r - u$, and let $u_d = 0$ in Figure 7-1. Then, with $u = K_l u_c$, show that:

$$u = \frac{K_t}{K_t + 1}\, u_r \qquad\qquad [7\text{-}3]$$

Suppose, now, that the *sensitivity* of the controlled element to disturbing influences could be varied (such as, for example, by γ-Innervation as described in Chapter 6), such that the *gain*, K_t, would not necessarily

have to be a constant. Then, if the reference signal *is* constant, show,
from equation [7-3], that:

$$\frac{\partial u}{u} = \frac{\partial K_t}{K_t} \frac{1}{1 + K_t} \qquad \text{[7-4]}$$

The right side of equation [7-4] defines the response of u to changes
in the gain, K_t, or in the sensitivity of the controlled element. Basically,
the quantity:

$$\frac{1}{1 + K_t} = Response \ Function$$

measures the amount by which u will differ from some nominal value
when K_t differs from *its* corresponding nominal value. To understand this
better, show, finally, that:

$$\frac{\partial K_t}{K_t} = \frac{\partial u_c}{u_c},$$

so that:

$$\frac{\partial u / u}{\partial u_c / u_c} = \frac{1}{1 + K_t} \qquad \text{[7-5]}$$

From which,

$$\frac{\partial u}{\partial u_c} = \frac{u}{u_r} = \frac{K_t}{1 + K_t}. \qquad \text{[7-6]}$$

Equation [7-5], which also defines the response function, tells us, for a
given value of K_t, how much of a percentage change in u we can expect
when u_c changes by a certain percentage. Thus, with the gain acting as
a parameter, one can ascertain from the response function how sensitive
to u_c the controlled signal, u, will be. This is also reflected in equation
[7-6].

****

Problem 7-2: In practice, the transfer function of a system is usually defined as the ratio of the *Laplace transform* of the output to the Laplace transform of the input. Recalling the definition of the Laplace Transform (see problem 3-4), *prove* that the transformed equation [3-14] defining the passive rheologic behavior of striated skeletal muscle can be written:

$$\overline{F}(s)\left[s + \frac{k_s}{c}\right] = \overline{\xi}(s)\left[s(k_s + k_p) + \frac{k_s k_p}{c}\right] + F(0) - (k_s + k_p)\xi(0) \quad [7\text{-}7]$$

Ignoring the terms $F(0)$ and $\xi(0)$ above due to initial values of F and ξ, what, then, is the Laplace Transfer Function $\overline{K}(s)$ of the muscle model depicted in Figure 3-1?

Show, now, that the *magnitude* of the Laplace Transfer Function, when s is replaced by $i\omega$, is precisely equal to Ck_p as defined in equation [3-28], i.e., *prove* that:

$$|\,K(i\omega)\,| = Ck_p,$$

so that,

$$F = |\,K(i\omega)\,|\,\xi_m \sin(\omega t + \phi) \qquad [7\text{-}8]$$

What you have just shown is that the steady-state response of a stable system to an input of the form: $\xi = \xi_m \sin \omega t$, is given by $\xi_m\,|\,K(i\omega)\,|\,\sin(\omega t + \phi)$, where $|\,K(i\omega)\,|$ is the magnitude of $\overline{K}(s)$ when s is replaced by $i\omega$, and ϕ is the argument of the complex quantity $K(i\omega)$. The magnitude $|\,K(i\omega)\,|$ is usually called the *Gain* of the system (the magnitude of the complex transfer function) and, together with ϕ, defines the *system frequency response* (for example, see Figure 3-4 which is called a Bode Plot).

****

Problem 7-3: With $\xi = \xi_m \sin \omega t$, solve equation [7-7] $\{F(0) = 0\}$ to show that the *Transient Response* of the model in Figure 3-1 is given by:

$$F = -\frac{k_s}{k_p}\frac{k_s}{c\omega}\frac{k_p\xi_m}{\left(\frac{k_s}{c\omega}\right)^2 + 1}\, e^{-\frac{k_s}{c}t} \qquad [7\text{-}9]$$

We see, then, that the decay time constant, τ_d for striated skeletal muscle is also equal to c/k_s, which, as was given in Chapter 3, is equal to $\frac{1}{15} = 0.0667$ seconds. The decay time response constant determines how fast u in Figure 7-1 will come however close we desire to u_r *without* over-shooting, which defines an *overdamped* feedback control system satisfying the response function:

$$u = u_r(1 - e^{-\frac{t}{\tau_d}}) \qquad [7\text{-}10]$$

Note from equation [7-10] that $u = 0$ when $t = 0$ (at which time the system is commanded to take on the value u_r); and, although *hypothetically* $u \to u_r$ exponentially as $t \to \infty$, *realistically* $u = 0.99u_r$ by the time $t = 5$ decay time constants (~ 0.33 seconds in this case). Thus, the smaller is the value of τ_d, the faster will u approach u_r.

For: $\frac{k_s}{c} = 15$, $\frac{k_s}{k_p} = 10$, and $f_\omega = 6$ cycles/sec, plot equation [7-9] as nondimensionalized force, $F/k_p\xi_m$, versus nondimensionalized time, t/τ_d, for $0 \leq \frac{t}{\tau_d} \leq 5$ and *discuss* your results. Then multiply $\frac{F}{k_p\xi_m}$ as defined in equation [7-9] by $\frac{F}{k_p\xi_m}$ as defined in equation [3-28] and plot the product of these two vs, $\frac{t}{\tau_d}$ for the same range (i.e., 0 to 5). Once again, discuss your results within the context of feedback control theory.

****

The Alpha Motor Neuron: Controlling Element of the System

Mathematical Analysis of the Stretch Reflex

Recalling that the main objective of the Myotactic Reflex Arc is to allow a muscle to maintain a relatively constant length, let us consider the length, ℓ, of a muscle fiber to be the monitored output, u, of a servomechanism that operates through the muscle spindle. We may consider the spindle equator (of variable length, ℓ_e, see Figure 6-1) to be the Feedback Element or sensor that is monitoring u at all times, such that the transduced primary feedback signal, u_p, thus becomes the combined firing rate of the type I_a and type II sensory nerves. For simplicity, let us examine the reflex early in the response range, where f_{II} is small compared with f_{I_a} and so may be neglected (c.f., Figure 6-2). Moreover, let us again assume that the alpha-motoneuron receives *only* inputs from the annulospiral nerve endings. Therefore, from equation [6-1], $f_\alpha = f_{I_a} = u_p$, which is proportional to ℓ_e, which, in turn, is a measure of $\ell = u$.

The "desired" length (u_r) of the muscle fiber may be taken to correspond to any spindle equator length less than ℓ_t, since, as can be seen from Figure 6-2, there will be no response to stretch unless $\ell_e \geq \ell_t$. Thus, ℓ_t becomes the reference length against which ℓ_e is being compared. At, or above this reference length, the I_a fibers are causing the α-motoneuron to put out a primary command signal, $u_c \geq f_t$.

As mentioned earlier, the controlling element of this servomechanism is actually the α-motoneuron, which acts as a "comparator" in the sense that it will not fire the motor unit until $\ell_e > \ell_t$, whereupon $f_\alpha > f_t$. The alpha-motoneuron really does not *compare* the actual length of the spindle equator with the reference length of same, in the strict sense of the word, but it does this *in effect* by not firing the motor unit until a threshold number of impulses per second are delivered to the motor end plate. Thus, the controlling signal, u_c in this system is f_α and the controlled element is the motor unit (muscle fiber) itself.

Finally, the disturbing signal, u_d, can be a passive stretch of the muscle tendon, or an active pull on the spindle equator (by gamma-motoneuron activity), or both. The activity of the γ-motoneurons simply controls the *sensitivity* of this servo-system to stretch, thus dictating how close to some reference length the actual motor unit fibers are to be kept. Observe that this feedback control model of the myotatic reflex is a simple on/off model, contracting the muscle when $f_\alpha = f_{I_a} \geq f_t$ and doing nothing otherwise. In that sense, this particular feedback control mechanism is *not* trying to get *u* to *equal* u_r. The reference signal in this case is not the *desired* value, per se, but, rather a *critical* value for which some response will be manifest; and the control signal is not strictly a function of $(u - u_r)$ in the traditional servomechanism sense (c.f., Schneck, D. J., 1990).

In summary, then, and bearing the above in mind, we can fit the Myotactic Reflex Arc into the schematic representation shown in Figure 7-1 by letting:

$u_r = f_t$ $u = f_{I_a} = u_p$ $u_c = f_\alpha$
$u_d = f_\gamma$ (active, sensitivity) $+ \xi$ (passive, stretch)
Comparator and Controller of System $= \alpha$-motoneuron
Controlled Element of System $=$ Motor Unit

and noting that:

$$u = u(u_d, \ u_c) = f_{I_a} = u(f_\gamma, \ \xi, \ f_\alpha).$$ [7-11]

Then, differentiating equation [7-11] by the chain-rule, one can write:

$$df_{I_a} = \frac{\partial u}{\partial f_\gamma} \, df_\gamma + \frac{\partial u}{\partial \xi} \, d\xi + \frac{\partial u}{\partial f_\alpha} \, df_\alpha$$ [7-12]

Letting, $\frac{\partial u}{\partial f_\gamma} = K_\gamma$, $\frac{\partial u}{\partial \xi} = K_\xi$, and, $\frac{\partial u}{\partial f_\alpha} = -K_\alpha$, where the respective K's represent the transfer functions corresponding to the appropriate suffix, equation [7-12] becomes:

$$df_{I_a} = K_\gamma df_\gamma + K_\xi d\xi - K_\alpha df_\alpha$$ [7-13]

Equation [7-13] is a mathematical description of how the rate of firing of the I_d fibers will change as a function of changes in the sensitivity of the spindle equator (df_γ), the state of stretch of the muscle fibers ($d\xi$) and/or the state of contraction of the muscle (df_α). The last term in the equation is negative because, as the muscle contracts, it shuts off the spindle mechanism, thereby decreasing the firing rate of the I_a fibers. The first two terms define the state of stretch $d\ell_e$, of the spindle equator.

If we knew the values of the various transfer functions, equation [7-13] would allow us to predict how the I_a fibers would respond to changes in any of the other variables. Unfortunately, rather few sophisticated attempts (see below) have been made to model the spindle equator in quantitative terms, so, at this time, it is not possible to define the appropriate transfer functions listed above. Furthermore, what few models there are tend to be linear lumped-parameter descriptions that do not isolate the specific effects of gamma-innervation, passive stretch or active contraction. Thus, what we present here is a *technique* for formalizing the description of muscle spindle behavior, with the hope that it will stimulate further research in this very interesting area.

Since we are on the subject, it should be pointed out further that even equation [7-13] is greatly simplified, for it leaves out at least three known facts: (1) the fact that there are *two* types of intrafusal fibers, *each* innervated by type I-a annulospiral nerves. This would necessitate writing:

$$df_{I_a} = df_{I_a}^{\text{Nuclear Bag}} + df_{I_a}^{\text{Nuclear Chain}} \qquad [7\text{-}14]$$

and introducing separate transfer functions (for a total of six altogether) for the Nuclear Bag (rate-dependent) and Nuclear Chain (amplitude-dependent) IF fibers, in accordance with equation [7-13]. In fact, there have actually been defined *three* types of IF fibers: *Dynamic* Nuclear Bag Fibers (at least one per spindle), *Static* Nuclear Bag Fibers (at least one per spindle), and the "traditional" nuclear chain fibers -- suggesting (even if no additional types of IF fibers remain to be discovered) the need for nine separate transfer functions, at least; (2) the fact that there are *two* types of γ-innervation of the spindle poles, which have been tacitly lumped together in this analysis. This would necessitate writing:

$$df_\gamma = df_\gamma^{\text{Plate}} + df_\gamma^{\text{Trail}} \qquad\qquad [7\text{-}15]$$

and introducing separate transfer functions for γ-plate and γ-trail innervation, thereby increasing still further the number of transfer functions that would be needed just to account for the firing frequency of the I-a fibers.

Moreover, as discussed in Chapter 6, a single muscle spindle may be innervated by as many as six γ-motoneurons, some innervating either the nuclear chain fibers (γ-trail) alone or *both* the nuclear chain and the static nuclear bag fibers (so-called γ-plate-static axons), and others innervating only the dynamic nuclear bag fibers (so-called γ-plate-dynamic axons); and (3) the fact that the response of the I_a fibers is a function not only of muscle stretch and/or tension development, but also of the *rate* of muscle stretch and/or tension development (velocity) and the acceleration associated with such tension development.

Thus, it has been found that the spindle actually responds *instantaneously* to *rates* of change of muscle length (so-called *phasic* changes), but it adapts within a few seconds, and its degree of response thereafter is determined by the *amount* of change of muscle length (so-called *tonic* changes). This can be incorporated into the mathematical model by writing equation [7-11] in the form:

$$f_{1_a} = u(f_\gamma,\ \dot{f}_\gamma,\ \ddot{f}_\gamma,\ \xi,\ \dot{\xi},\ \ddot{\xi},\ f_\alpha,\ \dot{f}_\alpha,\ \ddot{f}_\alpha),$$

which, obviously, makes the problem much more complicated, if not impossible to handle.

And speaking of time-dependence and complications, one might also note that synaptic delays are involved in all of the neural pathways discussed, so that transmission time-delays (and associated time constants) between muscle stretch and other inputs, and contractile response and other outputs, should also be incorporated into any realistic description of the muscle spindle mechanism. In other words, the response is not purely elastic, but viscoelastic, so one should set up the mathematical model to include appropriate time constants. These would indicate that the servomechanism *approaches* reference quantities with some phase lead or lag.

Finally, to make matters still worse, there is increasing evidence that muscle spindles react with significant amplitude and velocity-dependent nonlinearities, which suggest that simple, linearized, single-input single-output models may have limited usefulness in a generalized sense. This problem is circumvented in practice by keeping the peak-to-peak stretch of the spindle very small and allowing the stimulus to change slowly in experiments designed to establish the input/output characteristics of the spindle. Stretch amplitudes on the order of a few microns, up to one millimeter, applied at frequencies not exceeding 30-50 cycles/sec thus allow the techniques of linear analysis to be used to derive transfer functions describing the spindle response (see below). It is desirable to operate in the response range of the spindle receptors at 0.2 mm sinusoidal stretch amplitudes and 1 Hz or less cycles per second.

What all of this amounts to, is the realization that neuromuscular systems offer a real challenge to the control engineer. Not only do they involve time-dependent responses that transpire through a network of complex, multiple physiologic pathways, but the various information channels that bridge receptors to actuators are to date not very well defined, and there is a great deal of uncertainty as to whether or not all of these channels have even been identified (i.e., discovered) as yet. Nevertheless, engineers, by definition, are problem solvers and there is every reason to believe that the established field of control theory can make significant contributions to the study and understanding of biological servomechanisms.

With this in mind, we comment further that relationships such as equations [7-11] to [7-15] can also be written for the Flower Spray sensory nerve fibers. These also respond to the state of stretch of the spindle equator (although at considerably higher lengths), and these also turn off as the muscle contracts. Thus,

$$df_{II} = K^*_{\gamma} df_{\gamma} + K^*_{\xi} d\xi - K^*_{\alpha} df_{\alpha} \qquad [7\text{-}16]$$

where the starred quantities represent transfer functions characteristic of the Type II, rather than the type I_a fibers.

Note that equations [7-13] to [7-16] are written for *Homonymous* inputs to the ipsilateral flexors -- or *Agonist* muscles. By this, we mean that the inputs are being administered to the motor neuron supplying the same muscle *from which* the afferent Group I_a volley originates. One could now write a corresponding matching set of equations for inputs to this same motor neuron that originate in ipsilateral extensors -- or *Antagonist* muscles. These are called *Heteronymous* inputs, i.e., inputs from *other* than the muscle being innervated by the given motor neuron -- and, in this case, those inputs would be exactly opposite in sign to the values given in equations [7-13] to [7-16]. This is in accordance with our previous discussions (Chapter 6) of reciprocal inhibition and excitation by *Antagonist* muscles.

And finally, one can also write corresponding sets of equations for the excitatory synapses associated with ipsilateral motor units that are progressively *recruited* as necessary, and for the excitatory activity of the ipsilateral *synergist* muscle groups that participate in the accomplishment of a certain task. All of these various muscle units have type I_a and II sensory nerve fibers that respond basically the same way to stretch and to contraction. Furthermore, they all have associated transfer functions to describe these responses -- although the functions may as yet be unknown.

****

Problem 7-4: In a manner similar to that by which the Myotatic Reflex was made to fit into the scheme illustrated in Figure 7-1, show how the Inverse Myotatic Reflex can also be made to fit this scheme by identifying: u_r, u, u_c, u_d, the comparator and controller, and the corresponding controlled element of the system that operates through the Golgi Tendon Organs to control active muscle force output.

Based on your definition of the various parameters in Figure 7-1, describe how the system operates. Then derive the corresponding system equation similar to equations [7-11] to [7-13].

****

TRANSFER FUNCTIONS FOR THE STRETCH REFLEX

Many investigators have compiled a fairly impressive amount of experimental data in an effort to describe the input/output characteristics of the various reflex mechanisms that control muscular contraction. Despite all of this data, however, few satisfactory dynamic mathematical models have surfaced to quantify these mechanisms, although some common features *have* emerged in all of the reflex pathways thus far examined. For example, they all apparently exhibit response characteristics that are typical of critically over-damped, second-order physical systems (Schneck, D. J., 1990). This means, that, when disturbed, they regain their equilibrium position in the shortest possible time *without* significant oscillation.

Also, these biological servomechanisms tend to be more sensitive to *rates* of change of disturbing signals, rather than to magnitudes, per se. Thus, the ability of these transducers to respond rapidly without overshooting is generally limited to a particular range of frequencies of a disturbing signal. Moreover, the control systems typically have characteristic low-frequency responses and high-frequency responses that are quite different (for example, refer back to Figure 3-4 and the associated discussion on pages 101-118). The low frequency response is generally demarcated by a lower "break" or "corner" frequency, f_L, below which the system is essentially insensitive to change. That is to say, below f_L the rate of change of the disturbance is so slow that each increment essentially brings the system to a quasi-steady equilibrium long before the next change occurs. Thus, the transducer, being primarily *rate-sensitive*, adapts rather quickly to a new reference quantity and no control signal is generated to affect a response to change which would bring the system back to its original reference configuration. Essentially, the system "drifts" randomly with the disturbance, the latter acting like a floating setpoint, and no particular feedback control is in evidence below f_L.

For a range of frequencies above f_L, biological transducers become responsive in such a way that the strength of the response is in some sense proportional to the frequency of the disturbance, although not necessarily in phase with it. Typically, the response is defined by means of an open-loop transfer function of the form:

$$\overline{K}(s) = \frac{K_1(1 + sT_1)(1 + sT_2)(1 + sT_3) \cdots}{s^N(1 + sT_A)(1 + sT_B)(1 + sT_C) \cdots}$$ [7-17]

where: $\overline{K}(s)$ is the LaPlace transfer function (replace s by $i\omega$ to get frequency response), K_1 is the loop gain of the open-loop transfer function, the terms in the numerator of the equation define the "zeroes" of the transfer function (i.e., at what frequencies $\overline{K}(s)$ goes to zero), and the terms in the denominator define the "poles" of the transfer function (i.e., at what frequencies $\overline{K}(s)$ goes to infinity). The exponent N is an arbitrary integer and the system has corner or break frequencies at $\omega = (1/T_1)$; $\omega = (1/T_2)$; $\omega = (1/T_3)$; $\ldots$; $\omega = (1/T_A)$; $\omega = (1/T_B)$; $\omega = (1/T_C)$; $\ldots$. The corner frequencies can be most easily determined by plotting the nondimensionalized gain, in decibels, against the logarithm of circular frequency. From equation [7-17], we have:

Decibels $= 20 \log_{10} \dfrac{|K(i\omega)|}{K_1} = 20[\log_{10} | (1 + i\omega T_1) | + \log_{10} | (1 + i\omega T_2) |$

$+ \log_{10} | (1 + i\omega T_3) | + \cdots - N \log_{10} | i\omega |$

[7-18]

$- \log_{10} | (1 + i\omega T_A) | - \log_{10} | (1 + i\omega T_B) |$

$- \log_{10} | (1 + i\omega T_C) | - \cdots]$

For purposes of illustration, let:

$$N = 0 = T_2 = T_3 = T_A = T_B = T_C = \cdots = 0.$$

Then, equation [7-18] reduces to:

$$\text{Decibels} = 20 \log_{10} |(1 + i\omega T_1)|, \qquad\qquad \text{[7-19]}$$

since all the rest of the terms on the right of the equation become zero, or $\log_{10} 1 = 0$. Now, for very, very low frequencies ($\omega T_1 << 1$), equation [7-19] reveals that Decibels $= 20 \log_{10}(1) = 0$, so, for very low frequencies, the nondimensionalized gain in decibels will be essentially equal to zero. At the other extreme, for very high frequencies ($\omega T_1 >> 1$), equation [7-19] essentially reduces to Decibels $= 20 \log_{10}(\omega T_1)$ which plots as a straight line on logarithmic axes. This line cuts the Decibels $= 0$ axis at $\omega T_1 = 1$, thus intercepting the low-frequency curve ($dB = 0$) at this point and defining the lowest breakpoint frequency at the point $\omega = (1/T_1)$. At this corner frequency, the slope of the gain curve changes from zero to $+20$ decibels per decade for the case under consideration, i.e., for any two values of Decibels, and $\omega T_1 >> 1$,

$$(\text{Decibels})_2 - (\text{Decibels})_1 \approx 20[\log_{10}(\omega_2 T_1) - \log_{10}(\omega_1 T_1)]$$

$$= 20 \log_{10} \frac{\omega_2 T_1}{\omega_1 T_1} = 20 \log_{10} \frac{2\pi f_2}{2\pi f_1} \qquad\qquad \text{[7-20]}$$

and, for a decade change in linear frequency, $f_2 = 10 f_1$, so,

$$(\text{Decibels})_2 - (\text{Decibels})_1 = 20 \log_{10}(10) = 20 \text{ per decade.}$$

Having thus located (or defined) a lower breakpoint frequency at which the system gain response essentially begins, let us examine the next more complicated case where T_1 and T_A are the only parameters different from zero in equation [7-18]. Also, we assume that $(1/T_1) < (1/T_A)$. Since equation [7-18] is linear, the gain curve for this case may be obtained by simply adding to the gain curve obtained above for only $T_1 \neq 0$, the gain curve obtained by considering the situation where only $T_A \neq 0$. That is, we already know that the plot of equation [7-19] may be approximated by the line (Decibels) $= 0$ until $\omega = (1/T_1)$, and then by a straight line of slope 20 decibels per decade for $\omega > (1/T_1)$. Using similar reasoning, a plot of:

$$\text{Decibels} = -20 \log_{10} |(1 + i\omega T_A)| \qquad [7\text{-}21]$$

may be approximated by $\log_{10}(1) = 0$ for ω small, and a straight line of slope -20 decibels per decade for $\omega >> (1/T_A)$. The *composite* curve, then, of equations [7-19] and [7-21] will consist of $db = 0$ up to $\omega = (1/T_1)$, followed by a straight line of slope $+20$ db/decade, followed by a horizontal straight line again at $\omega = (1/T_A)$, where the curve of slope $+20$ db/decade now adds to (and cancels with) a curve of slope -20 db/decade. This is quite similar to the curve of amplitude C vs. frequency given in Figure 3-4 for the linear viscoelastic rheologic model of muscle tissue -- where the lower breakpoint frequency corresponding to T_1 was calculated (page 112) to be 1.3636 radians/second, and the upper breakpoint frequency corresponding to T_A was calculated (page 113) to be 15 radians/second, some 1.1 decades later. A straight line of slope $+20$ db/decade connecting these two extremes represents an *approximate* linear regression to the *actual* curve (equation [3-28] for C as a function of ω) which defines this region.

And so it goes -- every term in the *numerator* of equation [7-17] adding a break frequency at the corresponding point, $\omega = (1/T_i)$, $i = 1, 2, 3, \ldots$, and, adding a component to the gain curve consisting of a line of *positive* slope $+20$ db/decade; and every term in the *denominator* of equation [7-17] adding a break frequency at the corresponding point, $\omega = (1/T_i)$, $i = A, B, C, \ldots$, and, adding a component to the gain curve consisting of a straight line of *negative* slope -20 db/decade.

Each flat portion of the total gain curve between break frequencies defines an interval of frequency for which $\Delta db = 0$, i.e., so-called "flat-frequency-response-intervals" in the gain curve. Each sloping portion of the total gain curve between break frequencies defines an interval of frequency during which the transducer is responsive to a disturbance, hence defining the so-called "response-range" for the system. Ultimately, the high frequency response is generally demarcated by an uppermost break frequency, f_U, above which the rate of change of the disturbance is so rapid that the transducer has no *time* to respond effectively. In this limit, events happen basically faster than the response characteristics of the receptor, so the feedback element essentially does not even know anything is happening -- hence, again, no control signal is generated. The difference, $f_U - f_L$, (or, sometimes, the interval from 3 db below that corresponding to f_L to 3 db above that corresponding to f_U), defines the total *bandwidth* of the system, i.e., the total range of frequencies of disturbing signals over which the system will respond "satisfactorily" (see Schneck, D. J., 1990).

Finally, as already mentioned, biological transducers have amplitude-and-velocity-dependent nonlinearities which render simple linearized, single-input-single-output models relatively useless in a generalized sense. However, the servomechanisms do lend themselves to the techniques of linear analysis so long as the peak-to-peak amplitude of the disturbance is kept relatively small and the frequencies of the disturbance are kept low. Under these conditions, one may write simple transfer functions which, for critically over-damped, second-order physical systems, frequently take a general form such as:

$$\bar{K}(s) = \frac{\bar{g}(s)}{(1 + \tau_U s)(1 + \tau_L s)} \qquad [7\text{-}22]$$

where: $\tau_U = \frac{1}{\omega_U}$ and $\tau_L = \frac{1}{\omega_L}$ are time constants associated with the upper (U) and lower (L) break frequencies, respectively.

Several transfer functions which conform to the general idea of equation [7-22] have been proposed for the Stretch Reflex (see, for example, the work of Houk, et al., 1962, Houk and Stark, 1962, Gottlieb, et al., 1969, Poppele and Bowman, 1970, Baran, 1974, Baran, et al., 1975, Baran, 1976, Stein and Oğuztöreli, 1976, and others). This reflex pathway appears to exhibit a linear response for peak-to-peak stretch stimuli that have amplitudes on the order of a few microns on up to one millimeter, and that excite the spindle at frequencies not exceeding about two cycles per second (i.e., for slowly changing, low stretch velocities). For this situation, for example, Baran (1976) has proposed the following transfer function for the muscle spindle:

$$\overline{K}_{\mathfrak{s}}(s) = \frac{K_2(s + 0.06)}{(s + 74.05)(s + 14.86)} \qquad [7\text{-}23]$$

where K_2 is an arbitrary Gain Constant between 86 and 120 reciprocal seconds. Equation [7-23] is based on a viscoelastic muscle spindle model which was proposed by Gottlieb, et al., in 1969, and is reproduced here in Figure 7-2A.

The mammalian nuclear bag and chain region at the spindle equator (which is believed to be elastically stiffer and less viscous than the intrafusal spindle pole fibers themselves) is represented by a simple Voigt Body having an elastic constant k_b and a dashpot (viscous) constant B_b. The contractile regions at the spindle poles are represented by a Voigt Body having a (lower) spring constant, k_f, and a (higher) dashpot constant, B_f, in parallel with a contractile (γ-innervated) component represented by the active element, $F^*{}_m$. The tendinous attachments of the muscle spindles to the surrounding extrafusal fibers are represented by a simple elastic attachment lumped into the spring constant, k_e.

Tendons, Poles and Equators are attached in series, such that the total force, F_2, in each loop is the same, but they can deflect different amounts due to the viscous and elastic elements that are present. The individual deflections are designated X_1 for the tendinous region alone, X_2 for the combined tendons plus poles and X_m for the tendons plus poles plus equator (i.e., the total spindle motion).

As was done in Chapter 3 for the viscoelastic model of striated skeletal muscle, so, too, can this viscoelastic model of muscle spindles be viewed as a superposition of purely passive behavior ($F^*{}_m = 0$) and purely active behavior (i.e., isometric, with $X_m = 0$). The total transfer function is then obtained by adding the individual transfer functions for each case,

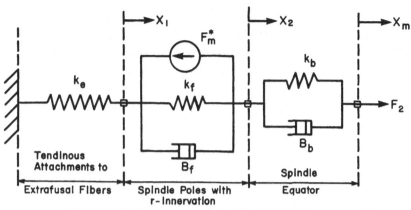

PART A: Viscoelastic Model of the Mammalian Spindle ($k_e > k_b > k_f$); $B_b < B_f$; Single Input-Output System.

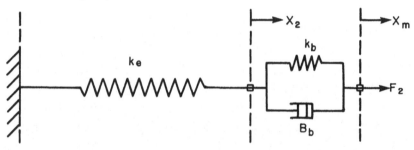

PART B: Standard Mechanical Lead Network:
$\tau_1 > \tau_2$ $\quad \frac{X_2}{X_m}(s) = K \frac{(1+\tau_1 s)}{(1+\tau_2 s)}$

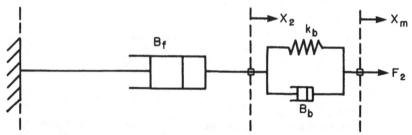

PART C: Standard Mechanical Lag Network:
$\tau_1 < \tau_2$ $\quad \frac{X_2}{X_m}(s) = K \frac{(1+\tau_1 s)}{(1+\tau_2 s)}$

Figure 7-2 Viscoelastic Model of the Mammalian Muscle Spindle, Compared With a Standard Mechanical Lead Network and a Standard Mechanical Lag Network

with X_1, X_2, and X_m being measured from the rest condition when $F_2 = 0$ and $F^*_m = 0$. Since superposition is implied based on linear systems analysis, one may consider one physical process at a time. Thus, in LaPlace notation, we first assume $F^*_m = 0$ and examine the passive spindle behavior:

$$F_2 = k_e X_1 \qquad \qquad \text{[7-24]}$$

$(F^*_m = 0)$:

$$F_2 = (k_f + B_f s)(X_2 - X_1) \qquad \qquad \text{[7-25]}$$

and:

$$F_2 = (k_b + B_b s)(X_m - X_2) \qquad \qquad \text{[7-26]}$$

From [7-24], $X_1 = \dfrac{F_2}{k_e}$, so that [7-25] becomes:

$$F_2\left[1 + \frac{k_f}{k_e} + \frac{B_f}{k_e} s\right] = (k_f + B_f s)X_2. \qquad \qquad \text{[7-27]}$$

Substituting this last equation for F_2 into equation [7-26], and rearranging, one obtains:

$$\frac{X_2}{X_m} = \frac{(k_b + B_b s)(k_e + k_f + B_f s)}{k_e(k_f + B_f s) + [(k_b + B_b s)(k_e + k_f + B_f s)]} \qquad \text{[7-28]}$$

The *net* deflection of the spindle equator, to which the sensory afferent nerves (in this case, only the I_a fibers were examined relative to the nuclear bag IF fibers) are sensitive, is given by $(X_m - X_2)$, so one may define a passive transfer function, $\overline{K}_X(s)$, as:

$$\overline{K}_X(s) = \frac{X_m - X_2}{X_m} = 1 - \frac{X_2}{X_m} \qquad \qquad \text{[7-29]}$$

Using equation [7-28], then, (with considerable algebraic rearranging), equation [7-29] becomes:

$$\overline{K}_x(s) = \frac{k_e}{B_b} \left\{ \frac{\left(s + \dfrac{k_f}{B_f}\right)}{s^2 + s\left[\dfrac{k_eB_f + k_eB_b + k_fB_b + k_bB_f}{B_bB_f}\right] + \dfrac{k_ek_f + k_ek_b + k_bk_f}{B_bB_f}} \right\}$$

[7-30]

Now, let:

$$\frac{1}{\tau_L} + \frac{1}{\tau_U} = \frac{k_eB_f + k_eB_b + k_fB_b + k_bB_f}{B_bB_f},$$

$$\frac{1}{\tau_L\tau_U} = \frac{k_ek_f + k_ek_b + k_bk_f}{B_bB_f},$$

$$K_2 = \frac{k_e}{B_b}, \quad \text{and,} \quad \frac{1}{\tau_3} = \frac{k_f}{B_f}.$$

Then,

$$\overline{K}_x(s) = K_2 \frac{\left(s + \dfrac{1}{\tau_3}\right)}{s^2 + s\left(\dfrac{1}{\tau_L} + \dfrac{1}{\tau_U}\right) + \dfrac{1}{\tau_L\tau_U}} = K_2 \frac{\left(s + \dfrac{1}{\tau_3}\right)}{\left(s + \dfrac{1}{\tau_U}\right)\left(s + \dfrac{1}{\tau_L}\right)}$$

$$= K_2 \frac{\tau_L\tau_U}{\tau_3} \frac{(1 + s\tau_3)}{(1 + s\tau_U)(1 + s\tau_L)}$$

[7-31]

which is in the form given by equations [7-22] or [7-23] for a critically over-damped, second-order physical system. This transfer function thus describes such a system and predicts the existence of three critical breakpoint or corner frequencies at the circular frequencies $(1/\tau_3)$, $(1/\tau_U)$ and $(1/\tau_L)$, in accordance with our previous discussion.

****

Problem 7-5: Assume now that $X_m = 0$ but $F^*_m \neq 0$. For this case, write the set of governing equations of motion corresponding to equations [7-24] to [7-26] written for the previous case (based on the phenomenological model depicted in Figure 7-2-A). Solve these equations simultaneously to define an *active* transfer function,

$$\overline{K}_F(s) = -\frac{X_2}{F^*_m} = \frac{\tau_L \tau_U K_2}{B_f(1 + s\tau_L)(1 + s\tau_U)} = K_y \qquad [7\text{-}32]$$

The total transfer function for the model is obtained by combining equations [7-31] and [7-32]:

$$X_m - X_2 = \overline{K}_X(s)X_m + \overline{K}_F(s)F^*_m \qquad [7\text{-}33]$$

Observe that equation [7-33] reduces to [7-31] for $F^*_m = 0$, and to equation [7-32] for $X_m = 0$. Compare equation [7-33] also with [7-13] in general form.

****

Problem 7-6: Following a method similar to that used in formulating equation [7-31] for the passive behavior of the model depicted in Figure 7-2A, *derive* a system transfer function for the passive behavior of the muscle model depicted in Figure 3-1.

From this transfer function, derive, further, expressions for the system break-point frequencies, and compare your results with those given in Chapter 3, (c.f. also, problem 7-2).

****

The model proposed by Baran, which shall be discussed below and is given by equation [7-23], actually corresponds to the *passive* behavior of the muscle spindle, as defined by equation [7-31]. Baran did not consider the active behavior of the tissue, but Gottlieb, et al., (1969) did propose an active transfer function of the form:

$$\overline{K}_F(s) = \frac{3200}{(s + 182)(s + 16.7)} = K_y \qquad [7\text{-}34]$$

for the mammalian spindle.

Now, replacing s in equation [7-23] by $i\omega$, as was done in problem 7-2 for the viscoelastic muscle model, one can write the associated transfer function in terms of a phase angle, ϕ_1, and a scaled amplitude, D_1, where:

$$\phi_1 = \text{Tan}^{-1}\frac{D_2}{D_3}$$

$$D_1 = \frac{\sqrt{D_2^2 + D_3^2}}{D_4 D_5}$$

$D_2 = 1095.0484\omega - \omega^3$
$D_3 = 66.02298 + 88.85\omega^2$
$D_4 = 220.8196 + \omega^2$
$D_5 = 5483.4025 + \omega^2$

and,

$$\frac{K_X(i\omega)}{K_2} = D_1 e^{i\phi_1} \qquad\qquad [7\text{-}35]$$

The modulus, D_1, in decibels is plotted in Figure 7-3 as a function of linear frequency, $\omega/2\pi$, on a log scale. The dotted points shown are actual values of $20\log_{10}D_1$ calculated from equation [7-35]. The solid lines are approximations used to locate the break frequencies of the re- sponse curves. Thus, a line of positive slope $+20$ db/decade approxi- mates the upsloping portion of the gain curve; a line of negative slope -20 db/decade approximates the downsloping portion of the gain curve; and two horizontal lines approximate the essentially flat frequency- response portions of the gain curve. In this way, three distinct corner frequencies are defined -- one at about $\omega = 0.06$, one at $\omega = 74.05$, and one at $\omega = 14.86$.

Note that there is an excellent correspondence between the actual values of Gain and the straight-line approximation, which, of course, is the key reason for the use of this type of diagram to define the corner frequencies. The errors are on the order of 3 decibels or less at any given point -- at best 3 db out of about -85, or some 3.5% at the low end of

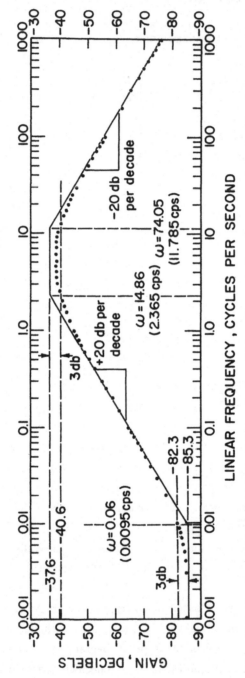

Figure 7-3 Non-dimensionalized Gain, in Decibels, vs. the Log of Linear Frequency, in cycles per second, for the Viscoelastic Model of the Mammalian Muscle Spindle Illustrated in Figure 7-2. This Graph is for Passive Behavior Only, and is based on Single-input-single-output Model Characteristics

the gain curve, and at worst, 3 db out of about −40, or some 7.5% at the high end of the gain curve. For instance, if we let $\omega = (1/T_1)$ in equation [7-19], we get: Decibels $= 20\log_{10}|(1 + i)| = 20\log_{10}\sqrt{2} = 3$ db as the "actual" value of gain at this corner frequency, compared with the "approximate" value of $20\log_{10}(1) = 0$ which was assumed for small frequencies.

Bearing this in mind, the modulus, D_1, and Phase Angle, ϕ_1 have been plotted against linear frequency on a log scale in Figure 7-4. To the left of the frequency labelled 5.2666 cps, note the similarity in shape between these curves and the corresponding ones plotted for the viscoelastic muscle model in Figure 3-4. That is to say, there is a phase lead that starts small, increases to some maximum value and then returns to zero, and this is accompanied by a corresponding increase in Gain of about an order of magnitude.

The curves to the right of the frequency labelled 5.2666 cycles per second enter into the picture now because equation [7-35] describes a viscoelastic *network* (Figure 7-2-A), as opposed to equation [3-28], which describes the simple first-order system shown in Figure 3-1. Thus, we see that the phase lead crosses over the axis to become a phase lag and the amplitude modulus returns to zero as second-order-like effects start to dominate the frequency-response of the spindle (see below). This occurs at the *crossover frequency*, $f = 5.2666$ cps, which corresponds to the *resonance frequency* of a spring-mass-dashpot system (c.f., Problem 3-6), for which system the resonance frequency at which the amplitude-response peaks is equal to the square-root of k_p/m, in radians per second.

From the numerator of equation [7-23], and Figure 7-3, we see that the lowest corner or break frequency associated with the spindle response is located at $\omega = 0.06$ radians per second, which corresponds to a linear frequency of 0.00955 cps or approximately 1.75 minutes per cycle. At this frequency, $D_1 = 7.71 \times 10^{-5}$ (−82.26 db) and $\phi_1 = +44.72°$. The value of D_1, in decibels is some 3 decibels above the value that D_1 has at a linear frequency of 0.00046 cps (1.656 cycles per hour), i.e.,

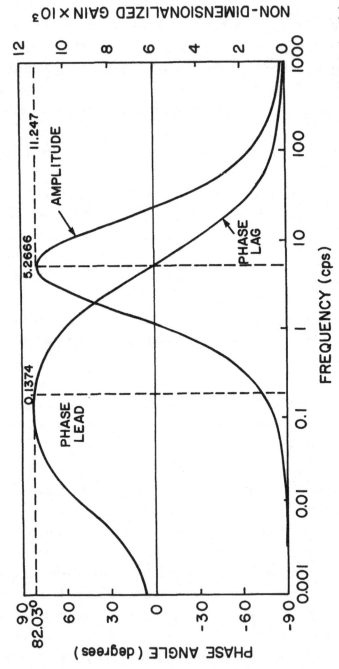

Figure 7-4 Nondimensionalized Modulus, D_1, and Phase Angle, ϕ_1, vs. Linear Frequency illustrate the Passive Viscoelastic Behavior of the Phenomenological Model Illustrated in Figure 7-2 for the Mammalian Muscle Spindle

$D_1 = 5.459 \times 10^{-5} = -85.26$ db, for which value of frequency the phase angle is equal to a very small $+ 2.74°$.

In other words, again we see that the amplitude response begins about three decibels above where the phase angle response begins, so that the two have essentially a flat frequency response from 3 decibels below the lower breakpoint frequency on down to zero cycles per second (see also Figure 7-3). This means that it takes a minimum disturbance of just over one and one-half cycles per hour to deform the spindle equator enough (passively) to excite the I_a fibers. Anything slower than that will elicit essentially no response, in the sense that an input X_m to the model depicted in Figure 7-2-A will be followed almost instantaneously by a corresponding and equal displacement of X_2, such that $X_m - X_2 = 0$ (essentially no Gain) at low frequencies. Stated another way, dashpots B_f and B_b are passively unresponsive at low frequencies, and for $k_e > k_b > k_f$, X_2 moves essentially in phase with X_m ($\phi_1 = 0$) and the difference $X_m - X_2$ is negligibly small ($\overline{K}_x(s) = 0$) for disturbances on the order of one and one-half cycles per hour. In a practical sense, anything slower than ten times that amount will really provide no significant output, as seen in Figure 7-4.

As frequency increases, dashpot B_b starts to become responsive. Since B_f is bigger than B_b and k_f is relatively small compared with k_e and k_b, with $F^*_m = 0$ the center loop of Figure 7-2-A is essentially not there yet and Figure 7-2-A can be drawn as in Figure 7-2-B. This, we recognize as a standard mechanical *lead* network, with X_m (input) leading X_2 (output). As the frequency continues to go higher, X_m leads X_2 by more and more, the phase lead angle going on to peak at a value of $82.03°$ for a linear frequency of 0.1374 cycles per second (about 8.25 cycles per minute), for which frequency $D_1 = 7.85 \times 10^{-4}$ (-62.1 db). As B_f now starts to become responsive, the phase lead angle begins to come down, returning to a value of $+44.72°$ at a linear frequency of 1.756 cps, for which $D_1 = 7.96 \times 10^{-3}$ (-41.98 db).

Note how, as the phase angle passes through $+44.72°$ at the lowest corner frequency, then through its maximum value of $+82.03°$, and finally back to the value of +44.72° that it had at the lowest corner frequency, the scaled amplitude D_1 increases at each point by about an order of magnitude $(5.459 \times 10^{-5} = -85.26$ db; $7.85 \times 10^{-4} = -62.1$ db; $7.96 \times 10^{-3} = -41.98$ db), equivalent to about $20 \log_{10}(10) = 20$ db; and, the frequency increases by about a decade $(0.00955 \approx 0.01$ cps to $0.1374 \approx 0.10$ cps to $1.756 \approx 1.00$ cps), at least in order of magnitude. Thus, as already discussed, the mean slope of the gain curve is about $+20$ decibels per decade in this frequency range (c.f., Figure 7-3), which is how the lower corner frequency is actually determined.

Moreover, it can also be seen that the maximum phase shift position ($+82.03°$ at 0.1374 cps) corresponds to the midpoint of the upward slop-ing portion of the gain curve (around -61.5 db in Figure 7-3). Finally, for a phase-lead network, the sine of the maximum phase lead angle may be written in terms of a parameter α_1, such that:

$$\operatorname{Sin}(\phi_1)_{max} = \frac{1 - \alpha_1}{1 + \alpha_1} \qquad\qquad \text{[7-36]}$$

For the transfer function given by equation [7-23], $(\phi_1)_{max}$ is calcu-lated to be 82.03°, so, from equation [7-36], $\alpha_1 = 0.004853$. Then,

$$\omega_{max} = \frac{\omega_{lower\ corner}}{\sqrt{\alpha_1}}$$

$$= 0.86128 \text{ radians per second}$$
$$= 0.1371 \text{ cycles per second,}$$

which is very close to the value indicated on Figure 7-4 (i.e., 0.1374).

Furthermore, an upper corner frequency is defined by,

$$\omega_{upper\ corner} = \frac{\omega_{lower\ corner}}{\alpha_1} = \frac{0.06}{0.004853}$$

$$= 12.3635 \text{ rad/sec}$$
$$= 1.9677 \text{ cycles/sec,}$$

which is just slightly higher (by about 0.21 cycles per second) than the value of 1.756 cps given for $\phi_1 = +44.72°$ the second time.

As B_f continues to become more and more responsive with increasing frequency, it becomes so effective as a damper that k_e effectively never "sees" the motion taking place at X_m and X_2. Since k_f is also small and $F^*_m = 0$, Figure 7-2-A reduces in essence to Figure 7-2-C, which is a standard mechanical lag network. The phase angle continues to decrease to zero as the gain reaches *its* maximum value of 1.1247×10^{-2} (-38.98 db) for a linear frequency of 5.2666 cps (33.09 radians per second).

Observe that this maximum occurs another 3 decibels above the value that D_1 had when ϕ_1 was again equal to $+44.72°$ at $\omega = 11.033$ rad/sec (1.756 cps). Thus, this behavior is consistent with the corresponding discussion in Chapter 3, relative to the frequency response characteristics of the model depicted in Figure 3-1. That is to say, the gain is essentially zero from 3 db below the lower corner frequency ($\omega = 0.06$) on down to zero cycles per second, and it reaches its maximum value some 3 db above the upper corner frequency ($\omega = 11.03$). The maximum value of the gain curve corresponds to the resonance frequency of the transducer, and the numerator of the transfer function describes the basic phase-lead characteristics of the transducer.

The phase-lag characteristics of the spindle are defined from information contained in the denominator of equation [7-23]. Thus, the next corner frequency, at $\omega = 14.86$ rad/sec (2.365 cps), for which $D_1 = 9.36 \times 10^{-3}$ (-40.573 db) and $\phi_1 = 33.42°$ locates the beginning of the frequency range for which the gain response of the transducer is again essentially "flat" (see Figure 7-3). The linear approximation line of increasing slope $+20$ db/decade has a corresponding value of -37.6 db at this linear frequency, which is 3 db above -40.6, and meets a line of decreasing slope -20 db/decade at this break frequency (2.365 cps).

Also significant about this particular corner frequency is the fact that it locates the lower limit of the frequency range within which the phase angle decreases almost linearly from a *lead* of about $+33.7°$ to a *lag* of about $-33.7°$ at a nearly constant rate of about $-7°$ per 1.00 cycle per second increase in frequency (see Figure 7-4). The *upper* limit of this frequency range corresponds to the other corner frequency given in the denominator of equation [7-23], i.e., $\omega = 74.05$ radians per second (11.785 cps), for which frequency $D_1 = 9.36 \times 10^{-3}$ (−40.573 db) again and $\phi_1 = -33.7°$ At this "roll-off" break frequency, the gain also stops being flat and becomes a pure lag decreasing at the rate of −20 db/decade as a function of the log of frequency (see Figure 7-3).

Thus, the two corner frequencies determined from the denominator of equation [7-23] bracket the frequency range (2 - 12 cps) over which decade (i) the transducer characteristics change almost linearly from phase lead to phase lag; (ii) the gain passes through its maximum minus about 1.6 db on either side of the maximum -- with an essentially "flat" frequency response in this range; (iii) the phase angle passes through zero at a cross-over frequency for which the gain reaches its maximum; and (iv) the phase angle decreases linearly from a lead of 33.7° to a lag of 33.7°.

Note further that, while the maximum phase lead occurred at the midpoint of the upward sloping linear portion of the db-gain curve in Figure 7-3, the maximum gain occurs at the midpoint of the downward sloping linear portion of the phase-angle curve in Figure 7-4. Going one step further, the phase lag passes again through 44.72° (but this time negative) at a frequency of 15.7645 cps (99.05 rad/sec), for which frequency $D_1 = 7.996 \times 10^{-3}$ (−41.94 db), or, some 3 db below its maximum. And finally, the maximum phase lag approaches 90° as $\omega \to \infty$ ($\alpha \to 0$ in equation [7-36]) and D_1 approaches zero as the effect of k_b in Figure 7-2-C is essentially negated by the high-frequency response of B_b (causing X_2 and X_m again to move by corresponding amounts). Indeed, from equation [7-23] we see that the limit of $K(i\omega)/K_2$ as ω gets very large is basically $(1/i\omega)$, which goes to zero as $\omega \to \infty$.

In summary, we conclude that the frequency response range for the typical muscle spindle gain is from about 0.01 cycles per second to 1000 cycles per second (some five decades), with a peak (and brief plateau) occurring at around 7 ± 5 cycles per second. The transducer shows phase lead characteristics for about the first two and one-half decades of its response range (the reflex sensitivity is greatest from about 0.9 to 1.8 cycles per second), and phase lag characteristics for the last two and one-half decades of its response range, with a flat frequency response in the mid-decade of 2 - 12 cps.

If we compare this model with Figure 3-4 for the muscle tissue itself, we see that the latter gain response is from about 0.10 cycles per second to 100 cycles per second (only three decades), with a peak occurring at around 15 cycles per second. It is thus feasible to conclude that the spindle responds passively to stretch sooner than does the muscle tissue itself -- or is certainly more sensitive to stretch than are the corresponding extrafusal muscle fibers. The increased sensitivity of the spindle seems to be about an order of magnitude on either end of the corresponding muscle frequency scale -- gain response starting at 0.01 cps for the spindle (as opposed to 0.10 for the EF fibers) and dying away at 1000 cps for the spindle (as opposed to 100 for the EF fibers). These effects may be explained primarily by the differences in the mechanical parameters defining the models in Figure 3-1 vs. Figure 7-2-A:

$$k_e = 2.00 \times 10^3 \text{ dynes/cm} \qquad c = 6.313 \times 10^7 \text{ dynes/cm/sec}$$
$$\text{(average value)}$$
$$k_f = 0.09 \times 10^3 \text{ dynes/cm} \qquad B_b = 0.024 \times 10^3 \text{ dynes/cm/sec}$$
$$k_b = 0.80 \times 10^3 \text{ dynes/cm} \qquad B_f = 0.026 \times 10^3 \text{ dynes/cm/sec}$$
$$k_s = 1.40 \times 10^8 \text{ dynes/cm} \qquad k_p = 5.200 \times 10^6 \text{ dynes/cm}$$
$$\text{(average)} \qquad\qquad\qquad \text{(average)}$$

Note how much stiffer (k_s and k_p vs. k_e, k_f and k_b) and more viscous (c vs. B_b and B_f) the extrafusal muscle fibers are relative to the muscle spindle tissue. The same reasoning carries over to the phase angle response, which peaks at 0.1374 cps for the spindle, compared with 0.721 cps for the EF fibers.

Characteristic break-point, or corner frequencies for the spindle occur at 0.00045 cps (beginning of phase-lead response), 0.00955 cps (beginning of gain response, 3 db above beginning of phase-lead response), 1.756 cps (3 db below the maximum gain), 2.365 cps (beginning of decreasing linear response range for phase angle and flat frequency response range for gain), 11.785 cps (end of linear response range for phase angle and flat frequency response range for gain), 15.7645 cps (where the gain is again 3 db below its maximum), and some 200 cps (where $D_1 = 7.94 \times 10^{-4} =$ −62 db, or, about 20 db below −41.94; $\phi_1 =$ 85.95°, and both are relatively insensitive to further changes in frequency).

These frequencies for the spindle compare with the following values obtained for the extrafusal muscle fibers: 0.015 cps (beginning of phase-lead response), 0.2170 cps (beginning of gain response, 3 db above beginning of phase-lead response), 2.3873 cps (3 db below the maximum gain), and 15 cps (beyond which both the magnification factor and the phase angle become essentially insensitive to frequency). The differences in response characteristics between the spindle and the EF fibers are consistent with the role of the spindle in control of muscular contraction.
****

Problem 7-7: In 1976, Stein and Oguztöreli proposed the following model for the muscle spindle:

$$\overline{K}(s) = K_o e^{-s\tau_o}(1 + s\tau_1)(1 + s\tau_2) \qquad \text{[7-37]}$$

where: K_o is an arbitrary Gain Constant, $\tau_o = 0.025$ seconds = the time delay associated with the reflex pathway, $\tau_1 = 0.100$ seconds = the time constant associated with the velocity sensitivity of the muscle spindle, and $\tau_2 = 0.023$ seconds = the time constant associated with the acceleration sensitivity of the muscle spindle. In equation [7-37], substitute $i\omega$ for s and write the corresponding transfer function in terms of a phase angle and a scaled amplitude, as was done above in the text. Then plot phase angle and scaled amplitude vs. frequency for the range of frequencies from 0.01 cycles per second up to 25 cycles per second. Compare the results you get with those of Figure 7-4 and note (and try to explain) any significant differences.

****

As indicated in equation [7-37], time delays are represented in the frequency domain in the form: $e^{-\tau_o s}$, where τ_o is the reflex system delay time. The total reflex loop time delay usually includes the following elements:

1. response time of primary spindle receptors, approximately 1 - 2 msec;
2. afferent and efferent fiber conduction velocity delays, 25 - 28 msec;
3. spinal cord monosynaptic delay, no more than 1 msec;
4. neuromuscular synapse transmission time delay, 50 μsec to as much as 1 msec;
5. delay from alpha-motoneuron signal to initiation of mechanical contraction, on the order of 10 msec.

The total spindle loop delay is thus from 27 - 31 msec (Stein and Oguztöreli use 25 msec) and, considering the total reflex delay to the actual initiation of mechanical contraction, the reflex system delay is then approximately 37 - 42 milliseconds.

Transfer Functions for the Inverse Myotatic Reflex

Compared with the volume of information that has accumulated on the muscle spindle, there is significantly less published literature on the dynamic characteristics of Golgi Tendon Orgaons. One transfer function that has been proposed to describe these organs (at least in the case of the soleus muscles in cats) is due to the work of Houk and Simon (1967) and takes the form;

$$\bar{K}(s) = K_o \frac{(1 + 0.063s)(1 + 0.69s)(1 + 6.5s)}{(1 + 0.027s)(1 + 0.50s)(1 + 5.0s)} \qquad [7\text{-}38]$$

where: $K_o = 40$ pulses per second per kilogram of body weight.

Note the increased complexity of equation [7-38] compared, for example, with equation [7-23] for the muscle spindle; and, realizing that each additional term in the numerator or denominator contributes another corner frequency to the response curves, we comment further that the more break frequencies that are associated with a transfer function, the more complex is the corresponding model that is represented by the transfer function. This particular model, then, contains several springs, dashpots (and even masses) that are combined in series/parallel arrangements, to give the system different response characteristics depending upon the frequency range within which it gets excited.

Thus, equation [7-38], where s has been replaced by $i\omega$, and plotted in Figure 7-5, shows the typical "wiggles" or "humps" that correspond to points of inflection where the system response characteristics change due to its associated phenomenological physical model. However, note the similarity in general shape among the Bode plots illustrated in Figures 3-4, 7-4 and 7-5, and bear in mind from the response characteristics shown in Figure 7-5 that this (as in Figure 3-4) model for the Golgi Tendon Organ has a phase angle that stays positive (indicating a lead) throughout the response range, and a Gain that does not return to zero.

Substituting $i\omega$ for s in equation [7-38], one can again write the associated transfer function in terms of a phase angle, ϕ_2, and a scaled amplitude, D_9, where:

$$\phi_2 = \text{Tan}^{-1} \frac{D_7}{D_6}$$

$$D_9 = \frac{\sqrt{D_6^2 + D_7^2}}{D_8}$$

$D_6 = 1 + 32.5\omega^2 + 11.027\omega^4 + 0.019\omega^6$
$D_7 = 1.726\omega + 7.868\omega^3 + 0.415\omega^5$
$D_8 = 1 + 25.25\omega^2 + 6.268\omega^4 + 0.0046\omega^6$

and,

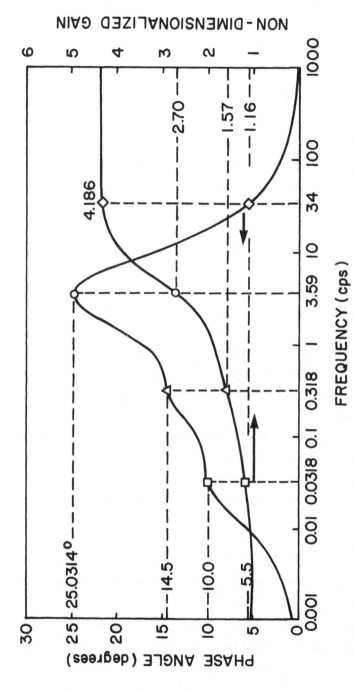

Figure 7-5 Nondimensionalized Modulus, D_9, and Phase Angle, ϕ_2, vs. Linear Frequency for a Linearized Model of the Golgi Tendon Organ, illustrating some key breakpoint Frequencies and corresponding Amplitudes

$$\frac{K(i\omega)}{K_o} = D_9 e^{i\phi_2} \qquad\qquad [7\text{-}39]$$

From the numerator of equation [7-38], we see that the lowest corner frequency for the Golgi Tendon Organ occurs at a linear frequency of some 0.0245 cycles per second, which demarcates the beginning of the Gain response range ($\omega = 1/6.5$ radians per second). At this corner frequency, the nondimensionalized gain ($K(i\omega)/K_o$) has a magnitude of 1.124 (1.015 db), and the corresponding phase lead is 9.41 degrees.

In contrast to the previous models which we have examined, the lowest corner frequency for *this* model is only about one decibel above where the phase lead response curve begins, the latter occurring at a linear frequency of approximately 0.00245 cps ($\omega = 1/65$), for which value the gain is 1.002 (0.018 db) and phase angle a scant 1.511°. At a frequency of 0.0245 cps the gain response essentially begins, but does not get too far before it encounters a second break frequency at 0.0318 cps ($\omega = 1/5 = 0.20$ radians per second from the denominator of equation [7-38]), where the gain has only reached the value of 1.165 (1.327 db) and the phase lead is 9.99 degrees. This latter break frequency demarcates one of those "wiggles" in the frequency response curves, which indicate the activation of another dashpot or spring in the associated phenomenological physical model.

There *is* another corner frequency approximately 3 decibels above the beginning of the phase lead response, and this occurs at 0.2307 cycles per second ($\omega = 1/0.69$ in the numerator of equation [7-38]), where the gain is 1.488 (3.452 decibels) and the phase angle has a value of + 13.85°. Again, the gain does not get very far beyond this frequency before it encounters another corner frequency at 0.3183 cps ($\omega = 1/0.50$ in the denominator of equation [7-38]), for which the gain is 1.573 (3.9373 db) and the phase lead is 14.47°.

The maximum nondimensionalized gain amplitude predicted by equation [7-39] is 4.186 (12.436 db), and the break frequency three decibels below this is at 4.716 cycles per second, for which the gain is 2.9635 (9.436 db) and the phase angle is +24.312°. This linear frequency corresponds to an angular frequency of 1/0.034, which is close to the value of 1/0.027 given in the denominator of equation [7-38]. Going one step further, the phase angle has a value equal again to +24.312° for a break frequency located at 2.712 cycles per second, for which frequency the gain is 2.3831, or 7.543 decibels. This linear frequency corresponds to an angular frequency of 1/0.059, which, again, is close to the value of 1/0.063 given in the denominator of equation [7-38].

Interestingly, the two corner frequencies at 1/0.50 and 1/5.0 are close to those representing three-decibel decrements from the point where the phase angle first reaches +24.312°. That is, 3 db below 7.543 (where $\phi_2 = 24.312°$), the gain is 1.687 (4.543 db) and the phase angle is 14.88° at an angular frequency of 1/0.324 (0.4913 cps), which is close to 1/0.500; and 3 db below *that*, i.e., below 4.543, the gain is 1.194 (1.543 db) and the phase angle is 10.20° at an angular frequency of 1/4.155 (0.0383 cps), which is close to 1/5.00. Equation [7-38], then, locates corner frequencies associated with the same types of "land marks" that were defined in conjunction with Figures 3-4, 7-4, and 7-5, but adds others associated with changes in the curvature of the Bode plots due to more complicated physical models of the behavior of the system. To what extent these added complications enhance our understanding of the behavior of the *in vivo* system is a matter that is still not resolved.

Because the transfer functions developed thus far are linear, and most accurate in the low frequency ranges, let us compare, now, the relative behavior of muscle tissue, the muscle spindle, and the Golgi tendon organs in the frequency range below ten cycles per second. This is done in Table 7-I, where significant maxima, minima, and break-point frequencies for each of these systems are presented in a manner that allows easy qualitative comparison.

As might have been anticipated based on their respective function, the spindle, tendon organ and extrafusal muscle fibers show frequency response characteristics that illustrate a progressively decreasing sensitiv-

CHARACTERISTIC	TABLE 7-I MUSCLE TISSUE	SPINDLE	GOLGI TENDON ORGAN
Beginning of Phase Lead Response, cps	0.015	0.00046	0.00245
Beginning of Gain Response, cps	0.217	0.00955	0.0245
Maximum Phase Lead, Degrees	56.4427	82.0315	25.0314
Frequency at which Maximum Phase Lead Occurs, cps	0.721	0.1374	3.59
Frequency at which Maximum Gain Occurs, cps	15.0	5.2666	250.0
Corner Frequency 3 db Below Maximum Gain, in cycles/sec	2.3873	1.756	4.7162
Other Characteristic Corner Frequencies, in cycles/sec (See text for relevant discussion)		2.365 11.785 15.764	0.0318 0.0383 0.2307 0.3183 0.4913 2.5263 2.7115 5.8946

ity -- the spindle being *most* sensitive (phase lead response begins at 0.00046 cps, gain response begins at 0.00955 cps), followed by the Golgi Tendon Organ (phase lead response begins about an order of magnitude later at 0.00245 cps, and gain response begins somewhat later at 0.0245 cps), and finally by the extrafusal fibers themselves (phase lead *and* gain responses beginning still almost an order of magnitude later at 0.015 and 0.217 cycles per second, respectively). The Golgi Tendon Organ, how-ever, peaks much later than either of the two other transducers, reaching its maximum phase lead at 3.59 cps (compared to 0.1374 cps for the spindle and 0.721 cps for the EF fibers), and its maximum gain at 250 cps (compared to 5.2666 cps for the spindle and 15 cps for the EF fibers).

Other than these rather qualitative types of comparisons, which seem to be self-consistent when viewed in terms of physiologic function, the reader should not get too excited about information such as is presented in Table 7-1 or Figures 3-4, 7-3, 7-4, and 7-5, because, again, the results are so heavily based on linearizations and other dramatic assumptions that their quantitative significance leaves a great deal to be desired. With this point in mind, we move on to say just a few words about some of the other muscular control systems which have been analyzed in some rational manner based on systems control theory.

Transfer Functions for Some Other Reflex Pathways

A survey of the literature will reveal that virtually every one of the control mechanisms described in Chapter 6 has been examined to some extent from a control systems point of view. It is not the intent of this text, nor would it be particularly meaningful at this point, to document systematically the myriad of transfer functions that have been proposed for the (seemingly) myriad of control mechanisms involved in musculoskeletal mechanics. Indeed, the effort would be immense by comparison to the ultimate value of such an exercise. It is thus left to the reader to pursue the topic further based on his or her individual interests. In this section, however, some relevant comments are made to illustrate the types of studies that have been performed in dealing with selected reflex pathways.

For example, it has been reported that, when sinusoidal stretch at amplitudes within the linear response range of the I_a primary endings (0.2 mm at 1 Hz) is applied to primary and secondary endings, the Bode plots of the frequency response show a similar dynamic behavior of *both* endings -- except for a much higher level of absolute firing rate of the primary endings (see Figure 6-2). This corresponds to an overall gain between one and two orders of magnitude greater than that of the secondary endings (type II fibers), as reported by Matthews and Stein in 1969. Furthermore, Poppele and Bowman (1970) found that the frequency response (from Bode plots) of the secondary endings show a dependence on the carrier frequency (the mean discharge frequency of the modulated output signal) that does not appear in the response of the primary endings. According to these authors, the frequency response of the secondary endings may be described by a transfer function which contains the same terms as the transfer function obtained for the primary endings, minus a specific differentiating term which would truly characterize the primary endings, and plus the addition of a time delay which the secondary endings interpose because they work through a disynaptic pathway. Rudyard, in 1972, attempted to propose a transfer function model for the secondary endings of the muscle spindle.

Transfer function models have also been proposed for the behavior of Pacinian Corpuscles, suggesting breakpoint frequencies at about 1 Hz, 100 Hz, and 1000 Hz; for the Otolith Organs, suggesting breakpoint frequencies at about 0.1 Hz and 150 Hz; and for the Semi-circular Canals, suggesting breakpoint or corner frequencies at about 0.1 Hz and 265 Hz. These are of interest in terms of balance and equilibrium considerations, and in terms of modeling control of posture and locomotion. Thus, for example, u_r in Figure 7-1 may represent some conscious desire on the part of an individual to position one of his or her limbs in a prescribed anatomic configuration. A reference signal to this effect is delivered from the appropriate level of consciousness to the sensorimotor cortex, which, in this case, is the comparator and controller of the system. That is, the sensorimotor cortex is receiving a feedback control signal, u, from the joint receptors (in accordance with their corresponding transfer function) telling it in what spatial configuration the joint involved presently finds itself. If u does not match u_r, an error signal is generated. The latter takes the form of commands sent via descending pathways to the motor neurons of the appropriate positional control system in the spinal cord. Thus, the control signal for the positional control system is derived from the error signal of the voluntary control system. The subsequent movement of the joint in question will be continuously monitored by the joint receptors, and, if an error still exists, the descending signals will be further corrected by appropriate circuits in the cortex.

And so it goes, circuit after circuit, feedback pathway after feedback pathway, system after system -- delicately, deliberately, efficiently, effectively, beautifully -- control of muscular contraction manifests itself through the ingenious servomechanism designs of mother nature and father time.

To illustrate how complex the mathematical analysis of such systems can become, we can summarize *just* the neurologic extrinsic control of muscular contraction by developing the following model, which is based on the synopsis presented in Table 6-IV, and on the associated feedback control diagram illustrated in Figure 7-6. Basically, the model states that the ultimate frequency at which a given α-motoneuron will fire (u_c) depends on the sum of (or, more generally, is a *function* of) all of the excitatory ($+$) and inhibitory ($-$) influences that have been described in this and the preceding chapters. Thus, one can write the following expression:

$$f_\alpha = u_c \text{ [Autogenic Inputs, Ipsilateral Inputs (Agonist and Antagonist), Contralateral Inputs (Agonist and Antagonist), Inputs From Skin Receptors, Inputs From Higher Centers ...]} \qquad \text{[7-40]}$$

$$= u_c[f_{I_a},\ f_{I_b},\ f_{II},\ f_{\text{Renshaw}},\ f_{III},\ f_{IV},\ f_\delta,\ f_{\text{Contralateral III, IV, }\delta},$$

$$f_{\text{Synergist } I_a,\ I_b,\ II,\ \alpha\text{- and Renshaw Cells}},$$

$$f_{\text{Recruit } \alpha\text{- and Renshaw Cells}},$$

$$f_{\text{Ipsilateral Antagonist } I_a,\ I_b,\ II,\ \alpha},$$

$$f_{\text{Contralateral Antagonist } I_a,\ I_b,\ II},$$

$$f_{\text{Contralateral Agonist } I_a,\ I_b,\ II},$$

$$f_{\text{Hypothalamus}},\ f_{\text{Cerebral Cortex}},\ f_{\text{Sub-Conscious}},$$

$$f_{\text{Other Higher Centers}},\ \cdots\ ] \qquad \text{[7-41]}$$

Extrinsic Control of Muscular Contraction

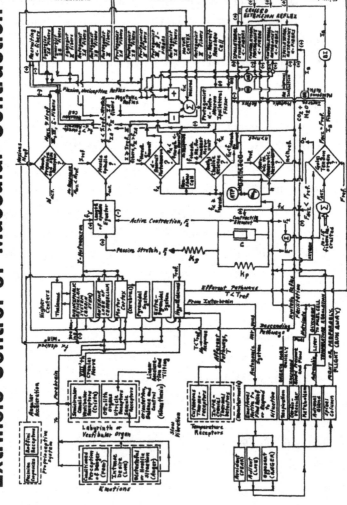

Figure 7-6 Schematic Flow Diagram, Illustrating Some of the Many Extrinsic Inputs To The Alpha-Motor-Neuron that either excite the latter, or inhibit it from discharging at a firing frequency of sufficient threshold so as to elicit a contractile response from the motor unit that the neuron controls.

Then, taking the differential of equation [7-41], one obtains:

$$df_\alpha = \frac{\partial u_c}{\partial f_{I_a}} df_{I_a} - \frac{\partial u_c}{\partial f_{I_b}} df_{I_b} - \frac{\partial u_c}{\partial f_{II}} df_{II} - \frac{\partial u_c}{\partial f_{\text{Renshaw}}} df_{\text{Renshaw}}$$

$$\left\{ \begin{array}{l} + \text{(Flexor)} \\ - \text{(Extensor)} \end{array} \right\} \frac{\partial u_c}{\partial f_{III,\ IV,\ \delta}} \left\{ \begin{array}{l} + \text{(Extensor)} \\ - \text{(Flexor)} \end{array} \right\} \qquad [7\text{-}42]$$

$$\times \frac{\partial u_c}{\partial f_{\text{Contralateral III, IV, }\delta}} df_{\text{Contralateral III, IV, }\delta} + \cdots$$

or

$$df_\alpha = K_1 df_{I_a} + K_2 df_{I_b} + K_3 df_{II} + K_4 df_{\text{Renshaw}} + \cdots \qquad [7\text{-}43]$$

or,

$$df_\alpha = \sum_{i=1}^{\substack{\text{total number} \\ \text{of inputs}}} K_i\, df_i \qquad [7\text{-}44]$$

For the various df_i in equation [7-44], one can substitute appropriate equations such as [7-13] for df_{I_a}, [7-16] for df_{II}, the results of Problem 7-4 for df_{I_b}, and so on, incorporating corresponding values of the various K_i's as discussed in earlier sections above. In each instance, one must, of course, have quantitative information about the transfer functions involved in the various reflex pathways. While much work remains to be done in this area, the examples presented above illustrate the types of results that are currently in the literature.

The greater the frequency of alpha-motoneuron action potentials in a muscle fiber, the greater the possible contractile force, F, that can be developed up to a saturation level called Tetanus. It has been shown by several investigators that the resultant contractile force in the muscle is indeed proportional to the frequency of α-motoneuron action potentials, f_α. It has even been suggested further that muscular activity depends as well on the *pattern* of f_α *pulse trains* -- such that (like the currently popular bar codes on super-market price labels and commercial mailing envelopes), not only the *value* of f_α, but also its spatial and temporal distribution into *signal bursts* may act to control muscular contraction. Carrying these ideas still further, then, it is one's ultimate goal to be able to write an expression at least of the form:

$$F = f(f_\alpha),   \text{[7-45]}$$

or,

$$dF = K_\alpha df_\alpha   \text{[7-46]}$$

where, df_α is defined by the relationships culminating in equation [7-44] above.

Since alpha-motoneuron activity can also be quantified in terms of its relationship to the average Electromyogram (EMG) amplitudes, E_m, one can write a corollary to equations [7-45] and/or [7-46], i.e., $F = K_m E_m$, where E_m is the average EMG amplitude, and K_m is a constant of proportionality. Recall, however, that threshold firing of an alpha motoneuron is only a *necessary* condition for the generation of F. It does not *guarantee* that a contraction will follow, in the sense that many events need to transpire within the *controlled system* before anything becomes manifest at the muscle tendons. Let us thus conclude our examination of neuromuscular control by saying a few words about what goes on in the box labelled, "Controlled Element of System," in Figure 7-1.

The Motor Unit: Controlled Element of the System

For purposes of analysis, one may envision that embedded within the large box labelled, "Controlled Element of System" in Figure 7-1 are *several* closed-loop feedback control systems, *each*, of which, itself, fits the canonical pattern illustrated in the figure. Moreover, in terms of control, one may develop a scenario whereby the motor unit "at rest" would prefer to *stay* that way, i.e., that the tissue does not inherently *intend* to contract, but would rather maintain a resting, equilibrated state. All of the "control systems" to be described below, then, are presumed to have as their ultimate objective a return of the anatomical architecture to some pre-existing resting configuration. The impulse from the alpha-motor neuron perturbs this resting state, and contraction results from a cascading series of disturbances that propagate faster than the embedded controlling signals can correct for them. For example, the sodium-potassium pump proceeds to repolarize the sarcolemma just as soon as the ACh causes a depolarization, and the Lohman reaction resynthesizes an ATP molecule on the myosin head just as soon as the cross-bridge is formed. With these preliminary considerations in mind, let us see how the material from Chapters 1 through 5 might be made to fit such a scheme.

Excitation
THE SYNAPSE

The first control system embedded into the anatomy of a motor unit actually involves the *synaptic region* -- which may be considered to be the *controlled element* of this system, near the motor end plate of the sarcolemma. Recall from Chapter 1 (section on *Excitation and the Establishment of an Active State*) that the arrival of an alpha motor neuron impulse at the terminal vesicles located just proximal to the myoneural junction triggers some 250 to 300 of these to liberate their contents -- about 20 to 25 thousand molecules of the transmitter substance Acetylcholine per vesicle -- into the synaptic region. This "*disturbing signal*" (f_α) thus results in the "squirting" of a sudden quantum of some 10^{-17} moles of ACh towards the motor end plate, per action potential arriving at the α-motoneuron terminals. The quantity of *Acetylcholine* actually present in the synaptic space at any given time, then, may be considered to be the "*controlled signal*" (or feedback signal, or output signal) of this system.

The α-motoneuron never actually makes direct contact with the muscle membrane, but its terminals are encapsulated by the latter via an indentation known as the synaptic trough. Within this series of indented regions of the sarcolemma are a number of subneural clefts, which are additional small membrane invaginations that increase the total surface area of the neuromuscular junction. A *basal membrane* within and lining these *subneural clefts* may be considered to be the *controlling element* of the system, in that this membrane contains the acteylcholinesterase enzyme that rapidly hydrolyzes the ACh almost as fast as it is liberated (c.f., Chapter 1). The products of this breakdown, i.e., Acetic Acid and choline, are resynthesized inside the nerve terminals, and are available for the subsequent action potential(s). To the extent that there is sufficient *Acetylcholinesterase* at each neuromuscular junction to hydrolyze about 10^{-14} moles of ACh in 5 milliseconds, the *activity* of this enzyme becomes, appropriately, the *"controlling signal"* for this feedback control system. And, finally, to the extent that this activity attempts to hydrolyze *all* of the ACh released by *each* α-motoneuron disturbance, the *"reference signal"* for this system may be taken to be zero.

As *also* discussed in Chapter 1, at the hydrolysis rate of 10^{-14} moles per 5 milliseconds, the 10^{-17} moles of ACh that is released by the synaptic terminals is present for only a fraction of a second (on the order of 5 microseconds) before it disappears from the neuromuscular junction. Thus, for any significant accumulation of ACh *above* 10^{-17} moles to occur, the α-motor neuron would have to fire at a frequency exceeding some 200,000 Hz. Since this never occurs in physiologic systems as we know them, ACh summation is nonexistent in normally functioning synapses. This means that the output, u, which is the amount of ACh released into the neuromuscular junction per second, can be modelled as a rapid sequence of exponentially decreasing ACh "spikes", each generated by a separate nerve action potential. One such mathematical model might take the form:

$$u = u(u_d, \ u_c, \ K_t) = \sum_{j=1}^{j=f_\alpha} 10^{-17} \ e^{-\frac{1}{\tau_s}(t - \frac{j-1}{f_\alpha})}$$

[7-47]

$$= \frac{\text{Synaptic Acetylcholine}}{\text{Spikes Per Second}} = u(t); \quad t \geq \frac{j-1}{f_\alpha}$$

The contribution of u_c to the model [7-47] appears through the exponential time constant, τ_s. That is to say, the rate-of-change of synaptic Acetylcholine for, say, $j = 1$ (the *first* of f_α spikes per second), is, at $t = 0^+$ (the instant immediately following the *release* ACh into the neuromuscular junction), from [7-47]:

$$\left[\frac{d(\text{ACh})}{dt} \right]_{\substack{j=1 \\ t=0^+}} = 10^{-17} \left(-\frac{1}{\tau_s} \right)$$

[7-48]

We may, as a simple first approximation, consider that equation [7-48] is governed by the activity of Acetylcholinesterase, and that this activity causes the synaptic quantity of ACh to *decrease* at the rate of 10^{-14} moles per 5 milliseconds -- eliminating 10^{-17} moles in about 5 microseconds. Thus,

$$u_c = u_c(u_r, \ u, \ K^*_c) = \frac{-d(\text{ACh})}{dt} \approx \frac{-10^{-14}}{5}$$

[7-49]

$$= \text{Activity of Acetylcholinesterase} \approx \text{Constant},$$

where: $u_r = 0 =$ "Desired" Synaptic ACh.

Substituting equation [7-48] into equation [7-49] yields the synaptic time constant, $\tau_s = 5$ microseconds. This time constant is, however, probably an order of magnitude too large, since, for $j = 1$ and $t = \tau_s$, equation [7-47] predicts that about one-third of the ACh released into the myoneural junction at $t = 0$ would still be there 5 microseconds later. Thus, as a better second approximation, we might assume τ_s to be on the order of 0.5 microseconds as the manifestation of the action of u_c on u, leaving behind only 0.0000454 of the quantity of ACh that we started with, essentially nothing, at the end of 5 microseconds.

The contribution of u_d to the model [7-47] appears, of course, through the excitation disturbance, f_α, i.e.,

$$u_d = f_\alpha,$$

where f_α needs to exceed at least 4 Hz in order to elicit a minimum muscular response. Furthermore, the forms of equations [7-47] through [7-49], as they relate to an input-output system such as is illustrated in Figure 7-1, suggest a response function for *both* the controlling element *and* the controlled element, satisfying an equation of the general type:

$$\frac{du}{dt} = Ku,$$ [7-50]

which has a solution: $u = e^{Kt}u_{\text{initial}}$ in the homogeneous case (Note: K could be negative).

For $u_r = 0$, in which case $u_c = K^*_c u$ (c.f., Figure 7-1), note in particular how well equation [7-50] fits the description of the controlling element of the system -- where, $u =$ Synaptic Acetylcholine, defined by equation [7-47], $u_c = \dfrac{du}{dt} =$ the activity of acetylcholinesterase, defined by equation [7-49], and $K^*_c = - K$ (see also problem 7-1). Thus, the transfer function for the controlling element could, in some sense, be defined in terms of the ratio of equation [7-49] to equation [7-47].

In the nonhomogeneous case,

$$\frac{du}{dt} - Ku = u^*(t), \quad u(0) = u_{\text{initial}}$$ [7-51]

the solution formula is:

$$u(t) = e^{Kt}u_{\text{initial}} + \int_o^t e^{K(t-\chi)}u^*(\chi)d\chi$$ [7-52]

For the case we are considering, if we take (for the moment) $u_{initial}$ equal to zero and consider the system to be in equilibrium with $u(t) \approx 0$ for $t \neq \frac{j-1}{f_\alpha}$ -- such system being subjected to a "sudden" impulse (10^{-17} moles ACh) each time $t = \frac{j-1}{f_\alpha}$, $j = 1, 2, 3, \ldots, f_\alpha$, -- so sudden, that during the time of disturbance the variation of χ in the exponential of equation [7-52] can be neglected, then the solution reduces, approximately, to:

$$u(t) = \int_o^t u^*(\chi)d\chi, \quad t \neq \frac{j-1}{f_\alpha} \qquad [7\text{-}53]$$

The accuracy of this approximation improves as the duration of the impulse $u^*(t)$ diminishes, and in the idealized limit of a *real* impulse of *zero* duration, the solution becomes exact -- but cannot be represented by a conventional function. Thus, for each $t = \frac{j-1}{f_\alpha}$, the solutions [7-47] or [7-52] may be modified to include the *Dirac Distribution*, or *Delta Function*, defined by the relation,

$$\int u^*(t)\delta\Big(t - \frac{j-1}{f_\alpha}\Big)dt = u^*\Big(\frac{j-1}{f_\alpha}\Big) \qquad [7\text{-}54]$$

where $u^*\Big(\frac{j-1}{f_\alpha}\Big) = 10^{-17}$ moles ACh, $j = 1, 2, \ldots, f_\alpha$. It is important to realize that the Dirac delta function is meaningful only under an integral sign, where limiting techniques can be employed. Thus, the complete solution for $u(t)$ involves *integrating* an equation such as [7-51], utilizing [7-54] for $t = (j-1)/f_\alpha$ and [7-47] for $t > (j-1)/f_\alpha$.

THE SARCOLEMMA AND T-SYSTEM

Based on the discussion above, and in previous chapters, we conclude that, in normally functioning muscle, (i) the frequency of Acetylcholine spikes (equation [7-47]) is equal to the frequency of stimulation, f_α, but *delayed* in time by some characteristic time constant -- on the order of 50 microseconds -- which is associated with the synaptic *transmission time* (Schneck, D. J., 1990); (ii) once the ACh *reaches* the sarcolemma, it "hangs" around for an additional 5 microseconds, or so, while it is being hydrolyzed by Acetylcholinesterase (secreted from the sarcolemma) into Acetic Acid and Choline; and, (iii) each quantum spike of ACh released by each α-motoneuron action potential is almost always sufficient to excite the muscle fiber to threshold, i.e., to generate a muscle action potential, m.a.p. -- but *NOT* necessarily sufficient to elicit a *contraction*. This is because to accomplish the latter, the amount of *calcium* released must reach a concentration threshold, and this does not normally occur until $f_\alpha = 4$ Hz, which, in a sense, is a measure of the activity of the calcium pump (see later).

Nevertheless, the Acetylcholine *output* (u) from the synaptic region becomes the "disturbing signal," u_d to the next feedback control system in the excitation sequence, the *"controlled element"* of which is the polarized Sarcolemma and T-system. It is believed that the muscle membrane end plate contains special protein molecules (as many as 10^4 receptors per square micrometer) -- called Acetylcholine receptors -- to which the ACh binds briefly before it gets hydrolyzed. This binding produces a conformational alteration that opens pores (as many as 40-200 per square micrometer) ranging in diameter from 6 to 7 Angstroms -- and increasing by some 5000-fold the membrane permeability. There results from this sudden increase in membrane permeability a rapid influx of Sodium ions and efflux of Potassium, which reverses the membrane polarity from its resting value of -90 mV to a peak of $+45$ mV over the next 980 or so microseconds. In fact, *most* of this voltage *reversal* takes place in the last 250 microseconds, the membrane potential rising at a nearly constant rate as high as 500 volts per second from -80 mV to $+45$ mV during this latter interval of time.

This observation brings up an interesting point: the Acetylcholine only "hangs around" for 5 or so microseconds, and is long gone by the time the sarcolemma reaches threshold (-50 mV) -- some 800 or more microseconds later. Obviously, then, the ACh cannot be *totally* responsible for the preliminary alterations in membrane permeability, but, rather, represents the "kick" that knocks over the first "domino," as it were. The subsequent inward rush of sodium that this kick triggers -- like people piling through an open door -- must then act as the "disturbance" that *keeps* the pores open for some time later once ACh "kicks it ajar" initially. The *number* of doors (pores) that the 250-300 "quanta" of ACh vesicles open must be sufficient to bring the membrane to threshold. If not enough pores are opened, the inward flux of sodium will not produce enough depolarization to bring the sarcolemma to threshold before the sodium pump (see later) begins to reverse things. But this is not normally a problem since ordinarily, *each* impulse that arrives at the neuromuscular junction creates an end-plate current flow about three to four times that required to bring the sarcolemma to threshold.

The latter has been measured to be a net movement of about 2.5×10^{-14} moles (1.5×10^{10} ions) of univalent ions per action potential, which, for a charge of 1.6×10^{-19} coulombs per univalent ion, corresponds to a charge of 2.4×10^{-9} coulombs per action potential. More accurately, this "disturbing" current flow, u_d, depends on the membrane depolarization, V_T, required to bring the controlled element to threshold (usually 40-50 millivolts from resting levels of around -90 mV), on the membrane resistance, R^*_m (typically on the order of 1000 ohms per cm^2 of surface area), and, on the membrane capacitance, C^*_m (some 1 to 10 microfarads per cm^2 of surface area) -- as reflected in the membrane time constant, $\tau^*_m = R^*_m C^*_m$. Thus, if τ^*_o represents the time interval necessary to depolarize the excitable membrane by a net voltage change V_T, the stimulus strength u_d required is given by (Schneck, D. J., 1990):

$$u_d = \frac{V_T}{R^*_m (1 - e^{-\tau^*_o / \tau^*_m})} \qquad [7\text{-}55]$$

If $V_T = 40$ mV, $R^*_m = 1000$, $\tau^*_o = 800$ microsec, $C^*_m = 6$ microfarads, and $\tau^*_m = 6$ milliseconds, equation [7-55] predicts that $u_d = 0.32 \times 10^{-3}$ amps, or, 320 microamps per square centimeter of motor end plate. This corresponds to 320×10^{-6} coulombs per second, per cm^2, or, 320×10^{-12} coul/microsec/cm^2, or, to 2.56×10^{-7} coul/cm^2 for the 800 microseconds required to bring the membrane to threshold (note: this time interval is called the *neuromuscular stimulation delay*). If the total area of the neuromuscular junction is on the order of 10^{-2} cm^2 (a "square" area roughly 1 mm on a side), then we get a net charge displacement of 2.56×10^{-9} coulombs, which agrees with the quoted measured value of 2.4×10^{-9} coulombs per action potential.

One could also work through the disturbing synaptic transmission events using Hatze's (c.f., Chapter 4) formulation as embedded into equation [4-36] for the end-plate potential, $\alpha^*(t)$. This formulation also takes into account the facts that during the fast sodium influx phase (i.e., the *absolute refractory period*, τ) of the muscle action potential -- when the membrane is completely depolarized -- and, up to about 4 or 5 msec thereafter (i.e., during the *relative refractory period*) -- when the membrane is recovering and repolarizing, it is difficult (or impossible) to elicit a response from the tissue to a second stimulus. However, at 5 msec per stimulus, they would have to be coming in at a frequency of 200 Hz or higher for this to be a problem. Almost *never* do the spinal nerves stimulate even the most active neuromuscular junctions more than 100 times per second, so, we may effectively dispense with stimulation constraints *in vivo* which have to do *either* with the absolute *or* the relative refractory periods of the tissue. For all intents and purposes, the motor end plate may be considered to be responsive to *each* stimulus that arrives.

The fast inward flux of sodium triggers a three-to-fourfold increase in the activity of the *Sodium Pump* (see Schneck, D. J., 1990) which, in *this* feedback control loop, is the *controlling element*. The sodium pump *actively* transports three sodium ions back to the outside of the sarcolemma for every two Potassium ions that it carries back in. This it does in an effort to restore the sarcolemma polarity back to its resting value of around -90 mV (u_r), as determined by the Goldman Equation (ibid.):

$$u_r = \frac{RT}{\bar{F}Z^*} \ell n \; \frac{P_K[K^+]_o + P_{Na}[Na^+]_o + P_{Cl}[C\ell^-]_i}{P_K[K^+]_i + P_{Na}[Na^+]_i + P_{Cl}[C\ell^-]_o}$$

$$\approx -90 \; mV \qquad\qquad [7\text{-}56]$$

where $\bar{F}$ is the Faraday Constant, 96,500 coulombs/mole; $Z^* = 1$; the various P's are permeability coefficients of the membrane to potassium, sodium, and chlorine; the subscript "o" refers to outside of the sarcolemma, and the subscript "i" to inside.

The activity, u_c, of the Sodium Pump may be written in terms of its ability to generate a *sodium efflux* from the interior of the sarcolemma, such efflux being also written as a current flow according to the relation (Schneck, D. J., 1990):

$$(u_c)_{max} = \frac{\varepsilon_3[Y_m]A\bar{F}Z^*}{\delta_m} \qquad\qquad [7\text{-}57]$$

where: ε_3 is the dissociation rate constant (sec^{-1}) between Sodium (the species being actively transported) and *carrier molecule*, Y; $[Y_m]$ is the total concentration (moles per liter) of Y in the sarcolemma membrane; A is the membrane area over which the transport takes place; and δ_m is the average membrane thickness. In general, when u_c is not at its maximum control level, it follows the principles that govern Michaelis-Menten active transport kinetics (ibid.). It should also be pointed out that the sarcolemma may contain as many as 100 to 200 Sodium-Potassium pumps per square micrometer of membrane surface; that the pump activity increases as the *cube* of intracellular sodium concentration; and that it is powerful enough to transport sodium ions against concentration gradients as high as 20 to 1. It thus acts as quite an effective controlling element as it completely repolarizes the sarcolemma within 5 milliseconds following the initial disturbance.

Since the motor end plate may be considered to be responsive to *each* stimulus that arrives, the transfer function of the sarcolemma converts the signals u_d and u_c described above into a net muscle action potential, u, the frequency of which is equal to the previously-defined frequency of action potential spikes.

****

Problem 7-8: Based on the discussions of this section, the muscle action potential, u, may be described as follows:

for $0 \leq t \leq 5$ microseconds (stimulation), $u = -90$ mV = constant;

for $5 < t \leq 810$ microseconds (depolarization to threshold), $u =$ an exponentially increasing function of time, which function has a slope of 500 volts/sec by the time $u = -50$ mV at $t = 810$ microseconds;

for $810 < t \leq 1000$ microseconds (fast sodium influx, fast potassium efflux), $u =$ a straight line of slope 500 volts/sec, reaching $u = +45$ mV at $t = 1$ msec; and,

for $1 < t \leq 5$ msec (Sodium pump recovery and fast chlorine influx), $u =$ an exponentially decreasing function of time, which function starts at $u = +45$ mV for $t = 1$ msec, and comes within 1% of its asymptotic value, $u = -90$ mV (resting potential) by the time $t = 5$ msec.

Derive a set of equations for $u(t)$ which satisfy the four conditions given above, and, from these, *Plot* the muscle action potential for one full "spike," assuming $f_\alpha = 100$ Hz (tetanic).

Also, based on the earlier discussion in this chapter, of the basic characteristics of feedback control systems, and on the results you obtained above, explain *why* the sodium pump (u_c) probably does not "kick in" to this system until $t > 0.5$ msec -- i.e., that the start of recovery actually lags the disturbance by about 500 microseconds.

****

Finally, one can again work through Hatze's (Chapter 4) formulation to recognize that the output u of *this* embedded feedback control loop actually corresponds to the solution for $\beta^*(t)$ in his equation [4-35]; and that the resulting action potential propagates all along the surface membrane of the muscle fiber, eventually depolarizing the T-system, as well.

Excitation-Contraction Coupling

SARCOPLASMIC RETICULUM CISTERNS

Proceeding in similar fashion, one now considers the *muscle action potential*, i.e., the *output* of the previous controlled element, to be the *disturbing signal*, u_d, of the next *controlled system*, which is the *terminal cisterns* (collectively) of the sarcoplasmic reticulum (c.f., Chapter 1). Here, the output, u, involves the release of calcium into the sarcoplasm as a result of permeability alterations which are induced in the cisterns by the m.a.p. of frequency f_α. Thus, analytic expressions for u might take the form of a sigmoidal function, like equation [1-2] (c.f., Problem 1-2), or Hill's equation [1-3] (c.f., Problem 1-3), or any of a number of other comparable forms -- not the least of which involve solutions to equations [4-33] and [4-34] in Hatze's formulation (c.f., Chapter 4). The point is that if appropriate mathematical forms for u_d, u_c, u_r, and u can be obtained as developed herein, one can apply equations such as [7-1] through [7-6], [7-10], and so on, to define the transfer function, phase, time-constant, and gain characteristics of the particular controlling or controlled element involved.

In this case, the *controlling element* involved is *also* an active pump mechanism -- but this time the ions involved, rather than being sodium and potassium, are calcium and magnesium. Thus, as soon as the Ca^{++} is released into the sarcoplasm, a *calcium pump*, operating in a manner analogous to the previously-described sodium pump, begins to transport Ca^{++} back into the terminal cisterns of the sarcoplasmic reticulum. The energy which drives this pump again comes from the breakdown of mg^{++}-ATP, with the ratio being 2 ions of calcium transported per molecule of ATP hydrolyzed; and the "controlling" signal obeys a relationship similar to equation [7-57].

Maximum uptake of calcium by the vesicles, i.e., $(u_c)_{max}$ appears to take place when the sarcoplasmic calcium concentration is around $10^{-5.54}$ molar (Bendall, J. R., 1969) which, from equation [1-2], corresponds to $f_\alpha = 5.3$ Hz, or, from equation [1-3], to $f_\alpha = 4.7$ Hz. Thus, we see that for $f_\alpha \approx 5$ Hz (on the average) -- just 1 Hz above the minimum threshold necessary to elicit a contractile response -- the pump is accumulating calcium ions back into the vesicles at a maximum rate. It therefore responds very quickly to sudden changes in calcium concentration as it attempts to return such concentration to the resting value, u_r, of 5×10^{-9} M. If one plots vesicular calcium uptake rate (in percent of maximum) vs. molar sarcoplasmic calcium concentration (in pCa), which is a measure of calcium-pump activity, u_c, one gets a curve which looks almost like a sine-wave (ibid.) -- symmetric about the horizontal ordinate axis corresponding to an uptake rate of 50%, with a maximum at around an abscissa of $10^{-5.5}$M and minima at 10^{-8} M (near the resting value) and 10^{-3} M (near the tetanic value). The curve is symmetric about the vertical abscissa axis corresponding to a sarcoplasmic calcium concentration of some $10^{-5.54}$ M (i.e., $(u_c)_{max}$).

We see, then, that when the frequency of stimulation is too large for the pump to handle, calcium summation will occur, and larger and larger amounts of calcium will accumulate in the sarcoplasm up to a tetanic contraction. The calcium pump also controls the *Protein Switch* (controlled system = Troponin-Tropomyosin Complex, c.f., Chapter 1), as it relates to the establishment of an *Active state* described, for example, in Hatze's formulation by equations [4-31] and [4-32]. It is left up to the reader to define, for *this* subsystem, the corresponding transfer functions and quantities u_r, u_c, u_d and u.

****

Problem 7-9: The muscle action potential *also* acts as the disturbance, u_d, that sets into motion the cascading sequence of biochemical reactions that are responsible for supplying (and replenishing) the energy that ultimately drives *all* of the ionic pumps and mechanical processes that are associated with a muscular contraction.

Working from Figure 1-8 and the discussions of Chapter 1, and following the philosophy developed in this chapter, work your way through the *hydrolysis* and *energy-release loops*, using as many subsystems, controlled elements and controlling elements as you feel are necessary to describe this aspect of muscular contraction. For each subsystem, *define* (and *quantify* to the extent that you are able) the corresponding variables u, u_d, u_c, and u_r. Make sure you include any factors (such as Lactic Acid) that may be acting to constrain any or all of the subsystems involved.

****

FINALIZATION OF THE ACTIVE STATE

Release of energy from the muscle fuel cell, together with activation of the Protein Switch, both act to *disturb* (u_d) the *resting state* of the discontinuous Actomyosin complex -- in which the *controlled element* is the HMM-S-1 "head" of the myosin *cross-bridge*. The output, u, then, of the *next* embedded feedback control system corresponds to the final manifestation of the *active state* of the muscle fiber, as reflected by the *number* of functional cross-bridge attachments formed between Actin and Myosin. Recall that this state is zero for the muscle at rest (which, in this case, may be taken to be the *reference signal*, u_r, for the subsystem under current examination), 100% for the muscle in a tetanic state, and, in between, follows the principles related to the *staircase effect* from a single twitch to a full tetanus. (c.f., Chapter 1). Thus, u, in some sense may be normalized to lie somewhere between 0 and 1, which lends itself to the type of statistical analysis proposed by Decraemer, et al., -- see, for example, equations [4-1] and [4-2] -- or, to the corresponding "weighting function", Ω, proposed in Hatze's formulation -- see, for example, equations [4-29] and [4-37].

In any case, the controlled signal is some sort of active filamentary overlap function. The *controlling element* for this subsystem is embedded into the sequence of events that constitute the *Lohman Reaction* -- wherein ADP picks up a phosphate group (from the breakdown of Phosphocreatine) to resynthesize ATP. As it reattaches itself to the globular head of the HMM-S-1 segment (the controlled element), the ATP thus formed simultaneously catalyzes the release of the myosin cross-bridges from the actin molecules. In that sense, the "relaxation" activity of ATP is embedded into u_c, which, quantitatively, may be calculated to be the Lohman reaction rate (which is catalyzed by the enzyme creatine kinase).

In the resting state, muscle has four to six times as much phosphocreatine as it does ATP, the latter amounting to about 5×10^{-6} moles per gram of tissue. However, despite this availability, the total supply of high-energy phosphates cannot sustain prolonged, intense muscular activity (when 10^{-4} to 10^{-3} moles of ATP may be consumed per minute, per gram of muscle) for more than a few seconds, at most -- which corresponds to perhaps 50 or so twitches. Thus, "back-up" systems in the form of glycolysis of stored glycogen into lactic acid help out as necessary. Anaerobically, contraction can continue until all the glycogen and phosphocreatine have disappeared, leaving behind lactic acid, creatine, and inorganic phosphate to accumulate along with an oxygen debt. If phosphocreatine and glycogen were not available, the total amount of ATP in muscle tissue would be used up after about 8 consecutive twitches -- not very much!

Contraction: The Development of a Power Stroke

At this point in the analysis, the picture gets somewhat fuzzy. That is to say, the identification of sequences of specific subsystems that cascade into one another to produce the "ratcheting action" which results in a contraction is not as uniquely defined as we would like it to be. This is because the fine details of the precise mechanisms taking place at the molecular level to produce the actual sliding filament scenario are still largely speculative, and under current scrutiny. As stated by Pate and Cooke (1989), "The crossbridge cycle in normally functioning muscle is obviously complex and insufficient experimental data are presently available to specify a model completely."

Clearly, the establishment of an *active state* "disturbs" (u_d) the *resting configuration* (u_r) of the Actomyosin Complex (the *controlled element* in this contraction phase). Perhaps this disturbance (as suggested by Hatze) sets up an electronic charge redistribution that, in turn, generates an oscillating electromagnetic field that, in turn, creates pulsating mechanical forces that, in turn, cause the high-frequency vibratory motion of the cross-bridges that, in turn, "*drags*" (u) the thin Actin filaments past the thicker Myosin filaments -- perhaps not. In fact, perhaps the entire sliding-filament mechanism is thermodynamic in nature (as suggested by Pate and Cooke, and others), rather than electromagnetic -- and then again, perhaps not. Maybe it is exclusively biochemical, involving sequences of enzymes and cis-trans isomerizations that have not even been identified yet.

Pate and Cooke (1989), expanding upon some earlier work done by other investigators, develop a five-state Kinetic model for the force-generating power stroke. The arrival of a muscle action potential is presumed to trigger the movement of the cross-bridges from one state to the next, each representing a (lower) relative free-energy minimum state for the fiber. Along the way, the force produced by an attached cross-bridge in state i ($i = 1, 2, 3, 4, 5$) is defined to be the spatial gradient of the Gibbs free energy function for that state.

Thus, state 1 (constant free-energy arbitrarily taken to define the datum plane for subsequent states) is the *Resting State*, wherein mg^{++}-ATP is attached to the Myosin head and the Actomyosin complex is discontinuous. State 2 (the slow, rate-limiting, exergonic hydrolysis step following the arrival of an action potential) is called the *Refractory State*, wherein the Actomyosin complex is *still* discontinuous, but the ATP on the Myosin head is now in the hydrolyzed form ADP-mg^{++}-P_i. State 3, called the *Weak Attaching State* marks the beginning of the actual *Power Stroke*. Here, the energy released by the hydrolysis of ATP provides the energy of activation that allows Actin to attach to Myosin, *forming* the Actomyosin complex:

$$\text{Actin} - \text{ Myosin} - \text{ ADP} - \text{ mg}^{++} - P_i,$$

but generating only a very *weak* contractile force in this state.

State 4 is the principal force-producing, or *Power State* of the cross-bridge cycle. It results from the *release* of the inorganic phosphate generated by the hydrolysis of ATP, leaving behind the Actomyosin-mg^{++}-ADP complex, and creating the largest free-energy drop -- on the order of 14 RT, compared with 2-3 RT for the other state-transitions -- in the power stroke cycle. Finally, as the ADP is further released to complete the fully-attached Actomyosin complex, the tissue drops to state 5, sometimes called the *Rigor State* or *Strong Attached State*. This is because at the end of the power stroke, Actin is now strongly bound to Myosin and will not release until the Lohman Reaction replaces the lost mg^{++}-ATP, which catalyzes this passive dissociation and brings the entire system back full circle to state 1 again.

Pate and Cooke then proceed to do a very elegant job of quantifying the Kinetics of their proposed 5-step power stroke cycle, and they *do* present very plausible results that are consistent with experimental observations. But the bottom line is that we *still* do not know *for sure exactly* what is going on -- not even if the filaments slide past one another the way we *think* they do. All we know is that the sliding-filament theory *thus far* appears to explain very nicely everything we know about muscular contraction, and it has not been in conflict with any known analytic or experimental findings, to date. So, we continue to explore the submicroscopic possibilities that may be responsible for generating the "ratcheting action" we call a "contraction."

However, let the record show that already some doubt has been cast on the exact role of the Tropohin-Tropomysin Complex, and the Protein Switch, in the contractile process. That is, some evidence has been reported (Chalovich, et al., 1981) which suggests that the troponin-tropomyosin complex does *not* inhibit the actin-activated ATPase activity by stereochemically preventing the binding of HMM-S-1 • ATP or HMM-S-1 • ADP ~ P$_i$ to Actin -- as has traditionally been assumed to be the case. Rather, these authors propose that the Protein Switch may act by blocking the *release* of inorganic phosphate from the

Acto-HMM-S-1 • ADP ~ P_i *complex.* In other words, even at rest, the Actomyosin cross-bridge configuration is intact, but nonfunctional because the energy required to drive it is "trapped" or blocked by the protein switch.

Similarly, we are unable to define clearly the *controlling element(s)* that attempt to bring u (the thin filaments being "dragged" past the thick filaments) back to the resting configuration u_r. Perhaps there *are* none, and that is why muscles must exist in opposing pairs -- the *antagonist,* in a sense, acting as the "controlling element" for the *agonist,* with u_c representing the *output* (force and/or displacement, or some combination of these and/or their respective derivatives) of the antagonist. On the other hand, *elastic restoring forces* are certainly a good candidate for u_c -- bringing the *cross-bridges* (at least) back to their equilibrium configuration in between each oscillation, as described in Chapter 1. In this case, the "controlling element" is manifest in actual material properties, the expression of which -- e.g., Young's Moduli, Poisson Ratios, and so on -- acts like a "Transfer Function" to convert actual deformation, ε, or u, into restoring forces, σ, or u_c.

Then, too, there is still the oscillating electromagnetic field theory, which asserts that restoring forces that return the cross-bridges to equilibrium are actually generated by *field* polarity reversals and, with them, cyclic variations in the forces driving the bridges. In this case, then, the active state of the muscle acts *either* as u_d (during the "power stroke" phase of the motion) *or* as u_c (during the "cross-bridge release" phase of the motion), depending on when it is examined. And finally, there is always the possibility that the answer may be, "all of the above" -- i.e., that some as-yet undefined *combination* of electromagnetic, biochemical, physico-elastic, and externally-mediated mechanisms may be driving the cross-bridges to generate a contraction.

Whatever the precise mechanism(s) might be, the *net* result of these cascading events, is an output, u, from the controlled element of Figure 7-1, which is in the form of an isometric, isotonic, isokinetic, ..., contraction that is an attempt to satisfy the "desired" u_r. This output, working against some external resistance, u_d, is fed back to the motor cortex of the brain for further evaluation. It *also* becomes the disturbance u_d that feeds into the various control mechanisms discussed in the first part of this chapter (e.g., equation [7-11], Problem 7-4, and so on) -- so that we have essentially come full circle. All that this analysis awaits, then, is further research to both *identify* and *quantify* (i.e., through input/output governing equations, transfer functions, mathematical models, and feedback-feed forward control theory) many of the intermediate pathways and mechanisms that still remain a mystery.

References

1. Allen, J. B., "Cochlear Micromechanics -- A Physical Model of Transduction," *J. Acoust. Soc. Am.*, Vol. 68, No. 6, Pages 1660-1670, December 1980.

2. Andrews, L. T., Iannone, A. M., and Ewing, D. J., "The Muscle Spindle as a Feedback Element in Muscle Control," In: *Proceedings of the Ninth Annual Conference on Manual Control*, National Aeronautics and Space Administration and Department of Transportation, NASA Conference Report Number CR-142295, NTIS Accession Number N75-19126, Pages 353-363, 1973.

3. Baran, E. M., "A Study of the Human Myotatic Reflex," M.S. Thesis, Drexel University, June, 1976.

4. Baran, E. M., "Mathematical Model of Human Myotatic Reflex," *Proc. 27th Annual Conference of Engineering in Medicine and Biology*, Paper #21.10, Page 182, October, 1974, Vol. 16.

5. Baran, E., Kresch, E., and Freedman, W., "Experimental and Theoretical Analysis of the Human Myotatic Reflex," *Proc. 28th Ann. Conf. Engrg. Med. & Biol.*, Bethesda, Maryland, Alliance for Engineering in Medicine and Biology, Paper Number A1.13, Page 15, 1975, Volume 15.

6. Barker, D., (Editor), *Symposium on Muscle Receptors*, Hong Kong, The Hong Kong University Press, 1962.

7. Barker, D., Hunt, C. C., and McIntyre, A. K., *Handbook of Sensory Physiology, Volume III, Section 2: Muscle Receptors*, Berlin, Springer-Verlag, 1974.

8. Bendall, J. R., *Muscles, Molecules and Movement: An Essay in the Contraction of Muscles*, London, Heinemann, 1969.

9. Best, W. II., "A Numerical Model for the Dynamic Response of the Human Otolith Organs," M.S. Thesis, Virginia Polytechnic Institute and State University, 1984.

10. Chalovich, J. M., Chock, P. B., and Eisenberg, E., "Mechanism of Action of Troponin-Tropomyosin," *J. Biol. Chem.*, Vol. 256, No. 2, pp. 575-578, Jan. 25, 1981.

11. Chaplain, R. A., Michaelis, B., and Coenen, R., "Systems Analysis of Biological Receptors, I. A Quantitative Description of the Input-Output Characteristics of the Slowly Adapting Stretch Receptor of the Crayfish," *Kybernetik*, Volume 9, Number 3, Pages 85-95, September, 1971.

12. Chen, W. J., and Poppele, R. E., "Small Signal Analysis of Response of Mammalian Muscle Spindles with Fusimotor Stimulation and a Comparison with Large-Signal Responses," *J. Neurophysiol.*, Vol. 41, Pages 15-27, 1978.

13. Cowherd, W. F., II, and Cadman, T. W., "Numerical Prediction of Transfer Functions," *Instruments and Control Systems*, Vol. 42, No. 5, Pages 109-113, May 1969.

14. Crosby, P. A., "Use of Surface Electromyogram as a Measure of Dynamic Force in Human Limb Muscles," *Medical and Biological Engineering and Computing*, Vol. 16, Pages 519-524, 1978.

15. Crowe, A., "A Mechanical Model of the Mammalian Muscle Spindle," *J. Theoret. Biol.*, Vol. 21, No. 1, Pages 21-41, October, 1968.

16. Del Toro, V., and Parker, S. R., *Principles of Control Systems Engineering*, New York, McGraw-Hill Book Company, Inc., 1960.

17. De Reuck, J., "Biometric Analyses of Spindles in Normal Human Skeletal Muscles," *Acta Neurol. Belg.*, Vol. 73, No. 6, Pgs. 339-347, Nov.-Dec., 1973.

18. Desmedt, J. E., (Editor), *Spinal and Supraspinal Mechanisms of Voluntary Motor Control and Locomotion*, Prog. Clin. Neurophysiol., Volume 8, Karger, Basel, 1980.

19. DiStefano, J. J., III, Stubberud, A. R., and Williams, I. J., *Theory and Problems of Feedback and Control Systems*, Schaum's Outline Series, New York, McGraw-Hill Book Company, Inc., 1967, Second Edition, 1990.

20. Downie, I. C., and Murray-Smith, D. J., "Stimulation of Systems Involving Pulse Frequency Modulation with Special Reference to Modelling of Muscle Spindle Receptors," *Proceedings of the 1981 UKSC Conf. on Computer Simulation*, Harrogate, May 1981, Westbury House, Guildford, Pages 143-153, 1981.

21. Eccles, J. C., Eccles, R. M., and Lundberg, A., "Synaptic Actions on Motoneurons Caused by Impulses in Golgi Tendon Organ Afferents," *J. Physiol.*, Vol. 138, Pages 227-252, 1957.

22. French, A. S., Holden, A. V., and Stein, R. B., "The Estimation of the Frequency Response Function of a Mechanoreceptor," *Kybernetik*, Vol. 11, Number 1, Pages 15-23, July, 1972.

23. Goodwin, G. M. Hullinger, H., and Matthews, P. B. C., "The Effects of Fusimotor Stimulation During Small Amplitude Stretching on the Frequency Response of the Primary Ending of the Mammalian Muscle Spindle," *J. Physiol. (London)*, Volume 253, Pages 175-206, 1975.

24. Gottlieb, G. L., and Agarwal, G. C., "Muscle Spindle Models: Multiple Input - Multiple Output Simulations," In: *Proceedings of the Eighth Conference on Medical and Biological Engineering*, Chicago, 1969.

25. Gottlieb, G., Agarwal, G., and Stark, L., "Studies in Postural Control Systems, Part III: A Muscle Spindle Model," *I.E.E.E. Transactions on System Science and Cybernetics*, Vol. SSC-6, No. 2, April, 1970.

26. Gottlieb, G., Agarwal, G., and Stark, L., "Stretch Receptor Models," *IEEE Transactions on Man-Machine Systems*, Vol. 10, No. 1, pp. 17-27, March, 1969.

27. Granit, R., *The Basis of Motor Control*, New York, Academic Press, 1970.

28. Granit, R., and Pompeiano, O., "Reflex Control of Posture and Movement," *Progress in Brain Research*, Vol. 50, Amsterdam, Elsevier Press, 1978.

29. Grodins, F. S., *Control Theory and Biological Systems*, New York, Columbia University Press, 1963.

30. Hasan, Z., and Houk, J. C., "Transition in Sensitivity of Spindle Receptors that Occurs when Muscle is Stretched More Than a Fraction of a Millimetre," *J. Neurophysiol.*, Vol. 38, Pages 673-689, 1975.

31. Houk, J., "A Viscoelastic Interaction which Produces One Component of Adaptation in Responses of Golgi Tendon Organs," *J. Neurophysiol*, Vol. 30, No. 6, Pages 1482-1493, November 1967.

32. Houk, J., and Henneman, E., "Feedback Control of Skeletal Muscles," *Brain Research*, Vol. 5, Pages 433-451, 1967.

33. Houk, J. C., and Stark, L., "An Analytical Model of a Muscle Spindle Receptor for Simulation of Motor Coordination," M.I.T. Re-

search Laboratory for Electronics, *Quart. Progr. Rept., No. 66,* Pages 284-289, Cambridge, Mass., July, 1962.

34. Houk, J. C., Jr., Sanchez, V., and Wells, P., "Frequency Response of a Spindle Receptor," M.I.T. Research Laboratory for Electronics, *Quarterly Progress Report Number 67,* Page 223, Cambridge, Massachusetts, October, 1962.

35. Houk, J. C., Cornew, R. W., and Stark, L., "A Model of Adaptation in Amphibian Spindle Receptors," *J. Theoret. Biol.,* Vol. 12, pp. 196-215, 1966.

36. Hulliger, M. Matthews, P. B., and Noth, J., "On the Response of I_a Fibres to Low Frequency Sinusoidal Stretching of Widely Ranging Amplitude," *J. Physiol. (London),* Vol. 267, No. 3, Pages 811-838, June, 1977.

37. Hulliger, M., Matthews, P. B., and Noth, J., "Effects of Combining Static and Dynamic Fusimotor Stimulation on the Response of the Muscle Spindle Primary Ending to Sinusoidal Stretching," *J. Physiol. (London),* Vol. 267, Number 3, Pages 839-856, June, 1977.

38. Hunt, C. C., and Perl, E. R., "Spinal Reflex Mechanisms Concerned with Skeletal Muscle," *Physiological Reviews,* Vol. 40, Pages 538-579, 1960.

39. Jöbsis, F. F., and O'Connor, M. J., "Calcium Release and Reabsorption in the Sartorius Muscle of the Toad," *Biochemical and Biophysical Communications,* Vol. 25, No. 2, pp. 246-252, 1966.

40. Jones, R. W., "Biological Control Mechanisms," In: Schwan, H. P., (Editor), *Biological Engineering,* New York, McGraw-Hill Book Company, Inc., Chapter 2, Pages 87-204, 1969.

41. Kalmus, H., (Editor), *Regulation and Control in Living Systems,* New York, John Wiley and Sons, 1966.

42. Koehler, W., and Windhorst, U., "Multi-Loop Representation of the Segmental Muscle Stretch Reflex: Its Risk of Instability," *Biol. Cybernetics,* Vol. 38, Pages 51-61, 1980.

43. Kostyukov, A. I., Bayev, K. V., and Vasilenko, D. A., "Regular Pulse Train Transformation by the Monsynaptic Connection: Neurophysiological Data and their Treating with Simple Stochastic Neuron Model," *Biological Cybernetics,* Vol. 24, Pages 219-226, 1976.

44. Kothiyal, K. P., and Ibramsha, M., "Fatigue in Isometric Contraction in a Single Muscle Fibre: A Compartmental Calcium Ion Flow Model," *J. Biomechanics,* Vol. 19, No. 11, pp. 943-950, 1986.

45. Loewenstein, W. R., and Skalak, R., "Mechanical Transmission in a Pacinian Corpuscle: An Analysis and a Theory," *J. Physiol. (London)*, Vol. 182, Number 2, Pages 346-378, January, 1966.

46. LoNigro, R., "An Analytic Evaluation of the Upper Break Frequency of the Human Otolith Organ," M.S. Thesis, Virginia Polytechnic Institute and State University, Department of Engineering Science and Mechanics, August, 1982.

47. Mansourian, P. G., "System Analysis of the Vestibulo-Ocular Control Mechanism," *Adv. Ophthalmol.*, Vol. 28, Pages 175-205, 1974.

48. Marsden, C. D., Merton, P. A., and Morton, H. B., "Servo Action in Human Voluntary Movement," *Nature*, Vol. 238, Pages 140-143, 1972.

49. Matthews, P. B. C., *Mammalian Muscle Receptors and their Central Actions*, Arnold Publishers, London, 1972, and Baltimore, The Williams and Wilkins Co., 1972.

50. Matthews, P. B. C., "Review Lecture: Evolving Views on the Internal Operation and Functional Role of the Muscle Spindle," *J. Physiol.*, Vol. 320, Pages 1-30, 1981.

51. Matthews, P. B. C., and Stein, R. B., "The Sensitivity of Muscle Spindle Afferents to Small Sinusoidal Changes of Length," *J. Physiol. (London)*, Vol. 200, Pages 723-743, 1969.

52. McRuer, D. T., Magdaleno, R. E., and Moore, G. P., "A Neuromuscular Activation System Model," *I.E.E.E. Transactions on Man-Machine Systems*, Vol. MMS-9, No. 3, Pages 61-71, 1968.

53. McRuer, D. T., Magdaleno, R. E., and Moore, G. P., "A Neuromuscular Actuation Model System," In: Iberall, A. S., and Reswick, J. B., (Editors), *Technical and Biological Problems of Control -- A Cybernetic View*, U. S. International Federation of Automatic Control, Pages 500-503, 1970.

54. Milhorn, H. T., Jr. *The Application of Control Theory to Physiological Systems*, Philadelphia, W. B. Saunders Co., 1966.

55. Milsum, J. H., *Biological Control Systems Analysis*, New York, McGraw-Hill Book Company, Inc., 1966.

56. Nightingale, J. M., "Automatic Control Systems," *Machine Design*, May 17, 1956, Pages 35-42, 1956.

57. Nightingale, J. M., "A Basic Outline of Servo Mathematics," *Machine Design*, June 28, 1956, Pages 74-81.

58. Nightingale, J. M., "Criteria for Evaluating Servo System Performance, Part I: Frequency Response and Stability, Nyquist Crite-

rion, Algebraic Criteria, Response Criteria," *Machine Design,* July 26, 1956, Pages 79-84.

59. Nightingale, J. M., "Criteria for Evaluating Servo System Performance, Part II: Steady-State Errors, Nyquist Plot, Transient Response, Relative Damping," *Machine Design,* August 9, 1956, Pages 106-110.

60. Nightingale, J. M., "Analyzing Servo Systems," *Machine Design,* November 1, 1956, Pages 87-91, 1956.

61. Nightingale, J. M., "Servo Feedback Systems," *Machine Design,* August 20, 1959, Pages 155-159, 1959.

62. Pate, E., and Cooke, R., "A Model of Crossbridge Action: The Effects of ATP, ADP and P_i," *J. Muscle Research and Cell Motility,* Vol. 10, Pages 181-196, 1989.

63. Poppele, R. E., and Terzuolo, C. A., "Myotatic Reflex: Its Input-Output Relation," *Science* (New York), Vol. 195, Pages 743-745, 1968.

64. Poppele, R. E., and Bowman, R. J., "Quantitative Description of Linear Behavior of Mammalian Muscle Spindles," *J. Neurophysiology,* Vol. 33, No. 1, Pages 59-72, January, 1970.

65. Reiner, J. N., *The Organism as an Adaptive Control System,* Englewood Cliffs, New Jersey, Prentice-Hall, Inc., 1968.

66. Riggs, D. S., *The Mathematical Approach to Physiological Problems,* Baltimore, The Williams and Wilkins Company, Inc., 1963.

67. Rosenberg, J. R., Murray-Smith, D. J., and Rigas, A., "An Introduction to the Application of System Identification Techniques to Elements of the Neuromuscular System," *Trans. Inst. Meas. and Control,* Vol. 4, No. 4, Pages 187-202, October-December, 1982.

68. Rosenthal, N. P., "A Linear Systems Analysis of the Myotatic Reflex and its Component," Ph.D. Dissertation, University of Minnesota, 1969.

69. Rudjord, T., "A Second-Order Mechanical Model of Muscle Spindle Primary Endings," *Kybernetik,* Vol. 6, Pages 205-213, 1970.

70. Rudjord, T., "Model Study of Muscle Spindles Subjected to Static Fusimotor Activation," *Kybernetick,* Vol. 10, No. 4, Pages 189-200, April, 1972.

71. Schneck, D. J., *Engineering Principles of Physiologic Function,* New York, The New York University Press, 1990.

72. Sejersted, O. M., "Maintenance of Na, K-Homeostasis by Na, K-Pumps in Striated Muscle," In: Skou, J. C., Norby, J. G.,

Maunsbach, A. B., and Esmann, M., (Editors), *The Na+, K+-Pump, Part B: Cellular Aspects*, New York, Alan R. Liss, Inc., 1988, pages 195-206.

73. Stein, R. B., "The Peripheral Control of Movement," *Physiological Reviews*, Volume 54, Pages 215-243, 1974.

74. Stein, R. B., and Oguztöreli, M. N., "Does the Velocity Sensitivity of Muscle Spindles Stabilize the Stretch Reflex?" *Biological Cybernetics*, Vol. 23, Pages 219-228, 1976.

75. Stein, R. B., and Oguztöreli, M. N., "The Role of y-Motoneurons in Mammalian Reflex Systems," *Biological Cybernetics*, Vol. 39, No. 3, Pages 171-179, 1981.

76. Stiles, R. N., "Mechanical and Neural Feedback Factors in Postural Hand Tremor of Normal Subjects," *J. Neurophysiol.*, Vol. 44, Pages 40-59, 1980.

77. Sumner, A. J., (Editor), *The Physiology of Peripheral Nerve Disease*, Philadelphia, W. B. Saunders, Inc., 1981.

78. Taber, L. A., and Steele, C. R., "Cochlear Model Including Three-Dimensional Fluid and Four Modes of Partition Flexibility," *J. Acoust. Soc. Am.*, Vol. 70, No. 2, Pages 426-436, August, 1981.

79. Taylor, A., and Prochazka, A., (Editors), *Muscle Receptors and Movement*, London, Macmillan, 1981.

80. Trimmer, J. D., *Response of Physical Systems*, New York, John Wiley and Sons, Inc., 1950.

81. Vodovnik, L., Lyman, J., and Reswick, J., "Neuromuscular Integration and Control," In: Brown, J. H. U., and Gann, D. S. (Editors), *Engineering Principles in Physiology*, New York, Academic Press, Volume I, Pages 99-118, 1973.

82. Yamamoto, W. S., and Brobeck, J. R., (Editors), *Physiological Controls and Regulation*, Philadelphia, W. B. Saunders Company, Inc., 1965.

83. Zwislocki, J. J., "Five Decades of Research on Cochlear Mechanics," *J. Acoust. Soc. Am.*, Vol. 67, No. 5, Pages 1679-1685, May, 1980.

Index

About The Author

Dr. Daniel J. Schneck is a Professor Of Engineering Science & Mechanics at Virginia Polytechnic Institute & State University, where he has been since 1973, and where he directs the Program In Biomedical Engineering administered by the Department of Engineering Science and Mechanics. Trained in both engineering and medicine, Dr. Schneck's research interests are in cardiovascular and musculoskeletal mechanics. In addition to this book, he is the author of *Engineering Principles Of Physiologic Function* (Volume 5 of this Biomedical Engineering Series), co-author (with Dr. Alan Tempkin) of *Biomedical Desk Reference* (Volume 3 of the N.Y.U. Monographs in Biomedical Engineering Series), editor of three other books, and sole-or-co-author of 150 refereed papers, technical reports, abstracts, book reviews, editorials, and shorter communications.

Dr. Schneck has served as chairman of the Biomedical Engineering Division of ASEE, international president of the Biomedical Engineering Society, and currently is completing a four-year term on the Montgomery County School Board. His concern for education is further evidenced by his numerous awards -- among them, the coveted Outstanding Biomedical Engineering Educator Award, presented by the Biomedical Engineering Division of ASEE; the prestigious W. E. Wine Award (the highest University-wide recognition of teaching excellence awarded at VPI), the "Outstanding Educator Of The Year Award," from the Engineering Science and Mechanics Society, and the "Outstanding Contribution To Engineering Education," award presented by the Instructional Unit of the Southeastern Section of ASEE.

Printed in the United States
By Bookmasters